Empirical Approaches to the
**VALIDATION OF
SPINAL MANIPULATION**

Empirical Approaches to the
VALIDATION OF
SPINAL MANIPULATION

Edited by

A. A. BUERGER, Ph.D.

and

PHILIP E. GREENMAN, D.O.

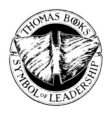

CHARLES C THOMAS • PUBLISHER
Springfield • Illinois • U.S.A.

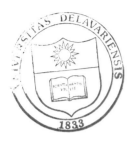

Published and Distributed Throughout the World by

CHARLES C THOMAS • PUBLISHER
2600 South First Street
Springfield, Illinois 62717

© *1985 by* CHARLES C THOMAS • PUBLISHER

ISBN 0-398-05086-4

Library of Congress Catalog Card Number: 84-16293

Printed in the United States of America
Q-R-3

Library of Congress Cataloging in Publication Data
Main entry under title:

Empirical approaches to the validation of spinal
    manipulation.

    Half-title: Validation of spinal manipulation.
    Based on a conference hosted by Michigan State University's
College of Osteopathic Medicine on the East Lansing campus,
Apr. 29-May 2, 1983.
    Includes bibliographies and index.
    1. Spondylotherapy--Congresses. 2. Backache--Treat-
ment--Congresses. 3. Manipulation (Therapeutics)--Con-
gresses. I. Buerger, A. A. II. Greenman, Ph. E.,
1928-   . III. Michigan State University. College of
Osteopathic Medicine. IV. Title: Validation of spinal
manipulation. [DNLM: 1. Backache--therapy--congresses.
2. Manipulation, Orthopedic--congresses. 3. Spine--
congresses. WE 725 E55 1983]
RZ399.S7E47   1985   617'.56   84-16293
ISBN 0-398-05086-4

DEDICATION

To J.S. Denslow, D.O. in recognition of his early efforts
in clinical research upon manual medicine and osteopathy.

CONTRIBUTORS

Gunnar B. Andersson, M.D., Ph.D.
Department of Orthopaedic Surgery I
Sahlgren Hospital
University of Goteborg
Goteborg, Sweden

Marianne Bergquist-Ullman, Ph.D., M.D.
Department of Orthopaedic Surgery I
Sahlgren Hospital
University of Goteborg
Goteborg, Sweden

A.A. Buerger, Ph.D.
Departments of Community Health Science
and Osteopathic Medicine
College of Osteopathic Medicine
Michigan State University
East Lansing, Michigan

M.S. Burke, M.B., B.Ch.
British United Providence Association Hospital
Cardiff, Wales
(Late of the University Hospital of Wales, Cardiff)

J. David Cassidy, D.C., B.Sc., F.C.C.S.(C)
Department of Orthopaedic Surgery
University Hospital
University of Saskatchewan
Saskatoon, Saskatchewan, Canada

C.E. O'Donoghue née Coxhead, M. Phil., M.C.S.P.
Royal Free Hospital
Harnstead, London, England

J. Shaw Dunn, M.B., Ch.B., Ph.D., F.R.C.S. (Glas.)
Department of Anatomy
University of Glasgow
Glasgow, Scotland

J. Dvorak, M.D.
Department of Neurology
University of Bern
Inselspital
Bern, Switzerland

D.P. Evans, M.Sc., M.D.
Department of Rheumatology
University Hospital of Wales
Heath Park
Cardiff, Wales

John H. Evans, Ph.D.
Bioengineering Unit
University of Strath-clyde
Glasgow, Scotland

Philip E. Greenman, D.O., F.A.A.O.
Department of Biomechanics
College of Osteopathic Medicine
Michigan State University
East Lansing, Michigan

Victor M. Hawthorne, M.D.
Department of Epidemiology
School of Public Health
University of Michigan
Ann Arbor, Michigan

William Johnston, D.O., F.A.A.O.
Department of Family Medicine
College of Osteopathic Medicine
Michigan State University
East Lansing, Michigan

Ayalew Kanno, Ph.D.
Bureau of Safety and Regulation
Michigan Department of Labor
Lansing, Michigan

W.H. Kirkaldy-Willis, M.A., M.D., FRCS(E&C)
Department of Orthopaedic Surgery
University Hospital
University of Saskatchewan
Saskatoon, Saskatchewan, Canada

M. McGregor, B.Sc., D.C.
Canadian Memorial Chiropractic College
Toronto, Ontario, Canada

James A.A. Miller, Ph.D.
Department of Mechanical Engineering
and Applied Mechanics
University of Michigan
Ann Arbor, Michigan

H-D. Neumann, M.D.
Buhlerstrasse 45
Buhl, West Germany

Craig Newell
Bureau of Safety and Regulation
Michigan Department of Labor
Lansing, Michigan

J.P. O'Brien, M.B., Ph.D., F.R.C.S. (Ed.), F.A.C.S.
Robert Jones and Agnes Hunt Orthopaedic Hospital
Oswestry, Scotland

Malcolm H. Pope, Ph.D.
Professor and Director of Research
Department of Orthopedics and Rehabilitation
University of Vermont
College of Medicine
Burlington, Vermont

G.G. Rasmussen, M.D.
Department of Rheumatology
Odense University Hospital
Odense, Denmark

Robert Soutas-Little, Ph.D.
Professor and Chairman
Department of Biomechanics
Michigan State University
East Lansing, Michigan

K.M. Tesh

Bioengineering Unit
University of Strath-clyde
Glasgow, Scotland

S.M.S. Young, M.C.S.P.

Physiotherapy Department
Royal United Hospital
Combe Park, Bath, England
(formerly Physiotherapist, Bristol Royal Infirmary, Bristol)

FOREWORD

THE field of manual medicine is receiving increased interest throughout the world, particularly during the past three decades. Although the field of manual medicine is probably as old as the history of medicine itself, it has been a discipline that has been the subject of relatively little research. Many advocates of the field feel that research is unnecessary, since the clinical effectiveness has been demonstrated for hundreds of years. Critics of the field state that such clinical experiences are only anecdotal and manual medicine should be subjected to the same scientific scrutiny as any other medical therapy.

Within the last decade there have been an increasing number of research studies concerning the validation of manual medicine in back pain. It is anticipated that other research efforts will increase within the next decade. Michigan State University's College of Osteopathic Medicine had the privilege of hosting a conference on the East Lansing campus April 29-May 2, 1983 which explored the issues surroundingthe research on the efficacy of manual medicine in back pain. Manipulative clinicians, epidemiologists, biostatisticians, biomechanical engineers and many others shared their interest and knowledge in their respective fields at this meeting. This volume contains the presentations at this meeting and we hope reflects the state of the art as of that time. It is our hope that the reader will gain a greater understanding of the multiple issues involved in the field.

Appreciation is expressed to all of the participants, the planning committee, and the support staff within the College of Osteopathic Medicine and at the Kellogg Center for Continuing Education at Michigan State University.

Myron S. Magen, D.O.
Dean
College of Osteopathic Medicine
Michigan State University

INTRODUCTION

LOW back pain continues as a major problem in our society. Approximately 80 percent of the general population will have at least one episode of acute low back pain in their life time. About one in four of the working population will have an acute episode each year. These episodes of low back pain contribute significantly to the cost of health care. Approximately 14 billion dollars are spent annually in the United States for low back costs both compensable and non-compensable. Low back pain is therefore a problem to the patient and to society at large (Snook, 1982).

Low back pain is also a problem to the health care practitioner. The natural history of low back pain is such that it is difficult to assume the effectiveness of therapeutic intervention. Some have stated that 90 percent of acute low back pain episodes recover without clinical intervention; 99 percent without hospitalization and 99.5 percent without surgical intervention. Because about 70 percent of patients with low back pain recover in three weeks, almost anything that is done during that three week period can be credited with the patient's successful recovery.

Manipulation has been utilized in patient care since before the time of Hippocrates. There appears to be clear evidence that Hippocrates utilized manipulation, primarily of the traction and compression type. Manipulation has continued as part of the armimentarium of the orthodox physician as well as many other health care providers up to the present (Schiotz and Cyriax, 1975).

Despite its long history of use, the effectiveness of manipulation have not been extensively researched. Within the past decade a number of researchers have attempted to validate the efficacy of manipulation. In this volume we will review the recently published results of clinical trials on manipulation and place them in perspective with the present knowledge of the epidemiology and biomechanics of back pain. This volume explores the problems presented in researching back pain and as well the difficulties in researching manipulation, such as the accuracy or inaccuracy of the diagnostic criteria utilized in defining a manipulable lesion and the absence of widely understood descriptions of the specific types of manipulative therapeutic interventions. The volume's contributors include nationally and internationally known experts in the field of biomechanics, epidemiology and manipulation. Representatives of most of the recently published clinical trials are included. The opinions expressed in each article are those of the individual authors.

We hope that this volume will provide an understanding of the present state of clinical trials on manipulation and also provide useful information for the design and implementation in future trials in this field, and also in research in epidemiology and biomechanics.

PROBLEMS OF TERMINOLOGY

Terminology in this field is not uniform. However there have been three recent efforts to begin to standardize terminology for both diagnostic and therapeutic techniques:

(1) The first effort was that by the Educational Council of Osteopathic Principles (ECOP). It is a group of faculty from all fifteen colleges of osteopathic medicine in America. The project director is Dr. Robert Ward from the College of Osteopathic Medicine at Michigan State University (Ward and Sprafka, 1981). The glossary originally compiled by ECOP is still under review and this group is also trying to expand it. This glossary is an attempt to standardize the terminology in the osteopathic profession in the United States.

(2) The second effort was that of the North American Academy of Manipulative Medicine (NAAMM) which is composed of allopathic and osteopathic physicians who use manual medicine mostly from the United States and Canada. NAAMM established a committee in 1982 to deal with the standardization of terminology from the perspective of North American M.D.s and D.O.s who use manual medicine. It utilized the language current within that organization and tried to cross-reference it to the ECOP glossary. ECOP and NAAMM use somewhat different terms and deal with somewhat different concepts but the NAAMM committee attempted to bridge between them. That terminology is now published and is under continuous review (Definitions/Glossary of Terms, 1982). It is shorter than the ECOP glossary in order to avoid replication.

(3) The third effort is that by the International Federation of Manual Medicine (FIMM). The FIMM group of which Dr. Neumann, who contributed to the final section of this volume, is now president has a scientific advisory committee which is attempting to achieve some standardization of terminology in the three languages used by FIMM because the official languages are English, French and German. Hence there are communication problems both within the field and also across languages.

However, the standardization of terminology was not an objective of this volume or of the conference which preceeded it, because it was too difficult to thrash out terminological differences during a conference aimed at placing the existing evidence from randomized clinical trials and other sources in perspective. Consider for example terms used by clinicians experienced in manipulation to describe the entity associated with back pain which they believe they treat, the *manipulable lesion*. Historically the chiropractors have termed it a *subluxation*. The American osteopathic physicians have termed it an *osteopathic lesion*, a *segmental dysfunction*, and most recently a *somatic dysfunction*. (The last term is the only one recognized within the International Classification of Disease.) Finally, until very recently most European manipulators have termed a manipulable lesion a *joint blockage*. Other terms are also in use. Hence in this volume we have not tried to force different authors to use the same terminology; but most of them tend to use somatic or segmental dysfunction as descriptions of the manipulable spinal lesion.

PREVIOUS WORK

It is essential to note that several somewhat similar strenuous efforts have preceeded this volume; they include Goldstein (1975), Buerger and Tobis (1977), Korr (1978), White and Gordon (1982), as well as many others. This volume must be viewed in the perspective supplied by this previous work.

CITATION OF REFERENCES

Our approach to the reference sections has been to supply to the reader the maximum amount of information available to us, especially in citations in languages other than English and in citations of publications by governments and international organizations. Hence, the citation formats are not always consistent, but we hope this approach will make location of the referenced publications as easy as possible.

SUMMARY

In summary, the major purpose of this book is to place in perspective the existing evidence from clinical trials on the effects of spinal manipulation upon low back pain. Therefore, sections on biomechanics and epidemiology and other characteristics of low back pain preceed sections on the evidence from uncontrolled and controlled clinical trials of spinal manipulation. These are followed by a section which attempts to place the available evidence in perspective from the viewpoints of both the clinical and basic sciences.

REFERENCES

Ad Hoc Committee on Definitions and Terminology, *Definitions/Glossary of Terms*, approved October 1982 by the North American Academy of Manipulative Medicine.

Buerger, A.A., Tobis, J.S. (eds.): *Approaches to the Validation of Manipulation Therapy*, Springfield, IL, Charles C Thomas, 1977.

Goldstein, M. (ed.); *The Research Status of Spinal Manipulative Therapy*. DHEW Publication No. (NIH) 76-998, 1975.

Korr, I.M. (ed.): *The Neurobiologic Mechanisms in Manipulative Therapy*. New York, Plenum Press, 1978.

Schiotz, E.H., Cyriax, J., *Manipulation Past and Present with an Extensive Bibliography*.

Snook, S.A. Epidemiology in *Low Back Pain* presented by Brigham and Women's Hospital and Harvard Medical School, November 29-December 1, 1982.

Ward, R., Sprafka, S.: Glossary of osteopathic terminology, *Journal of American Osteopathic Association*, Volume 80, no. 8, 552/119-567/134, April 1981.

White, A.A., Gordon, S.L., (eds.): *Symposium on Idiopathic Low Back Pain*. St. Louis, MO, C.V. Mosby, 1982.

ACKNOWLEDGMENTS

WE wish to thank Professor Robert Soutas-Little, Chairman of Biomechanics at this institution for preparing the introduction to the initial section of this volume.

We thank D. Thullen, for primary administrative responsibility for the organization of this volume, S. Kilbourn for primary responsibility for the conference which yielded this book and C. Burch for the heroic effort of typing and revising all the book's manuscripts superimposed on the normal load on her word processor.

We wish to thank Eberhard Mehling, M.D. for his aid especially with the German references and Wolfgang Gillar for his translation of significant portions of Dr. Dvorak's manuscript from German to English, B. Fortunate, D.O., for her supervision of the videotapes associated with this conference, and L. Behm for her invaluable library research.

We also wish to thank Ms. Betty Decker and the staff at the Instructional Media Center at this university for their help with many of the figures.

CONTENTS

Page

Introduction xiii

Section 1: THE BIOMECHANICS OF THE BACK

Chapter 1   *In vivo* Measurements of Loads on the Lumbar Spine in Some Basic
Postures and Work Activities. 5
G.B.J. Andersson

Chapter 2:   The biomechanics of the lumbar posterior elements and sacro-iliac
joints. 18
J.A.A. Miller

Chapter 3   Biomechanical properties of the intervertebral disk. 30
M.H. Pope

Chapter 4   The mechanical interaction between the thoracolumbar fascia
and the connective tissues of the posterior spine. 42
K.M. Tesh, J.H. Evans, J. Shaw Dunn, and J.P. O'Brian

Section 2: SOME CHARACTERISTICS OF BACK PAIN

Chapter 5   Epidemiology of low back pain. 53
G.B. Andersson

Chapter 6   An overview of the incidence of compensable occupational
back injuries in Michigan: 1970-1981 71
C. Newell and A. Kanno

Chapter 7   Differential diagnosis of back pain. 87
P.E. Greenman

Section 3: SOME CHARACTERISTICS OF SPINAL MANIPULATION

Chapter 8   Inter-rater reliability in the selection of manipulable patients. 106
W.L. Johnston

Chapter 9 Spinal manipulation for the treatment of chronic low back
          and leg pain: An observational study. 119
              J.D. Cassidy, W.H. Kirkaldy-Willis, and M. McGregor

Section 4:   RANDOMIZED CLINICAL TRIALS
OF MANIPULATION FOR LOW BACK PAIN

Chapter 10 The randomized controlled trial and low back pain:
           An introduction. 151
               V.M. Hawthorne
Chapter 11 Low back pain in industry: A randomized clinical trial. 164
               M. Bergquist-Ullman
Chapter 12 A randomized clinical trial of manipulation: Diagnostic criteria
           and treatment techniques. 174
               G.G. Rasmussen
Chapter 13 The selection and treatment of patients to be included in clinical
           trials of lumbar manipulation. 179
               M.S. Burke
Chapter 14 Controlled trials of mobilization and manipulation for general
           practitioner and hospital patients. 185
               S.M.S. Young
Chapter 15 A "double-blind" randomized clinical trial of rotational manipulation
           for low back pain. 193
               A.A. Buerger
Chapter 16 A multicenter trial of the physiotherapeutic management
           of sciatic symptoms. 208
               C.E. O'Donoghue née Coxhead
Chapter 17 The design and results of clinical trials of lumbar manipulation:
           A review. 228
               D.P. Evans

Section 5:   OVERVIEWS

Chapter 18 Neurological and biomechanical aspects of back pain. 241
               J. Dvorak
Chapter 19 A concept of manual medicine 267
               H-D. Neumann

CONCLUSION 273
INDEX. 277

Empirical Approaches to the
VALIDATION OF
SPINAL MANIPULATION

Section 1
THE BIOMECHANICS OF THE BACK

THE select group of biomechanical scientists participating in this volume took no position on the use of manipulation in treatment of low back pain and reviewed some of the basic research areas currently receiving attention.

There appears to be a gap between the basic and applied research of the biomechanical scientist and the clinical studies of the practitioner. This volume is one attempt directed at bridging this gap and increasing understanding. Within this volume are found differences in opinion which suggest the need to continue interaction and dialogue.

The papers in Section I are not meant to be a definitive treatment of the biomechanics of the back; they range from the general topic of spinal loads to a specialized area of the chronic effects of axial deceleration through impact on the spine. Presentations of the biomechanical properties of the tissues of the spine represent fundamental studies of the load-deformation properties of these materials. Increased understanding of these mechanical properties may lead to one explanation of the effectiveness of manual medicine.

During the past three decades, the science of biomechanics has assumed a role of major importance in medicine, being embraced by orthopedics, cardiology, human performance and sports medicine. Recently there has also been increased interest in the field of manual medicine in understanding the fundamental importance of the physical properties of the musculoskeletal system.

Robert Soutas-Little, Ph.D.
Professor and Chairman
Department of Biomechanics
Michigan State University
East Lansing, Michigan

CHAPTER ONE

IN VIVO MEASUREMENTS OF LOADS ON THE LUMBAR SPINE IN SOME BASIC POSTURES AND WORK ACTIVITIES

GUNNAR B.J. ANDERSSON, M.D., Ph.D.

THE influence of mechanical factors on low back pain is the reason why loads on the lumbar spine are measured, calculated and analyzed. It is widely believed that prevention of low back pain is possible — at least in part — through actions aimed at reducing these loads. To do so intelligently we need to know when the spine is loaded and to what degree. This chapter reviews selected papers in which loads on the lumbar spine in different postures and simple work activities were measured. Further information on load measurements and biomechanical spine models used to calculate loads can be found in book-chapters by Andersson (1982), Chaffin (1982), Pope et al. (1982), Schultz (1982) and White et al. (1982).

MEASUREMENT METHODS

Three methods will be discussed here; disc pressure measurements, electromyography, and intra-abdominal pressure measurements. All of these have been used extensively, but none is a direct measure of lumbar spine load.

Disc Pressure Measurement

The first paper on pressure measurements of the intervertebral disc was by Petter in 1933, who measured disc expansion (after disc removal and after sectioning of the annulus fibrosus) as well as the amount of pressure needed to reduce the expansion. Pressures within the disc were not measured until the early fifties when Naylor and Smare (1951) recorded pressure increases in healthy discs immersed in water and in isotonic saline. Following studies by Virgin (1951), Charnley (1952), Ott (1954), Hendry (1958), and Bush et al. (1956), the disc nucleus was postulated to have hydrostatic properties. These properties were explored and proved by Nachemson in 1960 using a pressure measurement needle and turning it in the three principal directions of stress while discs were loaded in vitro. Pressures in normal discs were found to be 1.3 to 1.6 times the vertically applied load and increased linearly with increasing compressive loads up to about 2000 Newtons. Tzivian et al. (1970) confirmed Nachemson's findings that the relationship between externally applied compressive loads and intradiscal pressures was linear. But, the conversion factor between the applied load per unit of cross-sectional area and the intradiscal pressure was not the same throughout the loading range; the higher the load, the lower the conversion factor.

Following these early studies which were all made on disc segments loaded in compression, Schultz et al. (1979), Berkson, Nachemson, and Schultz (1979) and Nachemson, Schultz and Berkson (1979) analyzed the mechanical behavior of 42 human cadaver motion segments under different loading conditions.

The pressure changes were relatively small in torsion, extension, and shear, but they were comparatively large in compression, flexion, and lateral bending. The ratio of intradiscal pressure to applied pressure was a function of the applied compressive load, decreasing monotonously from in the mean about 2.5 at 100 Newtons to 1.3 at 400 Newtons.

Schultz et al. (1979) concluded that it is reasonably accurate to interpret pressure changes in vivo as due to compressive load changes. In vivo measurements were first made by Nachemson and Morris in 1964, who inserted a membrane-covered, liquid-filled needle connected to a pressure transducer into a lumbar disc nucleus. The membrane needle has been replaced in subsequent studies by a semiconductor strain gauge transducer needle (Nachemson, 1976; Nachemson & Elfstrom, 1970).

Electromyography

The basis of electromyography is the electric activity generated by depolarization of the muscle cell membrane, resulting in a contraction. The precise relationship of the electric output and the mechanical output of a contracting muscle is still uncertain. The relationships are empirical and depend on many factors. It seems clear that a linear relationship cannot be expected over the entire force range of a muscle even during static conditions (isometric tension). In a dynamic situation the relationship is further complicated. On the other hand, neither in static nor in dynamic situations has a non-monotonic relationship ever been suggested, so a mechanical comparison of different loading conditions based on the myoelectric output is acceptable; an increased level of myoelectric activity means an increase of force but unknown magnitude. For the back muscles specifically, a close to linear relationship has been found over a reasonably large force range (Andersson, Herberts & Ortengren, 1976; Andersson, Ortengren & Herberts, 1977; Andersson, Ortengren & Schultz, 1980; Asmussen, Poulsen & Rasmussen, 1965; Chapman & Troup, 1969; Grieve & Pheasant, 1976; Schultz et al., 1982).

Intra-Abdominal Pressure

The idea that trunk-pressures might assist the trunk in postures of forward flexion was suggested in the early part of the century (Keith, 1923). Rushmer (1946) and Adno (1956) performed dog experiments to investigate how accurately intraintestinal pressures reflected pressures in the trunk cavities. Both concluded that intraintestinal pressures could be used to estimate variations in intraperitoneal pressure, but they also cautioned that the range of their studies was small. In 1956 Davis found that intragastric pressures did increase when the trunk moment was increased, and these findings were confirmed by Bartelink (1957). These early studies were followed by those of Morris, Lucas, and Bresler (1961) who at the same time recorded the myoelectric activities of several trunk muscles and the intrathoracic pressure and made a mathematical model of the forces acting on the spine.

Stubbs (1973) brought the measurement method to the workplace, and has, together with Davis, attempted to use intra-abdominal pressure to estimate safe levels of manual forces at work (Davis & Stubbs, 1977; 1978). Early measurements were made with rubber balloons. Watson, Ross and Kay (1962) introduced a pressure-sensitive radio pill, which transmitted intraintestinal pressures using telemetry. This method has been used extensively by Davis and coworkers. Other groups have employed strain gauge transducer catheters, which are either swallowed or inserted intrarectally. The two methods have been compared by Nordin et al. (1984) and appear to yield similar results.

The theory behind the supportive role of the trunk pressures is that when, for example, a weight is lifted, a flexion moment develops about the spine. This moment is counterbalanced by the posterior back muscles. The pressure in the trunk cavities assists in this respect, producing an extensor moment. The muscle contraction forces needed for equilibrium are reduced, which reduces the stress on the vertebral column. Studies performed in the laboratory have mainly aimed at assessing the load-relieving role of the intra-abdominal pressure during lifting and other physical activities (see Andersson, 1982; Morris et al., 1961).

POSTURAL INFLUENCE ON BACK LOAD

Standing and Sitting

Nachemson and Morris (1964) recorded disc pressures in standing, sitting and reclining postures. Pressures when standing were 30 percent higher than when sitting, while pressure when reclining were 50 percent less than when sitting. These results were confirmed by Nachemson and Elfstrom in 1970, when they published a comprehensive study of common movements, maneuvers and physical exercises. Standing and sitting postures were later studied in detail by Andersson (1974), Andersson et al. (1974), Andersson and Ortengren (1974). These studies also confirmed that the disc pressure was about 40 percent lower in standing than in unsupported sitting. The reason for this appears to be the increase in trunk load movement that occurs when the pelvis is rotated backwards in sitting, and the deformation of the disc caused by the associated lumbar spine flattening. When supports were added to the chair disc pressure was found to be influenced by the back rest, by the use of lumbar supports, and by arm rests. An increase in back rest inclination (seat-back rest angle) resulted in a lower disc pressure presumably because an increasing part of the trunk weight was transferred to the back rest. The lumbar support influences the posture of the spine reducing the pressure as the deformation of the disc is reduced, and arm rests support the weight of the arms, thus reducing the body weight above the disc.

The electromyographic activity (EMG) of the trunk muscles in erect standing and in sitting postures has been studied extensively. Much of this work has been summarized in previous papers and will not be repeated here (Ortengren and Andersson, 1977; Andersson, 1982). Some controversy exists over whether the back muscles are active in relaxed standing or not. Most authors have found slight activity, usually less in the lumbar and cervical regions than in the thoracic region.

The evidence today suggests that the back muscles are active in upright standing, but the level of activity is always low, and there are considerable interindividual variations. Concomitant with activities in the back muscles is slight activity in the vertebral portion of the psoas major muscle. The abdominal muscles are also slightly active during relaxed standing, particularly the internal obliques.

Although the activity in the lumbar region is similar in standing and in unsupported sitting, there is a somewhat higher level of activity in the thoracic region when sitting (Andersson, 1974; Andersson et al., 1974; Andersson & Ortengren, 1974; Floyd & Silver, 1955; Joseph & McColl, 1961; Lundervold, 1951; Rosemeyer, 1971). Some information is also available on abdominal muscle activity in sitting. Carlsoo (1963) recorded slight activity in the anterior oblique muscles, but the rectus abdominis and transverse muscles were not investigated. The iliopsoas muscle is also slightly active when a sitting posture is assumed (Andersson et al., 1974; Morinaga, 1973; Nachemson, 1966). There is general agreement that the myoelectric activity in sitting decreases when the back is slumped into full flexion; the arms are supported; and the back rest is used. The backrest inclination is important with electromyographic levels decreasing when the backrest is inclined further backwards, at least to 110 degrees. Placing a support in the lumbar region only reduces the muscle activity as much as a full back support.

Forward Flexion and Extension From a Flexed Position

Trunk forward flexion is a combined movement of the spine and the pelvis. The first 50 to 60 degrees are accomplished by motion of the lumbar spine and additional flexion mainly by rotation of the pelvis (Davis et al., 1965; Farfan, 1975). In extension, the reverse applies: at first the pelvis rotates backward, after which extension of the lumbar spine completes the movement.

The muscles of the trunk control this pattern of motion elegantly, as indicated by their electric activity. During the first portion of a flexion movement, strong activity is found in the pelvis and preventing motion at the hip joints. As flexion progresses, the increasing trunk moment is balanced by a corresponding increase in back muscle activity. In the fully flexed position, however, the activity ceases almost completely. Floyd and Silver (1955) hypothesized that the so-called flexion relaxion of the back muscles is due to reflex inhibition, but other explanations are also possible. In any case, in the fully flexed posture the trunk moment is resisted by structures other than active muscles. Most authors conclude that the ligaments provide the major share, together with stretched extensor muscles. Farfan and Lamy (1975), adopting this idea in a mechanical model, found stress on the ligaments to be considerable and close to their failure strength. Gracovetsky, Farfan, and Lamy (1977; 1980) have indicated the importance of the thoracolumbar fascia in these situations, Adams, Hutton and Stott (1980) the importance of the lumbar apophyseal joints. In the control of pelvic stability through the flexion movement the gluteus maximus has been found to relax as full flexion is approached, while the hamstring muscles are greatly active at first and remain active throughout the flexion movement. The abdominal muscles are active only during the first few degrees of flexion, that is, when the movement is initiated (Allen, 1948; Basmajian, 1978; Floyd & Silver, 1950; Ono, 1958). Apparently gravity forces alone thereafter cause the movement.

In studies of static positions of flexion, an increase in the myoelectric activity of the back muscles has been found, both when the angle of flexion is increased and when external loading is increased at a fixed angle of flexion (Andersson et al., 1977; Morris et al., 1962; Okada, 1970; Shultz et al., 1982). In attempted flexion resisted by external forces, on the other hand, there is a decrease in the activity in the lumbar part of the ESM (Jonsson, 1970).

When rising again from the flexed to the upright position, a reverse sequence is observed to that when bending forward (Allen, 1948; Donish & Basmajian, 1972; Floyd & Silver, 1950, 1955; Morris et al., 1962; Portnoy & Morris, 1956). The gluteus maximus comes into action early and probably initiates extension together with the hamstrings (Okada, 1970). The posterior back muscles become active only thereafter. This indicates that the extension movement starts with a fixation and posterior rotation of the pelvis. It is noteworthy that the extensor muscle activity is greater when the trunk is being raised than when it is being lowered, although in neither is it close to its maximum. The direction of the movement in relation to the weight forces is obviously important.

Disc pressure measurements in different angles of flexion have shown a linear relationship between the pressure and trunk moment when the sine of the angle is used to measure trunk flexion (Andersson et al., 1977; Schultz et al., 1982).

Pressures within the trunk were related to the trunk moment, increasing when the moment was increased (Asmussen & Poulsen, 1968; Bartelink, 1957; Davis, 1956; Eie, 1966). Andersson, Ortengren and Nachemson (1977) showed that the pressure-moment relationship was systematic and that the pressure in forward-flexed postures increased linearly with an increase in trunk flexion angle and an increase in external load. These findings were confirmed by Hemborg et al. (1984) who found, however, that the pressure increase was nonlinear at higher loads; a lower pressure increase than expected was found. Grew (1980) studied intra-abdominal pressures under isometric loading of the trunk. Several load directions and trunk postures were included and the pressure response related to the trunk moment. The response-moment relationship was linear in all tests, but the slope of the pressure-moment curve differed depending on the subject posture and mass, the direction of the load, and the load placement. The greatest slope (largest pressure increase per unit of moment) was found when extensor moments were applied, the lowest when the trunk was flexed. This can be explained by the actions of the abdominal muscles; they contract most vigorously when an extensor moment is applied.

Extension

When the trunk is extended from the upright position, myoelectric back muscle activity is found during the initial phase and in the position of full extension (Allen, 1948; Floyd & Silver, 1955; Morris et al., 1962; Pauly, 1966). Between these two extremes of the movement, there is only slight activity throughout the movement, particularly the rectus abdominis. Extension of the trunk against resistance results in a marked increase in the activity of the muscles of the lumbar region of the back (Jonsson, 1970; Morris et al., 1962; Pauly, 1966).

Lateral Flexion

When the trunk is flexed laterally, activity increases in the posterior back muscles on both sides of the spine. The main increase in activity in the lumbar region is on the contralateral side (Carlsoo, 1961; Floyd & Silver, 1955; Friedevold, 1958; Morris et al., 1962; Portnoy & Morris, 1956). When the trunk is loaded by the arm in lateral flexion, comparatively higher levels of activity are found on the contralateral side of the lumbar region and on the ipsilateral side of the thoracic region (Andersson et al., 1977). In the lumbar region the activity is higher when the electrodes are placed over more laterally located muscles. This is what can be expected from model calculations and from intramuscular electrode studies by Jonsson (1970). He found the iliocostalis and longissimus muscles to be active in lateral flexion, while the multifidi, which are closer to the spine, were usually inactive. The response of the back muscles to a loading condition where a weight is held in one hand in the upright posture is equivalent to that in lateral flexion; the contralateral muscles contract (Andersson et al., (1977; Floyd & Silver, 1955). The abdominal muscles also show activity in lateral flexion both ipsilaterally and contralaterally, the level of activity being higher on the contralateral side (Carlsoo, 1963).

In their study of working postures Andersson et al. (1977) included also twisting and lateral bending. By statistical analysis Ortengren et al. (1978) showed that the pressure increase in lateral bending was greater than in simple forward flexion, and that this was even more obvious when rotation was included. Intra-abdominal pressure measurements in lateral bending and rotation indicate that the pressure is quite insensitive to such postural changes. This is perhaps one weakness when using intra-abdominal pressure to study vocational activities.

Rotation

When the trunk is rotated, the back muscles are active on both sides of the spine. Although Portnoy and Morin (1956) and Carlsoo (1963) recorded similar levels of activity on both sides, differences were observed by Morris, Benner and Lucas (1962) and Donish and Basmajian (1972). The ipsilateral longissimus and iliocostalis muscles, as well as the contralateral multifidus and rotator muscles, were active in the lumbar region while activity was mainly symmetrical in the thoracic region. Similar observations were made by Jonsson (1970) in attempted rotation. Andersson, Ortengren and Herberts (1977) studied combined positions of lateral flexion and rotation with external load and recorded comparatively high levels of activity on the contralateral side of the lumbar region.

The abdominal muscles show an activity pattern similar to the back muscles but with much lower levels of activity (Carlsoo, 1963).

The disc pressure and intra-abdominal pressure responses have been discussed above.

LIFTING

Electromyographic Studies

The back muscles, the muscles of the buttocks, and the ischiocrural muscles are all active during a lift. The abdominal muscles are also active, but to a smaller degree. The levels of myoelectric activity in these various muscles are directly related to the trunk moment and therefore influenced by the weight of the burden, the body posture, and the distance between the mass center of the burden and the lumbar spine (See Andersson, 1982; Ortengren & Andersson, 1977).

The question of whether the spine should be flexed or straight during the lift has been the subject of electromyographic analyses. Generally, in these studies, either the back muscle activities are similar in a leg lift and a back lift or, more often, they are higher in the back lift (Andersson et al., 1977; Andersson & Schultz, 1979; Grieve, 1974; Morris et al., 1961).

Disc Pressures

Nachemson and Morris (1964) studied the effect of external loading on the pressure in upright postures. A load-related increase in pressure was found, and later confirmed by Nachemson (1965) in 20 degrees of flexion. Nachemson and Elfstrom (1970) studied lifting from a chair using leg- and back-lifting methods. With the leg-lifting method a lower pressure response was found. But, in the study the moment arms were not the same, so the result is difficult to interpret. Andersson, Ortengren and Nachemson (1976) studied pulling and lifting using leg- and backlifting techniques. The pressure values were about the same when pulling with the back straight and flexed. No differences were found between the two lifting methods used when dynamic lifts were performed with constant moment arms. When the moment arm was reduced a reduction in pressure followed also. It was concluded that the essential point in reducing the load on the back when lifting is to keep the trunk load moment low.

Trunk Pressures When Lifting

The typical pressure response to lifting is an initial peak and a lower sustained pressure while the load is raised (Davis, 1981). Davis (1956; 1981) showed in his measurements that there was an almost linear relationship between the maximum pressure induced in the trunk cavities and the angle between the trunk and the ground for a given weight. He concluded that in a stooping position larger compression forces on the spine would occur and that therefore the back should not be bent during a lift. Morris, Benner and Lucas (1962) performed dynamic lifting experiments, which showed that the intra-abdominal pressure increased when the lifted weight increased. The pressure was at its maximum immediately after the start of the lift and decreased as the trunk was raised. Higher pressure values were always found in leg lifting than in back lifting. Eie and Wehn (1962) on the other hand, found that back lifting resulted in higher pressure than leg lifting. Davis and Troup (1964) studied the effect of pulling, pushing, and lifting on the intra-abdominal pressure. They found that pulling was somewhat less likely to produce large pressure increases than pushing and lifting. The pressure values invariably increased in magnitude when the weights were increased. Davis and Troup (1964) concluded that stooping to lift introduces large pressures within the trunk cavities, and they emphasized the importance of holding the trunk vertically. No comparison between different methods of lifting was made in that study, however. In 1976 Andersson, Ortengren and Nachemson published a study in which the intra-abdominal pressure was measured together with the disc pressure and the myoelectric activity of several back muscles during static and dynamic loading. During a pull, the intra-abdominal pressure was found to be about the same when back lifting and leg lifting postures were adopted as long as the pull was performed with the trunk comparatively vertical. With the trunk in a more flexed position, the intra-abdominal pressure rose to considerably higher values when the leg lifting method was used.

In dynamic lifting situations the intra-abdominal pressure responded to lifts of 10 kg, but the pressure values recorded were low. No difference was found when the lift was performed using the leg lifting or back lifting method. In some experiments the subjects were asked to strain their abdominal muscles as hard as possible by holding their breath and tightening the abdominal wall (Valsalva maneuvers). While the abdominal pressure rose in excess of 10 kilograms no decrease was found in the simultaneously recorded intradiscal pressure.

In other experiments a clear relationship was found between the intra-abdominal pressure and the trunk moment when the moment arm of the weight was changed during a lift: the larger the moment arm, the greater the pressure.

Hemborg et al. (1984) compared leg lifting and back lifting techniques and found higher pressure values with the leg lift, irrespective of external load. The myoelectric activity of the oblique abdominal muscles was recorded at the same time as the intra-abdominal pressure. During back lifts the maximum value of the myoelectric activity was found at the start of the lift, and the peak intra-abdominal pressure was shortly after the midportion of the lift. In leg lifts the peak of the myoelectric activity curve was delayed 0.4 to 0.6 seconds, and the peak pressure occurred shortly thereafter (0.2 seconds). Systematic strengthening exercises for the abdominal and back muscles, but no increase in intra-abdominal pressure was found when lifting before and after the exercise period.

SUMMARY

A review was made of some studies in which the loads on the spine were measured indirectly. By combining measurements with biomechanical models an excellent estimate can be made of the total load on the lumbar spine. This knowledge can now be used to investigate exposure — effect and load-pain relationships and to prevent low back pain by interventions at the workplace. Information useful in the treatment of low back disorders has also been provided.

REFERENCES

Adams, MA; Hutton, WC; Stott, JRR: The resistance of flexion of the lumbar intervertebral joint. *Spine, 5*:245-253, 1980.

Adno, J.: Some aspects on the mechanics of the abdomen. *South African Med J, 30*:535-539, 1956.

Allen, CEL: Muscle action potentials used in the study of dynamic anatomy. *Br J Phys Med, 11*:66, 1948.

Andersson, GBJ: On Myoelectric Back Muscle Activity and Lumbar Disc Pressure in Sitting Postures, thesis, Goteborg, Gotab, 1974.

Andersson, GBJ: Measurements of loads on the lumbar spine. In symposium on *Idiopathic Low Back Pain* (ed. A.A. White III, S.L. Gordon). St. Louis, Mosby, 1982, pp. 220-251.

Andersson, GBJ; Jonsson, B; Ortengren, R: Myoelectric Activity in Individual Lumbar Erector Spinae Muscles in Sitting. *Scan J Rehabil Med, 3 (suppl)*:91, 1974.

Andersson, G; Ortengren, R; Nachemson, A; Elfstrom, G: Lumbar disc pressure and myoelectric back muscle activity during sitting. Part 1: Studies on an experimental chair. *Scand J Rehabil Med, 6*:104-114, 1974.

Andersson, GBJ; Herberts, P; Ortengren, R: Myoelectric back muscle activity in standardized lifting postures, in Komi PV (ed): *Biomechanics 5-A.* Baltimore, University Park Press, 1976, pp.520-529.

Andersson, GBJ; Ortengren, R: Myoelectric back muscle activity during sitting. *Scand J Rehabil Med, 3 (Suppl)*:73, 1974.

Andersson, GBJ; Ortengren, R; Herberts, P: Quantitative electromyographic studies of back muscle activity related to posture and loading. *Orthop Clin North Am, 8*:85-96, 1977.

Andersson, GBJ; Ortengren, R; Nachemson, A: Quantitative studies of back loads in lifting. *Spine, 1*:178-185, 1976.

Andersson, GBJ; Ortengren, R; Nachemson, A: Intradiskal pressure, intra-abdominal pressure and myoelectric back muscle activity related to posture and loading. *Clin Orthop, 129*:156-164, 1977.

Andersson, GBJ; Schultz, AB: Transmission of moments across the elbow joint and the lumbar spine. *J Biomech, 12*:747-755, 1979.

Andersson, GBJ; Ortengren, R; Schultz, A: Analysis and measurement of the loads on the lumbar spine during work at a table. *J Biomech, 13*:513-520, 1980.

Asmussen, E; Klausen, K: Form and function of the erect human spine. *Clin Orthop, 25*:55, 1962.

Asmussen, E; Poulsen, E: On the role of the intra-abdominal pressure in relieving the back muscles while holding weights in a forward inclined position. *Comm Dan Natl Assoc Infat Paral, 28*:3, 1968.

Asmussen, E; Poulsen, E; Rasmussen, B: Quantitative evaluation of the activity of the back muscles in lifting. *Comm Dan Natl Assoc Infat Paral, 21*, 1965.

Bartelink, DL: The role of abdominal pressure in relieving the pressure on the lumbar intervertebral discs. *J Bone Joint Surg, 39-B*:718-725, 1957.

Basmajian, JV: *Muscles Alive.* Baltimore, Williams & Wilkins, 1978.

Berkson, MH; Nachemson, A; Schultz, AB: Mechanical properties of human lumbar spine motion segments. Part II: Responses in compression and shear; influence of gross morphology. *J Biomech Engineering, 101*:53-57, 1979.

Bush, HD; Horton, WG; Smare, DL; Naylor, A: Fluid content of the nucleus pulposus as a factor in the disc syndrome. Further observations. *Br Med J, 2*:81, 1956.

Carlsoo, S: The static muscle load in different work positions: An electromyographic study. *Ergonomics, 4*:193, 1961.

Carlsoo, S: Table, Chair and Work Posture. A study promoted by Folksam and Facit AB, 1963 (in Swedish).

Chaffin, DB: Occupational Biomechanics of low back injury. In *Symposium on Idiopathic Low Back Pain* A.A. White III, S.L. Gordon (ed.). St. Louis, Mosby, 1982, pp.323-330.

Chapman, AE; Troup, JDG: The effect of increased maximal strength on the integrated electrical activity of lumbar erectors spinae. *Electromyography, 9*:263, 1969.

Charnley, J: The imbibition of fluid as a cause of herniation of the nucleus pulposus. *Lancet, 1*:124, 1952.

Davis, PR: Variations of the intra-abdominal pressure during weight lifting in various postures. *J Anat, 90*:601, 1956.

Davis, PR: The use of intra-abdominal pressure in evaluating stresses on the lumbar spine. *Spine, 6*:90-92, 1981.

Davis, PR; Stubbs, DA: Safe levels of manual forces for young males. *Applied Ergonomics, 8* (pt 1):141-150, 1977; *8* (pt 2):219-228, 1977; *9* (pt 3):33-37, 1978.

Davis, PR; Troup; JDG: Pressures in the trunk cavities when pulling, pushing and lifting. *Ergonomics, 7*:465-474, 1964.

Davis, PR; Troup, JDG; Burnard, JH: Movements of the thorax and lumbar spine when lifting: A chronocyclophotographic study. *J Anat, 99*:13, 1965.

Donish, EW; Basmajian, JV: Electromyography of deep back muscles in man. *Am J Anat, 133*:25, 1972.

Eie, N: Load capacity of the low back. *J Oslo City Hosp, 16*:73, 1966.

Eie, N; Wehn, P: Measurements of the intra-abdominal pressure in relation to weight bearing of the lumbosacral spine. *J Oslo City Hosp, 12*:205, 1962.

Farfan, HF: Muscular mechanism of the lumbar spine and the position of power and efficiency. *Orthop Clin North Am, 6*:135, 1975.

Farfan, HF; Lamy, C: *Human Spine in the Performance of Dead Lift*. Montreal, St. Mary's Hospital, 1975.

Floyd, WF; Silver, PHS: Electromyographic study of patterns of activity of the anterior abdominal wall muscles in man. *J Anat, 84*:132, 1950.

Floyd, WF; Silver, PHS: Function of erectores spinae in flexion of the trunk. *Lancet, 1*:133, 1951.

Floyd, WF, Silver, PHS: The function of the erectores spinae muscles in certain movements and postures in man. *J Physiol (Lond), 129*:184, 1955.

Friedebold, G: Die Aktivitat normaler Ruchenstreck-muskulatur im Elektromyogramm unter verschiedenen Haltungsbedingungen: Eine Studie zur Skelettmuskelmechanik. *Z Orthop, 90*:1, 1958 (in German).

Gracovetsky, S; Farfan, HF; Lamy, C: Mathematical model of the lumbar spine using an optimized system to control muscles and ligaments. *Orthop Clin North Am, 8*:135-153, 1977.

Gracovetsky, S; Farfan, HF; Lamy, C: The mechanism of the lumbar spine. Presented at the Conference on Engineering Aspects of the Spine, London, May 7-9, 1980.

Grew, ND: Intra-abdominal pressure response to loads applied to the torso in normal subjects. *Spine, 5*:149-154, 1980.

Grieve, DW: Dynamic characteristics of man during crouch and stoop lifting, in Nelson, RC, Morehouse, CA (eds): *Biomechanics*, ed 4. Baltimore, University Park Press, 1974, pp.19-29.

Hemborg, B; Morritz; U; Hamberg, J; Lowing, H; Akesson, I: Intra-abdominal pressure and trunk muscle activity during lifting—effect of abdominal muscle training in healthy subjects. *Scan J Rehab Med*, 1984. In press.

Hendry, NGC: The hydration of the nucleus pulposus and its relation to intervertebral disc derangement. *J Bone Joint Surg, 40-B*:132, 1958.

Jonsson, B: *The Lumbar Part of the Erector Spinae Muscle: A Technique for Electromyographic Studies of the Function of its Individual Muscles*, Thesis, Goteborg, Elanders, 1970.

Jonsson, B: Topography of the lumbar part of the erector spinae muscle. *Anat Entwicklungsgesch, 130*:77, 1970.

Jonsson, B: The functions of individual muscles in the lumbar part of the erector spinae muscle. *Electromyography, 10*:5, 1970.

Joseph, J; McColl, I: Electromyography of muscles of posture: Posterior vertebral muscles in males. *J Physiol (Lond), 157*:33, 1961.

Keith, A: Man's posture: its evolution and disorders. Lecturer IV: The adaptations of the abdomen of its viscera to the orthograde posture. *Br Med J, 1*:587-590, 1923.

Klausen, K: The form and function of the loaded human spine. *Acta Physiol Scand, 65*:176, 1965.

Lundervold, AJS: Electromyographic investigations of position and manner of working in typewriting. *Acta Physiol Scand, Supplementum 84*, 1951.

Morinaga, H: An electromyographic study of the function of the psoas major muscle. *J Jpn Orthop Ass, 47*:351-365, 1973.

Morris, JM; Benner, G; Lucas, DB: An electromyographic study of the intrinsic muscles of the back in man. *J Anat, 96*:509, 1962.

Morris, JM; Lucas, DB; Bresler, B: Role of the trunk in stability of the spine. *J Bone Joint Surg, 43-A*:327, 1961.

Nachemson, A: Lumbar intradiscal pressure. *Acta Orthop Scand, Supplementum 43*:1-104, 1960.

Nachemson, A: The effect of forward leaning on lumbar intradiscal pressure. *Acta Orthop Scand, 35*:314-328, 1965.

Nachemson, A: Electromyographic studies on the vertebral portion of the psoas muscle. *Acta. Orthop. Scand. 37*:177, 1966.

Nachemson, A: Lumbar intradiscal pressure, in Jayson, M (ed.): *The Lumbar Spine and Back Pain*. Kent, Pitman Medical Publishing Co Ltd, pp.257-269, 1976.

Nachemson, A; Elfstrom, G: Intravital dynamic pressure measurements in lumbar discs. A study of common movements, maneuvres and exercises. *Scand J Rehabil Med, Supplementum*: 1-40, 1970.

Nachemson, A; Morris, J: In vivo measurements of intradiscal pressure. *J Bone Joint Surg, 46-A*:1077-1092, 1964.

Nachemson, A; Schultz, AB; Berkson, MH: Mechanical properties of human lumbar spine motion segments. Influences of age, sex, disc level and degeneration. *Spine, 4*:1-8, 1979.

Naylor, A; Smare, DL: Fluid content of the nucleus pulposus as a factor in the disc syndrome. Preliminary report. *Br Med J, 2*:975, 1951.

Nordin, M; Elfstrom, G; Dahlquist, P: Intra-abdominal pressure measurements using a wireless radiopressure pill and two wire-connected pressure transducers: a comparison. *Scand J Work Environ Health*, 1984. In press.

Okada, M: Electromyographic assessment of muscular load in forward bending postures. *J Faculty Sci, (Univ Tokyo) 8*:311, 1970.

Ono, K: Electromyographic studies of the abdominal wall muscles in visceroptosis. *Tohuku J Exp Med, 68*:347, 1958.

Ortengren, R; Andersson, GBJ; Nachemson, A: Lumbar back loads in fixed spinal postures during flexion and rotation. In *Biomechanics VI* E. Asmussen and K. Jorgensen (eds), Baltimore, Univ Park Press, 1978, pp.159-166.

Ortengren, R; Andersson, GBJ: Electromyographic studies of trunk muscles, with special reference to the lumbar spine. *Spine, 2*:44-52, 1977.

Ott, A.: Quellungsversuche mit operative entfernten Bandscheibengewebe. *Ztschr f Orthop,*

84:577, 1954 (in German).

Pauly, JE: An electromyographic analysis of certain movements and exercises. I. Some deep muscles of the back. *Anat Rec, 155*:223, 1966.

Petter, CK: Methods of measuring the pressure of the intervertebral disc. *J Bone Joint Surg, 15*:365, 1933.

Pope, M; Wilder, D; Booth, J: The biomechanics of low back pain. in *Symposium on Idiopathic Low Back Pain* (ed. A.A. White III, S.L. Gordon). St. Louis, Mosby, 1982, pp.252-295.

Portnoy, H; Morin, F: Electromyographic study of postural muscles in various positions and movements. *Am J Physiol, 186*:122, 1956.

Rosemeyer, B: Electromyographische Untersuchungen der Ruchen- und Schultermuskulatur im Stehen und Sitzen unter Berucksichtigung der Haltung des Autofahrers. *Acta Orthop Unfallchir, 71*:59, 1971 (in German).

Rushmer, RF: Nature of intraperitoneal and intrarectal pressures. *Am J Physiol, 147*:242-249, 1946.

Schultz, AB: Mechanical factors in the etiology of idiopathic low back disorders. In *Symposium on Idiopathic Low Back Pain* (ed. A.A. White III, S.L. Gordon). St. Louis, Mosby, 1982, pp.201-219.

Schultz, AB; Warwick, DN; Berkson, MH; Nachemson, A: Mechanical properties of human lumbar spine motion segments. Part I: Responses in flexion, extension, lateral bending and torsion. *J Biomech Engineering, 101*:46-52, 1979.

Schultz, AB; Andersson, GBJ; Ortengren, R; Bjork, R; Nordin, M: Analysis and quantitative myoelectric measurements of load on the lumbar spine when holding weights in standing postures: *Spine, 7*:390-397, 1982.

Schultz, AB; Andersson, GBJ; Ortengren, R; Nachemson, A; Haderspeck, K: Loads on the lumbar spine: Validation of a biomechanical analysis by measurements of intradiscal pressures and myoelectric signals. *J Bone Joint Surg, 64-A*:713-720, 1982.

Stubbs, DA: Manual Handling in the Construction Industry. *Construction Industry Training Board Report*, 1973.

Tzivian, IL; Rayhinstein, VH; Mosolova, MD; Ovseychik, JG: Mechanical properties of the nucleus pulposus of the lumbar intervertebral discs. *Ortopedija Traumatologija, 1*:55, 1970 (in Russian).

Virgin, WJ: Experimental investigations into the physical properties of the intervertebral disc. *J Bone Joint Surg, 33-B*:607-611, 1951.

Watson, BW; Ross, B; Kay, AW: Telemetring from within the body using pressure-sensitive radio pill. *Cut, 3*:181, 1962.

White, AA III; Edwards, WT; Liberman, D; Hayes, WC; Lewinnek, GE: Biomechanics of the lumbar spine and sacroiliac articulation: relevance to idiopathic low back pain. In *Symposium on Idiopathic Low Back Pain* A.A. White III, S.L. Gordon (ed.) St. Louis, Mosby, 1982, pp.296-322.

CHAPTER TWO

THE BIOMECHANICS OF THE LUMBAR POSTERIOR ELEMENTS AND SACRO-ILIAC JOINTS

JAMES A.A. MILLER, Ph.D.

INTRODUCTION

IT is well established that the lumbar spine is placed under significant loads in daily activities. By and large these loads are in the form of compression and shear forces which arise from the active muscle contraction forces required to counteract moments due to body weight. At the same time the lumbar spine seems to be protected by trunk and spine muscle action from having to resist significant moment loads because otherwise its relatively low bending stiffness would lead to unacceptably large spine motions.

Having established the loads on the lumbar spine in daily activities (see Andersson in this volume), the next step is to understand how these loads are distributed among the passive tissues of the lumbar spine — the intervertebral disc with its adjacent longitudinal ligaments on the one hand and the posterior elements on the other. High levels of stresses or strains locally in any of these tissues can lead to tissue damage, inflammation, edema and consequent symptoms. Thus we seek to establish which local structures are at risk in a particular task or activity. This chapter will review the salient biomechanical characteristics of the posterior elements and sacroiliac joints.

The Posterior Elements

Anatomy

The posterior elements include all bony and ligamentous structures posterior to the posterior longitudinal ligament. In general after 9 years of age little change in the neural arch and vertebral foramen is apparent (Reichmann and

18

Lewin, 1971).The pedicles are longer and thinner in the upper lumbar spine than the shorter and more massive pedicles of the lower levels. However, the interpedicular distance remains fairly constant from L-1 to L-5. The spinous processes are well developed in the upper lumbar spine becoming smaller as one moves caudally to L-5. Morphometric studies of lumbar vertebrae have been performed for example by Lanier (1939) and Sand (1970). The relevant ligamentous structures are described in any anatomic text. However, three points are worth noting. First, the supraspinous ligament does not pass from L-5 to the sacrum (Rissanen, 1960). Secondly, the central part of the interspinous ligament is bifid in the lumbar spine passing bilaterally from either side of the spinous processes. The direction of the fibers in this ligament, shown incorrectly in texts, is caudo-dorsal (Heylings, 1978) this fiber arrangement facilitates flexion of the lumbar spine. A final point is the anatomy and organization of the thoracolumbar fascia. As Farfan (1973) and Fairbank and O'Brien (1980) have pointed out, the abdominal muscles originate from this fascia, which in turn is connected to the interspinous and supraspinous ligaments posteriorly, to the transverse processes, and to the quadratus lumborum. This arrangement theoretically allows the abdominal muscles to apply an extension moment to the spine via the lumbosacral fascia in certain lumbar configurations. If this is so, then the lumbosacral fascia could also be considered as part of the posterior element complex.

The zygoapophyseal or facet joints are diarthroidal synovial joints with a synovium and capsular ligaments which have their fibers oriented in a direction perpendicular to the plane of the joint. Farfan (1973) has described the approximate orientation and area of these joints. Detailed morphological studies arc provided by Lewin et al. (1962).

The blood supply to the facet joints, interspinous ligament and paravertebral muscles is via a branch of the lumbar artery that perforates the intertransverse ligament. Each facet joint is innervated bisegmentally by the dorsal rami of the two spinal nerves, (Lewin et al., 1962).

Biomechanics of the Posterior Elements

Some idea of posterior element function can be gained from studying the results of in vitro mechanical tests of motion segments with and without the posterior elements intact.

In these tests known forces are typically applied in turn in given directions to the upper vertebra while the lower is held rigidly. The resultant three dimensional motions are then measured (Schultz et al., 1979; Berkson et al., 1979). In anterior-posterior shear tests, the presence of the posterior elements restricted motions under known forces by up to 30 percent. In moment tests, the posterior elements decreased motions in extension and torsion by about 40 percent. In other test directions their contributions were significantly less. So, from these results, the posterior elements seem to play a role in controlling intervertebral displacements in shear, extension and torsion.

Posterior element function in extension was also examined in vitro by Lorentz et al. (1982) who inserted pressure sensitive film directly into the apophyseal joint space before loading the motion segment in compression and extension. They found peak pressures of 40 kp/cm² and total joint contact areas of about 2.0 cm² under a combined compression load of 1400 N and 7 Nm (which represents a reasonable estimate of typical in vivo loads on the upright spine). (See chapter by Andersson in this volume.)

The mechanical properties of the complete posterior elements were measured recently for the first time in our laboratory by Skipor (1983). When compared to isolated intervertebral disc properties (Schultz et al., 1979) the posterior elements were 45 percent as stiff as the disc in anterior shear, 10-20 percent in compression, posterior and lateral shear. In lateral bending and torsion their stiffness was found to be 30 percent that of the disc, while in flexion and extension the figure was somewhat less.

In general, stiffness is a measure of the load that can be resisted at a given displacement. As noted above, posterior elements have modest stiffness values compared to those of the disc, but it should be noted that in flexion-extension and torsion they act at a considerable distance from the disc center. If we make the simplistic assumption that rotary motion occurs about this center, then this long lever arm (30-40 mm) increases their contributions to resisting loads placed on the lumbar spine. However, the presence of this lever arm also implies that in large spine motions they can be subject to large strains or deformations with possibilities for concomitant pathology. The normal range of movement of the facet joints has been estimated at 5-7 mm in the superior-inferior direction (Lewin et al., 1962). However, more detailed studies of posterior elements kinematics in vivo would seem warranted using CT or stereophotogrammetric techniques.

In a study of vertebral geometry and its effect on load-sharing between the disc and posterior elements, Miller et al. (1983) noted that the superior-inferior facet joint location relative to the intervertebral disc center also played a role in determining how the disc and facet joints distributed an anteroposteriorly-directed shear load applied to the superior vertebral body of a motion segment. The more the facets were located inferior to the disc, the larger the shear load the disc had to resist and the less the resulting antero-posteriorly-directed compressive load the facet joints had to resist. By implication, people with more inferiorly-placed facet joints may routinely expose their discs to larger shear loads than is usual. Would vertebral morphology be something to investigate in acute low back patients without sciatic involvement?

Another aspect of facet joint morphology that can have a bearing on how the loads internal to the motion segment are shared is the orientation and form of the left and right articular surfaces. Farfan (1973) has pointed out that some

30 percent of the macerated specimens he examined in the transverse plane had a difference in inclination of 12 degrees or more, supporting earlier findings (Farfan and Sullivan, 1967). This lack of right-left symmetry (or articular tropism) has been shown to cause vertebral rotation to the side of the more oblique facet in combined anterior shear and compression loading (Cyron and Hutton, 1980). This has been hypothesized as a mechanism by which asymmetric loading of both the intervertebral disc and facet joints can occur. Whether or not this necessarily leads to unilateral degeneration of either structure is unknown, but it deserves further investigation, perhaps with the aid of clinical investigations using CT scans. Certainly articular tropism is not always related to low back symptoms, since Farfan noted asymmetry in 23 percent of patients with no low back symptoms. He did note however a high correlation between the side of sciatica and disc protrusion and the side of the more oblique facet in his material.

When intact motion segments are loaded in combined torsion and compression, it has been shown that the facet loaded in compression carries about twice as much load as that loaded in tension (Adams and Hutton, 1981). This suggests that in torsional loading both compaction of the bony structures of the compression facet and distraction of the capsule and lateral ligamentum flavum at the tension facet are possible injury modes. The effect of asymmetry in exacerbating or diminishing these possibilities by introducing additional shear forces has not been examined.

Posterior element mechanics are of interest in considering the cause of spondylolysis. One theory is that although the neural arch is strong and can support over 2000 N applied in the anterior-posterior directions at the level of the facet joints (Suezawa et al., 1980), it is susceptible to fatigue failure at submaximal loading levels (Hutton et al., 1977). If the rate of bone repair is slower than the accumulation of cyclical damage, say as might occur in repeated stooping and lifting, then the possibility of fatigue fracture of the pars interarticularis can arise. This type of failure could be replicated in 7 out of 8 young cadaver specimens under cyclic loading at only 25 percent of maximal static load levels (Hutton et al., 1977).

As in other joints it has been shown that reduced motions and abnormal loading can lead to facet joint degeneration. For example, it has been shown by Kahanovitz et al. (1983) in cases with internal fixation without arthrodesis that the facet joints one level above the lower Harrington hook showed areas of fibrillation, fissures and thinning of normal cartilaginous surfaces characteristic of osteoarthritis some 6-26 months after the operation.

Conclusions

In the last five years a number of studies have concentrated on how the posterior elements may be loaded in a given set of activities. More clinical data is clearly needed on variability in their morphology, and specific tests need to be designed that objectively test their function as completely as possible in the back pain patient.

Sacro-Iliac Joints

Anatomy

Most commonly, the first three sacral levels form the sacral part of the sacro-iliac joint (Paterson, 1893). In the fetus the joint is narrow, running parallel to the vertebral column axis with an area of about 1.5 cm^2 (Brooke, 1924). With growth it curves in the caudo-dorsal direction, increasing in width (Solonen, 1957). In the adult it has an area of about 18 cm^2 (Sashin, 1930).

A synovial membrane lines the joint capsule anteriorly, while posteriorly it blends with the fibers of the interosseus ligaments. Normally there is no free fluid in the joint. On the iliac side the articular cartilage is thin (0.5-2.0 mm) and striated, while on the sacral side it is smoother and two or three times thicker although somewhat thinner posteriorly and superiorly (Bowen and Cassidy, 1981).

Sacro-Iliac Ligaments: These were the subject of a careful study by Weisl (1954a) on some 92 specimens. He found that the capsular ligament completely surrounds the joint, being thinnest cranially, about 1 mm thick ventrally, and thickest caudally (15 mm wide and 3 mm thick). Dorsal to the joint are a number of substantial accessory ligaments arranged in three layers. The deep layer is comprised cranially of about thirteen sets of 8 mm long fiber bundles which are 3 mm in diameter passing dorso-laterally from sacrum to ilium. Caudally an equal number of bundles pass cranially from the sacrum; they are about 12 mm long and 2 × 4 mm^2 in area. An intermediate layer of interwoven fasciculi about 2-3 mm thick is directed dorsally and laterally together with the superior and laterale posticum ligaments. Superficially there are inconstant ligaments less than 1 mm thick from the caudal lateral sacral tubercle to the iliac crest, and a superficial part of the sacrotuberous ligament and ligamentum posterior longum (50 mm long, width 10 mm, thickness 1 mm) passing cranially from the S-3 and S-4 lateral tubercles to the posterior iliac spine.

In summary, this system of accessory ligaments has a unilateral cross-sectional area of over 300 mm^2, apparently to resist the ubiquitous shear loads placed on this joint. The sacrotuberous and sacrospinous ligaments provide ventral and lateral fixation of the caudal part of the sacrum (Slocum and Terry, 1926).

Articular Geometry: Great inter-individual variation is present in any geometric parameter used to describe these joints: the shape of the ventral and dorsal joint margins, the shape of the articular surfaces, or the relative orientation of these surfaces. No significant sex differences have been found in these parameters by Weisl (1954b), who reported an extensive study of sacroiliac geometry which will form the basis of the following review.

In general, the margins of the joint form the shape of an inverted "L," with the shape of the ventral and dorsal margins varying independently of one another. In both fetuses and adults the sacral joint surface is such that each arm of the "L" ends in an elevation bounding a central depression. The cranial elevation is the most prominent. The maximum mean difference in joint surface elevation is about 2 mm in the fetus and 11 mm in the adult. Often the central depression extends along the arms of the "L" to form depressions behind the elevation at the ends. In general, the corresponding iliac surface is not a true replica of the sacral geometry. After the second decade, geometric changes with age are common. Most commonly, smaller interlocking elevations and depression and ankyloses occur near the ventral margin of the joint. Bowen and Cassidy (1981) found that age-related changes typical of osteoarthritis affected the iliac cartilage more than the sacral cartilage; by the fourth and fifth decades osteophytes had often formed on the ventral margin of the joint. By the 6th decade 85 percent of the females and all of the male specimens examined by Sashin (1930) showed osteophyte formation.

Innervation of the Joint: A dissection study by Solonen (1957) in 18 specimens showed some variation in innervation patterns, but most frequently the vertebral, cranial and caudal aspects of the joint were innervated by the L-4, 5 spinal cord levels, whereas the dorsal aspect was innervated from the S-1 and S-2 levels.

Relative Location and Orientation of Joint Surfaces: The orientation and location of the right and left sacro-iliac joints relative to one another can be ascertained by averaging data provided by Solonen (1957). The distance between the most lateral points of each joint at the L-1 level was 110 mm with a standard deviation (SD) of 9 with a range from 95 to 129 mm. Separation of the most caudal points on each surface was 92 mm (SD = 5) varying from 83 to 101 mm. Weisl (1954) found that the overall width and length of the joints averaged 35 and 58 mm respectively.

In the frontal plane the sacrum is wedge-shaped at the L-1 and L-2 levels, but flairs laterally at S-3 (Table II-1). This data shows that the wedge forms an angle of about 10 degrees to the sagittal plane. Similarly, a cranial view of the sacrum in the transverse plane shows that at the S-1 and S-2 levels the anterior joint margins are more widely spaced than the posterior margins, yielding a wedge angle from 24-43 degrees (Table II-2). At the S-3 level the left and right joint surfaces are nearly parallel.

Muscle: Although no single joint muscles cross the sacro-iliac joint, contraction of any or all of the adjacent muscles such as the psoas, quadratus lumborum, abdominal oblique, lateral erector spinae or piriformis, the sacral portion of the gluteus major will place shear and moment loads on these joints in proportion to their contraction forces.

TABLE II-1

Level	Mean	Standard Deviation	Range	Number Observations
S1	9°	7°	− 5 to 23°	45
S2	10°	12°	− 12 to 40°	60
S3	− 7°	9°	− 25 to 13°	60

Angle in degrees which the sacroiliac joint surface makes with a caudally-directed axis in the frontal plane. The angle is positive where the tangent to the surface and axis meet below the sacrum, negative where it meets cranial to the joint. Data extracted for left and right sides and combined from Solonen (1957).

TABLE II-2

Level	Mean	Standard Deviation	Range	Number Observations
S1	43°	18°	0 to 64°	26
S2	24°	17°	− 6 to 62°	26
S3	11°	18°	− 45 to 37°	26

Angle in degrees between tangents through each joint surface in the transverse plane. A positive angle occurs when the tangents meet dorsal to the sacrum, a negative when they meet ventral to the sacrum. Data extracted from Solonen (1957).

Biomechanics of the Sacro-Iliac Joints

We know rather little qualitatively about how these joints are loaded in various body postures, such as upright standing, forward trunk flexion, bipedal or unipedal stances for example. By knowing both the forces and moments on each joint, their geometry and that of the pelvis, and their mechanical properties, analyses can be performed to estimate how they are loaded in any given task or body configuration, and which structures are most heavily or most frequently stressed. In such analyses it will be important to know the mechanical properties of the symphysis pubis and the geometry of the surrounding muscle origin and insertion points.

Kinematic Studies: In general these studies have been useful in showing that slight motion occurs in vivo in the sacro-iliac joint, decreasing with the age of the individual. Weisl (1955) showed radiographically that when subjects move from the recumbent to the standing position, the sacral promontory moved ventrally about 6 mm with an apparent axis of motion 5-10 cm below it, but the axis was highly variable. In another study of 12 subjects Colachis et al. (1963) reported 'small' movements but no absolute magnitudes of sacral motion was determined. In a single subject, changes of 1-5 mm in the separation between adjacent points on the sacrum and iliac crest were found when the legs were 'scissored' 30 degrees anteriorly and posteriorly in the sidelying position (Frigerio et al., 1974). Although these studies indicate motions between points on the three bones constituting the pelvic girdle can reach 25 mm, they do not yield any clear insight into how this structure functions as an entity under loading different situations.

Estimates of Loads on the Sacro-Iliac Joints: With the knowledge that the compression load on the lumbar disc is about 1000 N in relaxed standing, the downwards shear loads on each sacro-iliac joint will be about one half of this value. The joint may also be placed under bending moments in both the sagittal and frontal planes due to the moment exerted by trunk weight. These may be partially or totally balanced by moments generated by active muscle contractions depending on the circumstances. In the absence of muscle activity, however, the passive sacro-iliac structures must resist the moments alone. In the sagittal plane the superincumbent body weight acts about 5 cm anterior to the joint center, exerting flexion moment of 40 kg × 5 cm or 20 Nm divided between each joint. In the absence of extensor trunk muscle activity this moment must be resisted by the joint capsule, dorsal accessory ligaments and sacrotuberous and sacrospinous ligaments. It is this moment that probably gives rise to the anterior sacral promontory motion observed by Weisl (1955) in passing from the recumbent to the standing position.

In the frontal plane the joints lie about 10 cm closer together than the hip joints, whose spacing is about 20 cm. In biped standing the lateral flexion moment due to body weight alone will therefore be about 50 kg multiplied by 5 cm or 25 Nm. However, this moment is balanced by that due to the reaction force at the hip joint on the contralateral side of the sacrum. Thus in relaxed standing each joint is under a constant shear force of 500 N, and a flexion moment of about 20 Nm. Dynamic activities that introduce inertial effects may double these loads.

Maximal compression loads of 3500 N have been estimated at L-3 in lifting tasks (Nachemson, 1976), thus increasing these shear and bending moment loads on the sacroiliac joints, largely due to muscle contraction forces. Thus the shear on each joint will rise to 1750 N from the 500 N in relaxed standing. With the cross-sectional area of the dorsal accessory ligaments already established at about 300 mm², the maximum loading stress would be about 6N/mm². Typical failure stress for other spinal ligaments are about 20 N/mm² (Tkaczuk, 1968). At a length of 25 mm and with a modulus of elasticity approaching 600 N/mm² (Nordwall, 1973), the strain might lie around 20/600 or

3 percent, equivalent to an elongation of about 1 mm. If these ligaments are oriented craniolaterally then the sacrum is essentially suspended from each ilium. The horizontal component of the ligament tension (determined by ligament inclination) will compress the ilia against the sacrum, enhancing the effect of the joint surface irregularities in decreasing joint motion.

In one-legged standing, the lateral bending moment on the support side may change sign (Pauwels, 1980) and could reach 25 Nm, while both the flexion and shear loads will double. Indeed, Schunke (1938) noted the pubic bone moves forward in relation to that on the unsupported side; however, whether or not this is due to these increased loads remains to be determined.

In forward flexion of the trunk the sacrum is again suspended from the ilia. Assuming trunk weight (40 kg) acts at five times the lever arm of the gluteus muscle and sacrotuberous and sacrospinous ligaments (which will resist the flexion moment about the sacro-iliac joints (Lusskin and Sonnenschein, 1927), then the combined downward shear may reach 40 kg plus 5 multiplied by 40 kg, or 240 N on both joints in simple forward bending without weight holding or lifting. The dorsal accessory ligaments again are ideally oriented to resist such a ventrally-directed shear force.

Some insight into the mechanical strength of the sacro-iliac joints can be gained from the failure tests of Gunterberg et al. (1976). These investigators first noted that sacral and sacro-iliac joint resections as high as S-1 have been performed in tumor surgery with uneventful recoveries and subsequent ambulation. Using cadaver tests they demonstrated the mean axial "compressive" strength (actually the downward shear strength) was 4865 N for the combined intact joints. A resection which left the S-1 portion of the joints intact reduced the compressive strength by 30 percent, while a yet higher resection reduced it by 50 percent. Failures always occurred in the lateral part of the sacrum relatively close to the sacro-iliac joint. Hence the intact, and even the damaged joint, possesses a relatively large shear strength.

In summary, simple estimates of sacro-iliac loading place shear loads in the range 300-1750 N in daily activities with simultaneous flexion and lateral bending moments of 25-50 Nm not being uncommon.

Mechanical Properties of the Sacro-Iliac Joints: What kinds of motions may be expected under the above magnitudes of loads? The only study reported to date was that by Slocum and Terry (1926) who reported that sectioning the sacrospinous and sacrotuberous ligaments allowed a dorsal movement of the caudal sacrum of 1.1 mm under a compressive load of 750 N. This illustrates one function of these structures in limiting flexion movements of the loaded sacrum.

In a recent study, (Miller et al., submitted) preliminary results show single sacro-iliac joint shear stiffnesses of 200-1500 N/mm and moment stiffnesses of 12-30 Nm/degree depending on the test direction. The joint has roughly similar stiffnesses to lumbar motion segments in anterior-posterior and caudally-directed shear under 300 N, but was nearly 10 times stiffer in medial shear tests placing the entire joint capsule under direct tension. The sacro-iliac joints were twice as stiff as spine segments in torsion (12 Nm/degree), three times as stiff in cranially-directed tension, eight times as stiff in flexion and 15 times as stiff in lateral bending (29 Nm/degree).

Pregnancy results in a hormonally-mediated decrease in ligament stiffness after the fourth month, increasing this effect until parturition and returning to normal four months after birth (Brooke, 1924). Clearly, relaxation of the symphysis pubis and ventral sacro-iliac capsule will yield the largest increase in the birth canal diameter. Apparently this decrease in stiffness may approach about one-half the usual stiffness value.

Conclusion

These kinds of data on the magnitude and directions of the loads on the sacro-iliac joints, when coupled with information on the joint geometries and mechanical properties, will enable mathematical structural models to be designed to simulate how and when the sacro-iliac joints are loaded. These analyses may be carried out along much the same lines described elsewhere in this volume by Andersson in the lumbar spine. Studies analogous to the above load-sharing studies of the facet-joints, which require knowledge of tissue mechanical properties like those reported here, will allow the prediction of areas of high, possibly cyclic, strain and could improve our understanding of sacro-iliac joint mechanics. This in turn could lead to improved diagnostic and treatment modalities, since we will understand better how to alter or relieve the significant loads on these joints. Clearly much further research is warranted on all aspects of sacro-iliac joint function.

REFERENCES

Adams, M.A. and Hutton, W.C.: The relevance of torsion to the mechanical derangement of the lumbar spine. *Spine, 6*:241, 1981.

Berkson, M.H.; Nachemson, A.; and Schultz, A.B.: Mechanical properties of human lumbar spine motion segments, Part II: Responses in compression and shear influence of gross morphology. *ASME Journal of Biomechanical Engineering, 101*:53, 1979.

Bowen, V. and Cassidy, J.D.: Macroscopic and microscopic anatomy of the sacroiliac joint from embryonic life until the eighth decade. *Spine, 6*:620, 1981.

Brooke, R.: The sacroiliac joint. *Journal of Anatomy, 58B*:299, 1924.

Colachis, S.; Worden, R.; Bechtol, C. and Strohm, B.: Movement of the sacroiliac joint in the adult male: A preliminary report. *Archives of Physical Medicine, 44*:490, 1963

Cyron, B.M. and Hutton, W.C.: Articular tropism and stability of the lumbar spine. *Spine, 5*:168, 1980.

Fairbank, J.C.T. and O'Brien, J.P.: The abdominal cavity and thoraco-lumbar fascia as stabilizers of the lumbar spine in patients with LBP. Presented to "Engineering Aspects of the Spine", Abstract of Conference arranged by Institute of Mechanical Engineers, London, May 1979.

Farfan, H. and Sullivan, J.D.: The relation of facet orientation to intervertebral disc failure. *Canadian Journal of Surgery, 110*:179, 1967.

Farfan, H.: *Mechanical disorders of the low back.* Philadelphia, Lea and Febiger, 1973.

Frigerio, N.; Stowe, R. and Howe, J.: Movement of the sacroiliac joint. *Clinical Orthopaedics and Related Research, 100*:370, 1974.

Gunterberg, B.; Romanus, B. and Stener, B.: Pelvic strength after major amputation of the sacrum. An experimental study. *Acta Orthopaedica Scandinavica, 47*:635, 1976.

Heylings, D.J.: Supraspinous and interspinous ligament. *Journal of Anatomy (London), 125*:127, 1978.

Hutton, W.C.; Scott, J.R.R. and Cyron, B.M.: Is spondylolysis a fatigue fracture? *Spine, 2*:202, 1977.

Kahanovitz, N.; Bullough, P. and Jacobs, R.R.: The effect of internal fixation without arthrodesis on human facet joint cartilage. Presented at the International Society for the Study of the Lumbar Spine, Cambridge, U.K., May, 1983.

Lanier, R.R.: The presacral vertebrae of American white and negro males. *American Journal of Physical Anthropology, 25*:341, 1939.

Lewin, T.; Moffett, B. and Viidik, A.: The morphology of the lumbar synovial intervertebral joints. *Acta Morphologica Neerlando-Scandinavica, 4*:299, 1962.

Lorentz, M.; Patwardhan, A. and Vanderby, R.: Load bearing characteristics of lumbar facets in normal and surgically altered spinal segments. *Spine*, 1983, in press.

Lusskin, H. and Sonnenschein, H.: Low back sprain. The sacroiliac syndrome. *American Journal of Surgery, 3*:534, 1927.

Miller, J.A.A.; Andersson, G.B.J. and Schultz, A.B.: Mechanical properties of the adult sacroiliac joint. Submitted to Orthopaedic Research Society Meeting, 1984.

Miller, J.A.A.; Haderspeck, K. and Schultz, A.B.: Posterior element loads in lumbar motion segments. *Spine*, 1983, in press.

Nachemson, A.: The lumbar spine: an orthopaedic challenge. *Spine, 1*:59, 1976.

Nordwall, A.: Studies in idiopathic scoliosis. *Acta Orthopaedica Scandinavica, Supplementum 150*, 1973.

Pauwels, F.: *Biomechanics of the locomotor apparatus.* Berlin, Springer Verlag, 138, 1980.

Paterson (1893) cited by Solonen (1957).

Reichman, S. and Lewin, T.: Growth processes in the lumbar neural arch. *Zeitschrift fuer Anatomie und Entwicklungsgeschichte, 133*:89, 1971.

Risannen, P.M.: The surgical anatomy and pathology of supraspinal and interspinous ligaments of the lumbar spine, with special reference to ligament ruptures. *Acta Orthopaedica Scandinavica, Supplementum 46*, 1960.

Sand, P.G.: *The human lumbo-sacral vertebral column. An osteometric study.* Ph.D. Thesis, University of Oslo, 1970.

Sashin, D.: A critical analysis of the anatomy and pathologic changes of the sacro-iliac joints. *Journal of Bone and Joint Surgery, 12*:891, 1930.

Schultz, A.B.; Warwick, D.N.; Berkson, M.H. and Nachemson, A.L.N.: Mechanical properties of human lumbar spine motion segments—Part I: Response in Bending and Torsion. *Journal of Biomechanical Engineering, 101*:46, 1979.

Schunke, A.B.: The anatomy and development of the sacro-iliac joint in man. *Anatomical Record, 72*:313, 1938.

Skipor, A.F.: *Facet joint biomechanics in lumbar spine motion segments.* M.S. Thesis, Dept. of Materials Engineering, University of Illinois at Chicago, 1983.

Slocumb, L. and Terry, R.J.: Influence of the sacrotuberand and sacrospinous ligaments in limiting movements at the sacroiliac joint. *Journal of the American Medical Association (JAMA), 87*:307, 1926.

Solonen, K.A.: The sacroiliac joint in the light of anatomical, roentgenological and clinical studies. *Acta Orthopaedics Scandinavica, Supplementum 26*, 1957.

Suezawa, Y.; Jacob, H.A.C. and Bernoski, F.P.: The mechanical response of the neural arch of the lumbosacral vertebra and its clinical significance. *International Orthopaedics (Sicot)*, *4*:205-209, 1980.

Tkaczuk, H.: Tensile properties of human lumbar longitudinal ligaments. *Acta Orthoepaedica Scandinavica, Supplementum 115*, 1968.

Weisl, H.: Ligaments of the sacro-iliac joint examined with particular reference to their function. *Acta Anatomica, 20*:201, 1954.

Weisl, H.: The articular surfaces of the sacro-iliac joint and their relation to the movements of the sacrum. *Acta Anatomica, 22*:1, 1954.

Weisl, H.: The movements of the sacro-iliac joint. *Acta Anatomica, 23*:80, 1955.

CHAPTER THREE

BIOMECHANICAL PROPERTIES
OF THE INTERVERTEBRAL DISC

M.H. POPE, Ph.D.

SINCE Mixter and Barr's description (1934), herniated nucleus pulposus has been the most common indication for lumbar spine surgery. Degenerative intervertebral joint disc disease is stated by some (Beadle, 1931) to be the most common cause of low back pain. The peak incidence of disc herniations is between the ages of 30 and 40 (Hult, 1954). Herniations are found in 15% to 30% of pathological specimens and they are also found in normal individuals in myelographic studies. In general there was an increase in degenerative changes with age with all affected by the age of 60 (Farfan et al., 1972; Puschel, 1930).

ANATOMICAL CONSIDERATIONS

The intervertebral disc consists of three distinct anatomical parts. The first is the cartilaginous endplates of the vertebral bodies, the second the cartilaginous lamellae of the annulus fibrosus which connect the vertebrae and the nucleus pulposus and the third the nucleus pulposus. The annulus is comprised of collagen fibers in the form of concentric laminated sheets. The fibers are angled at about 20° to each other in the adjacent sheets. In the inner part of the disc, the collagen is attached directly to the cartilaginous endplates while in the outer area it is attached directly to the bone.

Up to the age of 30, the nucleus behaves like a sponge (Blumenkrantz, 1977; Bodine, 1980; Bonnaire, 1899). A degenerated nucleus is unable to sustain much fluid pressure. The end-plates are subjected to less central pressure and the loads are distributed peripherally. In the outer annulus of a degenerated disc there is less peripheral tension, more compressive stress, more expansion and thus higher fiber stresses (Farfan, 1973). These degenerate discs also demonstrate much greater dispersion of the instantaneous centers of motion (Rolander, 1966) and show a smaller strain to failure in torsion (Farfan, 1970, 1973, 1978). Degeneration and aging also result in decreased hysteresis, residual deformity (Farfan, 1973) and greater stiffness (Galante, 1967), and a change in creep properties (Kazarian, 1975). Galante (1967) also noted increases in the tensile properties of the disc up to the third decade, after which there was no significant change.

When the disc is subject to compression, pressure is exerted on the cartilage of the plates and on the nucleus pulposus. The nuclear pressure is converted into tensile strain on the lamellae of the annulus and results in lateral expansion and bulging. When the center of the load is outside the axis, the nucleus is reported to act as a fulcum and changes the distribution of stress along the circumference of the annulus. The means by which the intervertebral disc strains in flexion moments has been an enigma. Steindler (1955) suggested that the nucleus moves posteriorly during flexion with a radial bulge occurring anteriorly. Roaf (1960) used discograms and found no change in nuclear position while Shah (1978) used the same technique to confirm posterior motion of the nucleus. Brown (1957) suggested that the whole disc moves anteriorly with flexion. Recently, using radiopaque markers, we have shown that the disc moves as a unit with no net movement of the nucleus relative to the rest of the disc (Kelsey, 1975).

DISC BIOCHEMISTRY

Intervertebral discs contain both types I and II collagen. The nucleus pulposus contains only type II while as the annulus fibrosus shows a smooth change from type I to II going from outer to the inner regions. It is probable that the type II collagen, which are more highly hydrated are able to deform under load and thus absorb compression stresses applied to the tissues (Grynpas, 1980).

There are some changes with level in the spine. It has been shown that in thoracic discs there is a higher proportion of reducible cross-links than in the lumbar discs. This variation with locations may be due to the physical environment of the disc. It has been observed that in discs immediately above those that are diseased, there is a higher proportion of reducible cross-links (Herbert, 1975). There is biomechanical evidence to support this also. Stokes et al. (1981) have demonstrated by biplanar radiography an increased mobility of the disc immediately above the fusion site, also possibly indicating the increased content of collagen with fewer cross links. It has been demonstrated that although under normal conditions most collagen is stable, it is being degraded and replaced (Eyre, 1977; Grant, 1972; Hallen, 1962; Harris, 1954; Prockp, 1976). The quantity of hydroxylysine (Barnes, 1974; Royce, 1977) and glycosylated hydroxylysine (Barnes, 1974; Ghosh, 1977; Murai, 1975) in type I collagen decrease with age up to the age of about 25 years.

The other major component of disc cartilage is proteoglycans. The ratio of chondroitin-4 sulfate to chondroitin-6 sulfate is age dependent. By the sixth decade, chondroitin-6 sulfate is predominant (Mathews, 1967; Taylor, 1971). In young discs, the majority of proteoglycans possess a hyaluronic acid bonding region (Hardingham, 1976; Stevens, 1979). With aging, there is a deficiency of the hyaluronic acid binding region of the protein (Hardingham, 1976; Naylor, 1955; Stevens, 1979). There also appears to be a decrease in total glycosaminoglycan content (Happey, 1961; Hopwood, 1974; Naylor, 1976). The total glycosamine content reaches a maximum during the third decade (Adams, 1976; Hardingham, 1976) and decreases in the elderly (Emes, 1975; Hardingham, 1976; Hopwood, 1974).

BIOPHYSICS AND NUTRITION

The intervertebral disc is the largest avascular structure in the human body and depends totally on exchange via passive diffusion for its nutrition and disposal of metabolic waste products (Urban, 1977, 1978). Diffusion occurs at the periphery of the annulus and through the vertebral end-plate primarily. The blood supply at the end-plate stops at approximately 18 years of age and since prolapse is generally observed first with the 25-year-old age group, it has been suggested that decreased end-plate nutrition may be a primary event associated with the onset of the degenerative events of aging and disease (Diamant, 1968). Also, there is a correlation between decreased permeability of the central region of the end-plate and disc degeneration (Nachemson et al., 1970).

Kramer (1977) considered the intervertebral disc as an osmotic system in which intradiscal and extradiscal oncotic forces in addition to the ionochemical drives are taken into the intradiscal forces would comprise the sum of the hydrostatic forces of the swelling pressure of the nucleus pulposus plus the osmotic force due to solute concentration of the free water fraction. The extradiscal forces are due to pressure loads on the intervertebral disc and to the solute concentration in the extradiscal fluid. Thus, if there is a change in any of these factors, shifts in fluids and metabolic substances will result. Nachemson's work (1964) implies that there is an influx of fluid into the intervertebral disc when one is lying down and an outflow when one is standing, sitting, or carrying a load. The discs have been reported to narrow in the working day and recover during bed rest. Reversed flow has been experimentally established at approximately 700 to 800 N (Kramer, 1977).

INTRADISCAL PRESSURE

Intradiscal pressure measurements by the Gothenberg group have led to a better understanding of the role of posture, exercise and loads on the disc. According to Nachemson (Nachemson and Morris, 1964; Nachemson and Evans, 1968; Nachemson et al., 1970), the hydrostatic pressure that is generated in the nucleus pulposus approximates 1.5 times the mean applied pressure over the entire area of the end-plate. For equilibrium of forces there must be equal forces applied to both sides of the end-plate. If the area of the nucleus were half of the area of the end-plate, then the mean pressure between the annulus and end-plate would be half of the mean external applied pressure. Nachemson (1964, 1968,1969, 1970) has demonstrated that intradiscal pressure is higher in sitting than in standing. At the level of L-3 there was a disc load in standing corresponding to body weight. In the supine position, the load was about 50% lower, whereas lifting a 20 kg weight resulted in a load of three times greater. An increase of back-rest inclination led to a decreased pressure as did an increase in lumbar support. However, a thoracic support increased the disc pressure.

Simultaneous measurements of intra-abdominal pressure, intradiscal pressure, and EMG showed that the intradiscal pressure fell slightly when abdominal pressure was increased. However, this was not a consistent finding.

LOAD CAPACITY

Simple vector diagram to calculate the loads on the lumbar spine reveals that when one just bends over, the forces in the spine at the L3-4 level may be above those which cause fractures (Armstrong, 1952; Bayer, 1954, Geneis, 1939; Mattiash, 1956). However, normal lumbar spines can withstand around 10kN of vertical force before failure (Perey, 1957; Schultz, 1970). Some authors have suggested that the load is partially supported by an increased intra-abdominal pressure (Bartelink, 1957; Eie, 1966; Morris, 1961) although this has been disputed by Farfan (1978).

Virgin (1951) was the first to suggest that the nucleus pulposus hydrostatically pressurizes the disc. Nachemson also showed that a normal resting disc pressure of about $1.5N/m^2$ and the disc is prestressed by the tension of spinal ligament with the force of about $1.5N/m^2$ (Nachemson and Evans, 1968) and possibly by the psoas muscle (Nachemson and Morris, 1966). Under imposed loading the intradiscal pressure rises to approximately 1.5 times the applied loads (Nachemson, 1963). This indicates the nucleus is transforming the compression loads into radially directed tensile forces in the annulus. Sonnerup (1972) found that the pressure is maximum in the anterior and decreases to the periphery. Markolf demonstrated that the annulus also carries a significant amount of the compressive load to the disc (Markolf, 1971; Markolf and Morris, 1974). In the following sections we will discuss the particular effects of certain load vectors.

COMPRESSIVE LOADING

There appears to be a relationship between compression and the pathogenesis of disc degeneration (Hirsch, 1949; Hirsch and Nachemson, 1961). Lindholm (1952) demonstrated increased disc degeneration in rats subjected to asymmetrical compression loads. Obviously, this loading included flexion moments.

Bipedal rats were also found to encounter disc degeneration and herniation more frequently than controls. Even though there appears to be a relationship between compressive stress and disc degeneration, acutely compressive loading does not cause disc herniations. When a motion segment is loaded to failure in compression, the uniform result is an end-plate fracture (Evans, 1959). This is true even if the annulus is incised. Virgin (1951) made a longitudinal posterolateral incision and still found no disc herniation with compression. Similar findings are reported by Hirsch (1955) and Markolf (1971, 1974). Farfan (1972) reported that the degenerated disc was stronger than the normal disc in compression whereas Brown (1957) found no difference between normal and degenerated discs. Markolf (1974) compressed discs with a radial hole, discectomy, and an axial hole through the entire motion segment. Injury caused changes in the mechanical properties of the disc; however, by the third loading cycle the motion segment showed nearly normal behavior. Markolf (1974) suggested that there was some kind of self-sealing effect in the disc. It is probable that Schmorl's nodes may be due to healed microscopic end-plate fractures (Perey, 1957; Vernon-Roberts, 1973).

Several authors report that fluid runs out of a disc with compression and Virgin (1951) maintained that the fluid could only come from the disc. However, recent work has indicated that the vascular and lymphatic fluids are more easily forced out of the vertebral body. This raises the interesting possibility that it is the vertebral body that cushions the vertebrae rather than vice versa.

TORSIONAL LOADINGS

Farfan (1970, 1973) claimed that a small angular twist will produce a large loss of disc volume. He also demonstrated that a single high rate axial rotation of 15 to 20° produced annular injuries. Farfan (1973) believes that rotation is the clinical mechanism of nuclear extrusion. To mimic a fibrotic nucleus, Farfan (1973) injected Silastic into the disc. After 50 rotations, the Silastic had traced through the disc to the periphery and had extruded in many cases. Hirsch (1949, 1969) suggested that these kinds of extrusion are a relatively late phenomenon in the degenerative process due to the self-sealing effect of young discs. It is probable that annular protrusion occurs late in the disease process.

Sullivan and Farfan (1971) showed that experimental posterior facetectomy leads to disc degeneration in rabbits. This was thought to be caused by increased torsional loading. Farfan's (1973) experiments in human material show that the articular facets contribute to approximately ½ of the torsional strength of the motion segments and about ¼ of the remainder is contributed by the disc itself. Thus, the strength is reduced by a factor of ⅓ when the disc is generated.

FLEXION

Flexion extension and lateral flexion loads are of particular interest since they lead to bending of the disc. An experimental finding suggests that these are not compression loads that are the most damaging to the disc (1973). In flexion, the compressive stress on the anterior portion of the discs are increased. Brown et al. (1957) were unable to produce disc failure by bending in flexion and by lateral bending. However, after removal of the posterior elements failure did occur by means of avulsion from the vertebra. Adams and Hutton (1982) hyperflexed motion segments and found that 43% failed by posterior prolapse. Lower lumbar segments were more susceptible. Thus, it appears that this mechanism may be the most common mechanism of failure. In the industrial environment, picking up a heavy load to the side may be the most severe stress to the disc.

SHEAR LOADING

Markolf (1970) reported a high shear stiffness. The first step in shear failure is the failure of the facets (Lantz, 1978). After facet failure, the disc would be carrying 75% of the shear loading.

Motion segments with degenerated disc show increased shear when subjected to torsion. Stokes (1981) found that patients with a proven herniation showed asymmetric facet motion at the affected level. There was also increased shear, a result also reported by other authors. Farfan (1978) and others decreased motion at the affected segments (Begg, 1949; Hirsch, 1969; Manasor, 1959; Rolander, 1966).

TIME-DEPENDENT BEHAVIOR

Farfan (1973) found a rapid decay in the torque applied to the disc materials. The torques at rupture and the initial stiffness were found to be significantly higher in cycled than in uncycled specimens. Kazarian (1972) demonstrated increased deflections and creep with the application of vibration. These observations may be relevant to the risk of truck and tractor operators developing disc herniations (Kelsey, 1975; Kelsey and Hardy, 1975). The combination of cyclic loading and the posture probably places abnormal stresses on the lumbar spine.

Hirsch and Nachemson (1954) first reported creep and relaxation in the disc for higher loads which were said to produce greater deformation and faster creep rates (Bailey, 1974). Kazarian (1975) performed creep tests on degenerated motion segments and found that the nondegenerated discs creep slowly as compared to the degenerated ones. Thus, it is probable that degeneration results in discs that are less viscoelastic and have less ability to absorb shocks. Virgin (1951) found that the discs exhibit hysteresis. Hysteresis was found to vary with the magnitude of the load, the age of the disc and the level. Brown et al. (1957) did a disc fatigue test by applying an axial load and a repetitive forward bend. The disc showed signs of failure after 200 cycles and completely failed after 1000 cycles.

MECHANICAL PROPERTIES OF DISC TISSUE

The strength of disc materials was studied by cutting the disc and vertebrae into axial sections (Brown, 1957; Nachemson, 1962). The anterior and posterior regions were stronger than the lateral region and the central region was found to be the weakest. This is consistent with failure of the materials. Galante (1967) cut the disc annulus into thin samples. The tensile stiffness was found to vary as a function of orientation. The axial specimens were the most flexible; those at 15° to the horizontal plane were the stiffest. Wu and Yao (1976) measured the biomechanical properties and orthotropic nature of the annulus. Lin et al. (1978) used a finite element analysis to verify the experimenal data from a lumbar intervertebral joint. The material constants were ultimately determined by minimizing the error between the experimental data and the predicted deformations. It was shown that the orthotropic elastic moduli of the lumbar intervertebral disc were independent of segment level but decreased as a function of the severity of degeneration.

ANALYTICAL MODELS

Over the last decade there have been a number of attempts to model the spine (Orne, 1971; Schultz, 1970) and the motion segments. The first model was a discrete parameter, two-dimensional model devised by Orne (1971). This included the initial curvature of the spine, the variable geometry of the components of the spine and their material properties. Prasad (1971) extended this model to include the facet interaction. Schultz (1970) gave a three-dimensional quasi-static model with springs to represent the deformable elements of the discs and ligament. The model used nonlinear geometric configuration. More recently this group (Spilker, 1980) used an asymmetric finite element model which showed that disc geometry and material properties have a significant effect on disc bulge and vertical deflection. The disc height and radius were significantly changed by intradiscal pressure.

A simple model was presented by Hickey (1980) in which the fibers were considered to have the same mechanical properties as tendon. The model explained the observed function of failure of the disc in compression torsion, and the model was based on observed arrangements of the collagenous fibers in the annulus fibrosus. The structure of the disc was found to protect the collagen fibers in forward bending and torsion, and compression was predicted to cause end-plate fracture rather than annular failure.

CONCLUSIONS

A great deal of work has been done over the years on the intervertebral disc. Although not all clinical low back pain can be attributed to the disc, it is clearly an important area focus. Future work should concentrate on the relationships between disc biochemistry and biomechanics, on the development of more precise mathematical models, and on the predicted disc loading and different industrial loading circumstances.

REFERENCES

1. Adams, P. and Muir, H · Qualitative changes with age of proteoglycans of human lumbar discs. *Annals of Rheumatic Disease, 35*:289, 1976.
2. Adams, M.A. and Hutton, W.C.: Prolapsed intervertebral disc: A hyperflexion injury. *Spine, 7*:184, 1982.
3. Armstrong, J.R.: *Lumbar Disc Lesions.* Edinburgh, Churchill Livingstone, 1952.
4. Bailey, A.J., Robins, S.P. and Balian, G.: Biologic significance of the intermolecular crosslinks of collagen. *Nature, 251*:105, 1974.
5. Barnes, M.J., Constable, B.J. and Morton, L.F. and Royce, P.M.: Age-related variations in hydroxylation of lysine and proline in collagen. *Biochemical Journal, 139*:461, 1974.
6. Bartelink, D.L.: The role of abdominal pressure in relieving the pressure on the lumbar intervertebral discs. *Journal of Bone and Joint Surgery, 39-B*:718, 1957.
7. Bayer, H.: Mit welchen Kraeften wirken die Rueckenstrecker auf die Lendenwirbelsaeule ein? *Zeitschrift fuer Orthopaeidie, 84*:607-615, 1954.
8. Beadle, O.A.: The intervertebral disc: Observations on their normal and morbid anatomy in relation to certain spinal deformities. *London, Medical Research Council Report 161*, 1931.
9. Begg, A.C. and Falconer, M.A.: Plain radiography in intraspinal protrusion of lumbar intervertebral disks: A correlation with operative findings. *British Journal of Surgery, 36*:225, 1949.

10. Blumenkrantz, N., Slyvest, J. and Asboe-Hanson, G.: Local Low-collagen Content May Allow Herniation of Intervertebral Disc: *Biochemical Medicine, 18*:283-290, 1977.

11. Bodine, A.J., Brown, N., Hayes, W.C. and Jiminez, S.A.: The effect of sodium chloride on the shear modulus of articular cartilage. *Transactions of the 26th Annual Meeting of the Orthopaedic Research Society, 5*:37, 1980.

12. Bonnair, E. and Bue, V.: Influence de la position la forme et les dimensions du bassin. *Annales de Gynecologie et d'Obstetrie, 52*:296, 1899.

13. Brown, T., Hanson, R. and Yorra, A.: Some mechanical tests on the lumbo-sacral spine with particular reference to the intervertebral discs. *Journal of Bone and Joint Surgery, 39-A*:1135, 1957.

14. Diamant, B., Karlsson, J. and Nachemson, A.: Correlation between lactate level and pH of patients with lumbar rizopathies. *Experientia, 24*:1195, 1968.

15. Eie, N.: Load capacity of the low back. *Journal of the Oslo City Hospitals, 16*:73, 1966.

16. Emes, J.H. and Pearce, R.H.: The proteoglycans of the human intervertebral disc. *Biochemical Journal, 145*:549, 1975.

17. Evans, F.G. and Lissner, H.R.: Biomechanical studies on the lumbar spine and pelvis. *Journal of Bone Joint Surgery, 41-A*:278, 1959.

18. Eyre, D.R. and Muir, H.: Quantitative analysis of type I and II collagens in human intervertebral discs at various ages. *Biochimica et Biophysica Acta, 592*:29, 1977.

19. Farfan, H.F.: Experimental Surgery: Effects of torsion on the intervertebral joints. *Canadian Journal of Surgery, 12*:336, 1969.

20. Farfan, H.F.: *Mechanical Disorders of the Low Back*. Philadelphia, Lea & Febiger, 1973.

21. Farfan, H.F.: The biomechanical advantage of lordosis and hip extension for upright activity: Man as compared with other anthropoids. *Spine, 3*:336, 1978.

22. Farfan, H.F.: Cossette, J.W., Robertson, G.H., Wells, R.V. and Kraus, H.: The effects of torsion on the lumbar intervertebral joints: The role of torsion in the production of disc degeneration. *Journal of Bone and Joint Surgery, 52-A*:468, 1970.

23. Farfan, H.F., Heberdeen, R.M. and Dubow, H.J.: Lumbar intervertebral disc generation, the influence of geometrical features on the pattern of disc generation: A postmortem study. *Journal of Bone and Joint Surgery, 54-A*:492, 1972.

24. Fessler, J.H.: A structural function of mucopolysaccharides in connective tissue. *Biochemical Journal, 76*:124, 1960.

25. Galante, J.O.: Tensile properties of the human lumbar annulus fibrosis. *Acta Orthopaedica Scandinavica, Supplementum 5*:91, 1967.

26. Gallop, P.M. and Pax, M.A.: Post-translational protein modifications with special attention to collagen and elastin. *Physiological Reviews, 55*:418, 1975.

27. Geneis, H.: Experimentelle Beitrage zur Beckenmechanik. *Anatomischer Anzeiger, 88*:187, 1939.

28. Ghosh, P., Taylor, T.F.K. and Braund, K.G.: The variation of glycosaminoglycans of the intervertebral disc with aging: I. Chondrodystrophoid breed. *Gerontology, 23*:87, 1977.

29. Grant, M.E. and Prockup, D.J.: The biosynthesis of collagen: Part III. *New England Journal of Medicine, 286*:291, 1972.

30. Grynpas, M.D., Eyre, D.R. and Kirscher, D.A.: Collagen of the intervertebral disc: X-ray diffraction evidence for differences in the native molecular packing of types I and II collagens. *Transactions of the 26th Annual Meeting of the Orthopaedic Research Society, 5*:13, 1980.

31. Hallen, A.: Collagen and ground substance of human intervertebral disc at different ages. *Acta Chemica Scandinavica, 16*:705, 1962.

32. Happey, F., Wiseman, A. and Naylor, A.: A polysaccharide content of the prolapsed nucleus pulposus of the human intervertebral disk. *Nature, 192*:868, 1961.

33. Hardingham, T.E. and Adams, P.: A method for the determination of hyaluronate in the presence of other glycosaminoglycans and its application to human intervertebral disc.

Biochemical Journal, 159:143, 1976.

34. Harris, R.I. and Macnab, I.: Structural changes in lumbar intervertebral discs. *Journal of Bone and Joint Surgery, 36-B*:304, 1954.

35. Herbert, C.M., Lindberg, K.A. and Jayson, M.I.: Intervertebral disk collagen in degeneration disk disease. *Annals of Rheumatic Disease, 34*:467, 1975.

36. Hickey, D. and Hukins, D.: Relation between the structure of the annulus fibrosis and the function and failure of the intervertebral disc. *Spine, 5* (2):106:111, 1980.

37. Hirsch, C.: The reaction of intervertebral discs to compression forces. *Journal of Bone and Joint Surgery, 37-A*:1188, 1955.

38. Hirsch, C. and Friberg, S.: Anatomical and clinical studies on lumbar disc degeneration. *Acta Orthopaedica Scandinavica, 19*:222, 1949.

39. Hirsch, C., Jonsson, B. and Lewin, T.: Low back symptoms in a Swedish female population. *Clinical Orthopaedics, 63*:171, 1969.

40. Hirsch, C. and Nachemson, A.: A new observation on the mechanical behavior of lumbar discs. *Acta Orthopaedica Scandinavica, 23*:254, 1954.

41. Hirsch, C. and Nachemson, A.: Clinical observations on the spine in ejected pilots. *Acta Orthopaedica Scandinavica, 31*:135, 1961.

42. Hirsch, C. and Schajowicz, F.: Studies on structural changes in the lumbar annulus fibrosis. *Acta Orthopaedica Scandinavica, 22*:184, 1952.

43. Hopwood, J.J. and Robinson, H.C.: The structure and composition of cartilage keratin sulphate. *Biochemical Journal, 141*:517, 1974.

44. Hult, L.: The Munkfors investigation. *Acta Orthopaedica Scandinavica, Supplementum 16*:1, 1954.

45. Kazarian, L.: Dynamic response characteristics of the human vertebral column: An experimental study of human autopsy specimens. *Acta Orthopaedica Scandinavica, Supplementum 146*:1, 1972.

46. Kazarian, L.E.: Creep characteristics of the human spinal column. *Orthopaedic Clinics North America, 6*:3, 1975.

47. Kelsey, J.L.: An epidemiological study of acute herniated intervertebral discs. *Rheumatology Rehabilitation, 14*:144, 1975.

48. Kelsy, J.L. and Hardy, R.J.: Driving of motor vehicles as a risk factor for acute herniated intervertebral disc. *American Journal of Epidemiology, 102*:63, 1975.

49. Kramer, J.: Pressure dependent fluid shifts in the intervertebral disk. *Orthopaedic Clinics North America, 8*:211, 1977.

50. Lantz, S.H., Lafferty, J.F. and Bowman, D.A.: Response of the intervertebral disc to shear stress. Meeting of Air Force Physiology Research Group, Dayton, Ohio Wright Patterson Air Force Base, AFMRL, Oct., 1978.

51. Li, H.S., Liu, Y.K., Ray, G. and Nikravech, P.: Systems identification for material properties in the intervertebral disc. *Journal of Biomechanics, 11*:1, 1978.

52. Lin, H.S., Liu, Y.K. and Adams, K.: Mechanical response of the lumber intervertebral joint under physiological loading. *Journal of Bone and Joint Surgery, 60-A*:41, 1978.

53. Lindholm, K.: Experimental ruptures of intervertebral discs in rat's tails. A preliminary report. *Journal of Bone and Joint Surgery, 34-A*:123, 1952.

54. Markolf, K.L.: Stiffness and damping characteristics of the thoracic-lumbar spine. Proceedings of workshop of bioengineering approaches to the problems of spine. National Institutes of Health, September 1970.

55. Markolf, K.L.: Deformation of the thoracolumbar intervertebral joint in response to external loads and a biomechanical study using autopsy material. *Journal of Bone and Joint Surgery, 54-A*:511, 1971.

56. Markolf, K.L. and Morris, M.W.: Structural components of the intervertebral disc. *Journal of Bone and Joint Surgery, 56-A*:674, 1974.

57. Mathews, M.B.: Macromolecular evolution of connective tissue. *Biological Review, 42*:499, 1967.

58. Mattiash, H.H.: Arbeitshaltung und Bandscheibenbelastung. *Archiv fuer Orthopaedische Unfallchirurgie, 48*:147, 1956.

59. Menasor, M.V. and Duvall, T.: Absence of motion at the fourth and fifth lumbar interspaces in patients with and without low back pain. *Journal of Bone and Joint Surgery, 41-A*:1047, 1959.

60. Mixter, W.J. and Barr, J.S.: Rupture of the intervertebral disc with involvement of the spinal canal. *New England Journal of Medicine, 211*:210, 1934.

61. Morris, J.M., Lucas, D.B. and Bressler, B.: Role of the trunk in stability of the spine. *Journal of Bone and Joint Surgery, 43-A*.327, 1961.

62. Murai, A., Miyuhara, T. and Shiozowa, S.: Age related variations in glycosylation of hydroxylsine in human and rat skin collagens. *Biochimica et Biophysica Acta, 404*:345, 1975.

63. Nachemson, A.: Lumbar interdiscal pressure. *Acta Orthopaedica Scandinavica, Supplementum 43*, 1960.

64. Nachemson, A.: Some mechanical properties of the lumbar intervertebral discs. *Journal of the Hospital for Joint Disease, 23*:130-143, 1962.

65. Nachemson, A.: The influence of spinal movement on the lumbar intradiscal pressure and on the tensile strength in the annulus fibrosus. *Acta Orthopaedica Scandinavica, 33*:183, 1963.

66. Nachemson, A.: The load on lumbar discs in various postures. *Clinical Orthopaedics and Related Research, 45*:107, 1969.

67. Nachemson, A. and Elfstrom, G.: Intra-vital dynamic pressure measurements in lumbar discs. *Scandinavian Journal Rehabilitation Medicine, Supplementum 1*, 1970, pp. 1-40.

68. Nachemson, A.L. and Evans, J.G.: Some mechanical properties of the third lumbar interlamina ligament (ligamentum flavum). *Journal of Biomechanics, 1*:211, 1968.

69. Nachemson, A., Lewis, T., Maroudas, A. and Freeman, M.A.R.: In vitro diffusion of dye through the endplates and the annulus fibrosis of human lumbar intervertebral disk. *Acta Orthopaedica Scandinavica, 42*:589, 1970.

70. Nachemson, A. and Morris, J.M.: In vivo measurements of intradiscal pressure: Discometry, a method for the determination of pressure in the lower lumbar disks. *Journal of Bone and Joint Surgery, 46-A*:1077, 1964.

71. Nachemson, A. and Morris, J.M.: Electromyographic studies of the vertebral portion of the psoas muscle. *Acta Orthopaedica Scandinavica, 37*:177, 1966.

72. Nachemson, A.L., Schultz, A.B. and Berson, M.H.: Mechanical properties of human lumbar spine motion segments. Influences of age, sex, disc level and degeneration. *Spine, 4*:1, 1979.

73. Naylor, A., Happey, F. and MacRae, T.: Changes in the human intervertebral disc with age: a biophysical study. *Journal of the American Geriatric Society, 3*:964, 1955.

74. Naylor, A. and Shentall, R.: Biochemical aspects on intervertebral disk in aging and disease, in Jayson, M. (ed.): *The Lumbar Spine and Back Pain*, New York, Grune & Stratton, Inc., 1976, pp. 317-326.

75. Orne, D. and Liu, Y.K.: A mathematical model of spinal response to impact. *Journal of Biomechanics, 4*:49, 1971.

76. Perey, O.: Fracture of the vertebral endplates in the lumbar spine: An experimental biomechanical investigation. *Acta Orthopaedica Scandinavica, Supplementum 25*, 1957.

77. Prockp, D.J., Berg, R.A. and Kivirikko, K.I.: Intracellular steps in the biosynthesis of collagen, in Ramachondrom, G.N., Reddi, A.H. (eds): *Biochemistry of Collagen*, New York, Plenum Press, 1976, p. 163.

78. Prasad, P. and King, A.I.: An experimentally validated dynamic model of the spine. *Journal of Biomechanics, 4*:203, 1971.

79. Puschel, J.: Der Wassergehalt normaler und degenerierter Zwischenwirbelscheiben. *Beitraege zur Pathologischen Anatomie, 84*:123, 1930.
80. Putti, V.: New conceptions in the pathogenesis of sciatic pain. *Lancet, 2*:53, 1977.
81. Roaf, R.: A study of the mechanics of spinal injuries. *Journal of Bone and Joint Surgery, 42-B*:810, 1960.
82. Rolander, S.D.: Motion of the lumbar spine with special reference to the stabilizing effect of posterior fusion: An experimental study on autopsy specimens. *Acta Orthopaedica Scandinavica, Supplementum 90*:1-144, 1966.
83. Royce, P.M. and Barnes, J.M.: Comparative studies on collagen glycosylation in chick skin and bone. *Biochimica et Biophysica Acta, 498*:132, 1977.
84. Schultz, A.B. and Galante, J.O.: A mathematical model for study of the mechanics of the human vertebral column. *Journal of Biomechanics, 3*:405, 1970.
85. Shah, A.B., Hampson, W.G. and Jayson, M.I.: The distribution of surface strain in the cadaveric lumbar spine. *Journal of Bone and Joint Surgery, 60-B*:246, 1978.
86. Simounek, Z. and Muir, H.: Changes in the protein-polysaccharides of pig articular cartilage during prenatal life, development and old age. *Biochemical Journal, 126*:515, 1972.
87. Sonnerup, L.: A semi-experimental stress analysis of the human intervertebral disc in compression. *Experimental Mechanics, 142*:12(3), 1972.
88. Spilker, R.L.: Mechanical behavior of a simple model of an intervertebral disk under compressive loading. *Journal of Biomechanics, 13*:895-901, 1980.
89. Steindler, A.: *Kinesiology of the Human Body*. Springfield, IL, Charles C Thomas, 1955.
90. Stevens, R.L., Ewins, R.J.F., Revell, P.A. and Muir, H.: Proteoglycans of the intervertebral disc: Homology of structure with laryngeal proteoglycans. *Biochemical Journal, 179*:561, 1979.
91. Stokes, I.A.F., Wilder, D.G., Frymoyer, J.W. and Pope, M.H.: Assessment of patients with low back pain by biplanar radiographic measurement of the intervertebral motion. (Volvo Award Paper, ISSLS Meeting, 1980), *Spine, 6*:223-240, 1981.
92. Sullivan, J.D. and Farfan, H.F.: Pathological changes with intervertebral joint rotational instability in the rabbit. *Canadian Journal of Surgery, 14*(1)71, 1971.
93. Taylor, T.K.F. and Akeson, W.H.: Intervertebral disc prolapse: A review of morphologic and biochemic knowledge concerning the nature of prolapse. *Clinical Orthopaedics, 76*:54, 1971.
94. Urban, J.P.G., Holm, S. and Maroudas, A.: Diffusion of small solutes into the intervertebral disc: An *in vivo* study. *Biorheology, 15*:203, 1978.
95. Urban, J.R.G., Holm, S., Maroudas, A. and Nachemson, A.: Nutrition of the intervertebral disc: An in vivo study of solute transport. *Clinical Orthopaedics, 129*:101, 1977.
96. Vernon-Roberts, B. and Pirie, C.J.: Healing trabecular microfractures in the bodies of lumbar vertebrae. *Annals of Rheumatic Disease, 32*:406, 1973.
97. Virgin, W.J.: Experimental investigation into the physical properties of the intervertebral disc. *Journal of Bone and Joint Surgery, 33-B*:607, 1951.
98. Wu, H. and Yao, R.: Mechanical behavior of the human annulus fibrosus. *Journal of Biomechanics, 9*:1, 1976.

CHAPTER FOUR

THE MECHANICAL INTERACTION BETWEEN THE THORACOLUMBAR FASCIA AND THE CONNECTIVE TISSUE OF THE POSTERIOR SPINE

K.M. TESH, J.H. EVANS, J. SHAW DUNN, AND J.P. O'BRIEN

INTRODUCTION

MOTION of the lumbar spine is determined by the interaction of muscle and connective tissue. The effectiveness of these tissues in controlling spinal motion is dependent on their lever arms at the points of attachment. This study will investigate the contribution of the thoracolumbar fascia which, being the most dorsal structure associated with the spine, is in an advantageous position to resist flexion.

For many years it has been accepted that muscle contraction of the abdominal wall can generate an intra-abdominal pressure which may stabilize the spinal column during flexion. That the tensed abdomen can act as a support is understood if one considers a tube-shaped balloon wedged between the pelvic floor and the diaphragm in the abdominal cavity (Bartelink, 1957). The circumferential component of muscle action in the abdominal wall would squeeze the balloon, reducing its diameter, but simultaneously bulging the ends outward. The thrust on the diaphragm would be transmitted to the vertebral column via the rib cage. This antero-cranial force will produce both an extensor moment and a reduction in compressive load on the vertebral column.

In 1980 Fairbank and O'Brien carried out an experiment to simulate abdominal muscle action by pulling on the lateral margins of the thoracolumbar fascia. When the fascia was pulled the tips of the spinous processes approached one another resulting in extension of the lumbar spine. The posterior attachment of the fascia to the vertebral column would increase the load on the intervertebral disc.

Although both mechanisms described above produce an extensor moment on the vertebral column, the resultant axial loads counteract one another.

To explain the mechanism by which the thoracolumbar fascia extends the spine, Fairbank and O'Brien (1980) proposed that the ligamentous sheet interacted with the vertebral ligaments. The fiber orientation of the ligaments were thought to be such that extension of the lumbar spine could be achieved when acted upon by the thoracolumbar fascia. This mechanism would be in addition to the one proposed by Farfan (1973) which involved the thoracolumbar fascia deforming like a net under tension.

The anatomy of the thoracolumbar fascia and its attachment to the spinal column have not been described in sufficient detail to enable the various mechanisms to be tested. In view of the potential importance of the thoracolumbar fascia in spinal mechanics a detailed study of the anatomy and microstructure of the fascia and its interaction with the vertebral ligaments has been undertaken.

SOFT TISSUE MORPHOLOGY

Dissections in the lumbar region were carried out on 4 fresh and 4 embalmed cadavers to reveal the 3-dimensional anatomy of the following structures:

(1) the posterior layer of the thoracolumbar fascia,
(2) the junction at the midline of the posterior fascial layer with the supraspinous and bifid interspinous ligament, and
(3) the middle layer of the thoracolumbar fascia at its attachment to the transverse processes.

The microstructure of the posterior thoracolumbar fascial layer was studied using polarized light microscopy and conventional histology techniques on full thickness fascia samples. A series of transverse histological sections were made to examine the midline junction of the fascial layer and vertebral ligaments.

The posterior layer of the thoracolumbar fascia is composed of three laminae. Each lamina of the fascia displays collagen fibers in parallel array. Fiber direction alternates between laminae providing a network structure. The middle lamina is the major part of the posterior layer having a thick and closely packed fibrous structure. A sagittal section close to the midline reveals that in the thick midlamina the collagen fibers are arranged principally in a circumferential direction. The fibers in the superficial and deep laminae run predominantly longitudinally, and interweave with the midlamina at their junctions. (See Figure IV-1).

The three laminae of the posterior thoracolumbar fascial layer anchor onto

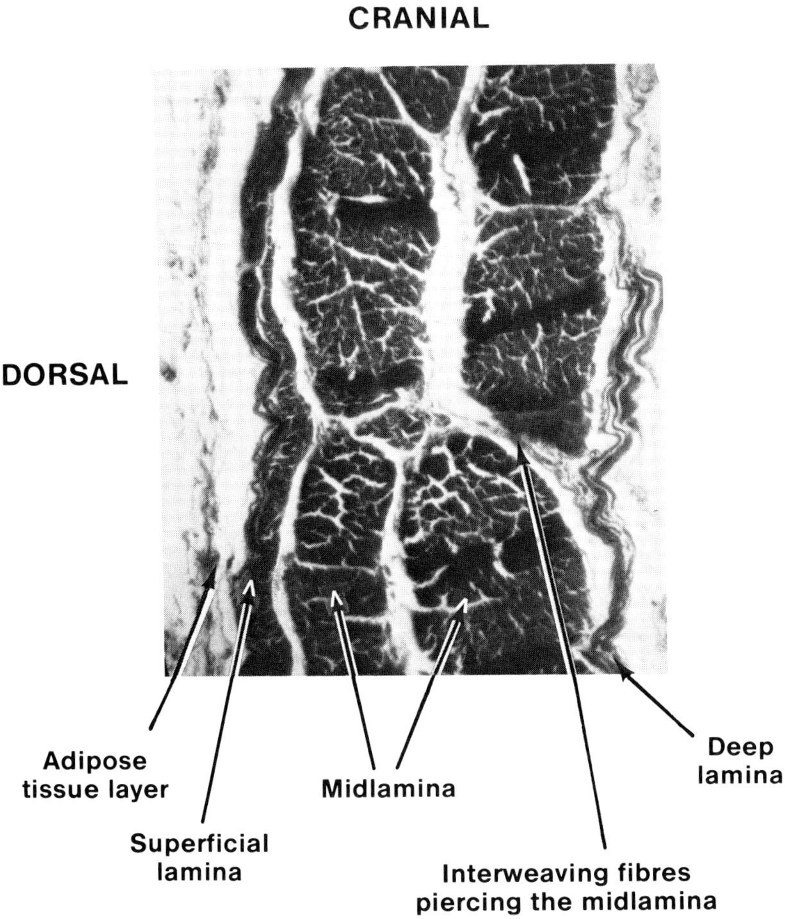

CRANIAL

DORSAL

Adipose
tissue layer

Superficial
lamina

Midlamina

Interweaving fibres
piercing the midlamina

Deep
lamina

Figure IV-1. A full thickness sagittal section of the posterior thoracolumbar fascia. (X160) (Specimen taken 3 cms from the midline at the L3-L4 level).

the tips of the posterior lumbar spines at the midline. Dissections carried out by Rissanen (1960)found the fascia attached to all the lumbar posterior spinous processes except for L5. Between the posterior processes the three laminae terminate at different sites in the interspinous space. (See Figure IV-2). The outer lamina runs into the superficial fibers of the supraspinous ligament. The middle lamina runs deeper along the side of the ligament and then splits into two branches; one branch running medially into the deep part of the supraspinous ligament while the other branch continues anteriorly towards the interspinous ligament. The inner lamina runs down the outside of the midline soft tissues, passing the supraspinous ligament, and merging with the interspinous ligament. The direction of the fibers in all three laminae is predominantly in an anterior-posterior direction.

The middle layer of the thoracolumbar fascia anchors onto the tips of the

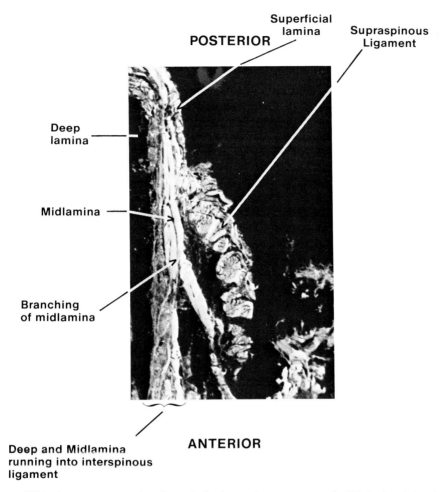

Figure IV-2. A transverse section through the interspinous space at the L3-L4 level showing the three laminae of the posterior thoracolumbar fascia entering the midline. (X16)

transverse processes and runs medially down to the base of the processes. Two sets of fibers radiate from the tips of the lower four transverse processes where the connective tissue is relatively thick and dense, whereas between the transverse processes the fascial sheet is thinner with no obvious fiber arrangement.

DISCUSSION

The interweaving arrangement between laminae in the posterior layer of the thoracolumbar fascia gives strong evidence for a net-type, deformable ligamentous sheet. In 1978, Bazergui et al. performed mechanical tests on whole sheets of thoracolumbar fascia. The ligamentous sheet was pulled longitudinally to simulate elongation during flexion maneuvers. At the highest loads, longitudinal extensions of 8% produced lateral contractions of 13% in the ligamentous sheet. The ratio of contraction to extension is typical of a net-like structure.

The thoracolumbar fascia could be expected to resist forward bending by its attachment to the ribcage above and to the pelvis below. However, a circumferential force at the lateral margins of the fascial sheet, set up by abdominal muscle tension, will prevent the width contracting and thus render it markedly more stiff in the longitudinal direction. The attachment of the fascia to the posterior spinous processes will restrain the sheet along the midline and transmit a longitudinal force to the spine drawing the processes together, resulting in extension of the lumbar spine.

Microscopic examination of the midline ligamentous structures revealed that the posterior layer of the thoracolumbar fascia interacts with the supraspinous and interspinous ligaments. The superficial and middle laminae of the fascia merge with both ligaments whereas the deep lamina interacts with the interspinous ligament only. The anterior-posterior orientation of collagen fibers in the fascia layer would suggest that tensing of the abdominal muscles would "bow-string" the vertebral ligaments posteriorly, drawing the processes together and bringing the lumbar spine into extension. Fairbank and O'Brien (1980) suggested that the thoracolumbar fascia attached onto each side of the bifid interspinous ligament and could cause extension of the lumbar spine when pulled laterally. Our findings have demonstrated that the fascia interacts with both the supraspinous and interspinous ligaments. Extension of the lumbar spine can still be produced by tension in the fascia, directed more posteriorly.

It is interesting to note that below the level of the posterior spinous process of L4 the superficial fibers of the thoracolumbar fascia decussate the midline without any attachment to the midline ligamentous structures. Heylings (1978) showed that the supraspinous ligament was absent at the L4-L5 interspace and this may account for the architectural change in the fascia at the midline.

The middle layer of the thoracolumbar fascia attaches directly to the vertebral column without involving the intertransverse ligaments. This finding conflicts with the ideas of Fairbank and O'Brien (1980) who suggested that the middle layer of the thoracolumbar fascia could stabilize the lumbar spine by maintaining a tension in the intertransverse ligament. However, the apparent lack of a ligament-fascia interaction does not detract from the stabilizing potential of the middle layer. The angled convergence of fibers onto the tips of the transverse processes may suggest that, when the middle layer is pulled laterally due to contraction of the abdominal muscles, there is not only a lateral pull on the transverse processes but also an angled force on the tips. This force acts behind the column's center of rotation and therefore its axial component is capable of extending the lumbar spine. In lateral bending however, the axial force components will be asymmetric due to differing fiber orientation and therefore a stabilizing moment will be generated in the coronal plane. The disposition of the fascia between the transverse processes could also prevent excessive lateral bending thereby maintaining a degree of stability in the coronal plane. The middle layer of the thoracolumbar fascia may thus help in stabilizing the spine in both the sagittal and coronal planes.

The aponeurosis of the latissimus dorsi muscle constitutes a part of the posterior layer of the thoracolumbar fascia. In electromyographic studies, carried out by Farfan (1977) in the compilation of a computer model of the lumbar spine, active potentials were measured in the latissimus dorsi muscle when the arms were tensed. During lifting maneuvers the arms will be tensed as the arm's inertia is overcome and an oblique force will be transmitted to the fascial sheet via the aponeurosis of the latissimus dorsi muscle. During lifting the thoracolumbar fascial sheet would be loaded in three directions: (1) longitudinally from the increased convexity of the spine, (2) circumferentially from abdominal muscle action, and (3) obliquely (60 degrees to the midline) from the latissimus dorsi muscle. The behavior of the ligamentous sheet under triaxial loading is likely to be markedly different from that detailed above under biaxial loading.

The attachment points of the posterior and middle layers of the thoracolumbar fascia allow it to act on a considerable lever arm which can generate large moments about the vertebral column when the fascia is put under tension. The skin, because it is furthest from the bending axis and because it presents a large cross sectional area, can generate an equally significant bending moment about the column when stretched at full flexion. Measurements by Tesh et al. (1983) of local skin compliance on volunteers predicted that normal skin can carry up to 5 percent of the bending moment due to body weight. As dermal scar tissue is markedly less extensible than normal skin (Figure IV-3) it can offer a higher resistance to forward bending, which may be clinically discernible and significant.

CONCLUSION

It has been demonstrated on the basis of dissections and histological observations that the muscles of the abdomen have the potential to stabilize the vertebral column through the action of the thoracolumbar fascia. This can be brought about by:

a. The intrinsic nature of the thoracolumbar fascia without direct involvement of the vertebral ligaments,

b. muscle contraction modifying longitudinal ligament tension via the thoracolumbar fascia, or

c. a combination of both mechanisms.

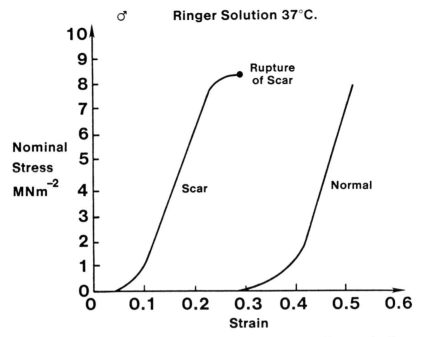

Figure IV-3. Stress-strain relation of dermal scar tissue compared with normal adjacent skin tissue (after Evans, 1973).

SUMMARY

During flexion of the lumbar spine the forces generated by external loads and body weight are balanced by the interaction of active and passive structures. As extreme flexion is approached, the contribution of the paraspinal muscles rapidly diminishes. However, the circumferential muscle components of the abdominal wall are active at this point and perhaps throughout the whole range of flexion.

In recent years it has been suggested that the spinal column may be motivated by abdominal muscles acting, via their aponeuroses, on the posterior ligamentous system. The net effect of the abdominal interaction of their aponeuroses with the posterior spinal structure. This paper examines the current hypotheses regarding the functional interrelation of thoracolumbar fascia and the spinal tissues in the light of a detailed anatomical study. These previously undescribed structural details may also be clinically relevant.

REFERENCES

Bartelink, D.L.: The role of abdominal pressure in relieving the pressure on the lumbar intervertebral discs. *Journal of Bone and Joint Surgery, 39B*:718-725, 1959.
Bazergui, A., Lamy, C., Farfan, H.F.: Mechanical properties of the lumbodorsal fascia.

Paper No. 1A-08. Proceedings of the 1978 Society for Experimental Stress Analysis Meeting. Wichita, Kansas, 1978.

Evans, J.H.: *Structure and Functionof Soft Connective Tissue*. Ph.D. Thesis, University of Strathclyde, Glasgow, 1973.

Fairbank, J.C.T., O'Brien, J.P.: The abdominal cavity and thoracolumbar fascia as stabilizers of the lumbar spine in patients with low back pain. Conference on: Engineering Aspects of the Spine, Paper no. C135/80, London, 1980.

Farfan, H.F.: *Mechanical Disorders of the Low Back*. Lea and Febiger, Philadelphia, 1973.

Farfan, H.F.: Mathematical model of the soft tissue mechanism of the lumbar spine. In Buerger, A.A., Tobis, J.S. (Eds.) *Approaches in the Validation of Manipulative Therapy*. Springfield, IL, Charles C Thomas, 1977, pp 1-41.

Heylings, D.J.A.: Supraspinous and interspinous ligaments of the human lumbar spine. *Journal of Anatomy, 125*:127-131, 1978.

Rissanen, P.M.: The surgical anatomy and pathology of the supraspinous and interspinous ligament of the lumbar spine with special reference to ligament ruptures. *Acta Orthopaedica Scandinavica, Supplementum 46.*, 1960, p 1.

Tesh, K.M., Evans, J.H., Shaw Dunn, J., O'Brien, J.P.: The contribution of skin, fascia and ligaments to resisting flexion of the lumbar spine. Conference on: Biomechanical Measurement in Orthopaedic Practice. Oxford, England, (in press), 1983.

Section 2

SOME CHARACTERISTICS OF BACK PAIN

T HE bulk of back pain is idiopathic (White and Gordon, 1982). By definition, this means that the majority of clinicians recognize that they do not know the origin(s) of most of the pathology of low back pain. The epidemiology and differential diagnosis of such a disease are particularly important and thorny problems, especially because they may supply clues to the biologic defects which underlie it. Hence the papers by Andersson and Kanno & Newell are of special interest, because they may spark investigations in these difficult areas.

REFERENCES

White, A.A., Gordon, S.L., (eds.): *Symposium on Idiopathic Low Back Pain.* St. Louis, MO, C.V. Mosby, 1982.

CHAPTER FIVE

EPIDEMIOLOGY OF LOW BACK PAIN

GUNNAR B.J. ANDERSSON, M.D., Ph.D.

INTRODUCTION

E PIDEMIOLOGY is the study of the distribution of a disease in a population and of those factors that influence this distribution. In this brief review of the literature on the epidemiology of low back pain I will try to first describe the frequency of back pain in the total population, and then the influence of individual and work related factors on the disease prevalence. An attempt of this nature is seriously hampered by difficulties in defining low back pain and classifying it into subgroups. Data must be interpreted with these factors in mind.

THE FREQUENCY OF LOW BACK PAIN

Information on the frequency of low back pain comes mainly from two sources: insurance statistics and cross-sectional prevalence studies. Because differences in insurance policies exist between countries, such data are not readily applicable to populations outside the country from which they were obtained.

National Statistics

Data from the United States have been summarized in a monograph by Kelsey et al. (1978) and in a recent paper based on that monograph (Kelsey and White, 1980). Impairments of the back and spine were the most frequent cause of activity limitation in persons under age 45, and the third most frequent cause in the 45-64 year age group. Per 100 subjects with ages between 25 and 44, a decrease in work capacity was caused by back pain with an average of

28.6 days a year; confinement to bed was necessary for about nine days. From 1963 through 1965, back pain was the diagnosis in 10 percent of all chronic conditions.

Benn and Wood (1975) found that 3.6 percent of all sickness absence days in Great Britain in 1969-70 had a diagnosis of back pain. The number of sickness absence episodes per 1,000 persons was 11 for women and 22.6 for men. The average absence period for men was 32.6 days. Wood (1976) has later attempted to calculate the impact of back problems on medical and social services (Table V-1). Other British surveys have shown that 25 percent of all working men are affected each year (Haber, 1971), that one man out of 25 change their work because of back pain (Taylor, 1976), and that 79,000 persons in Great Britain were chronically disabled in 1971 (Harris, 1971). Every single day there are as many as 0.05 percent of the British work force who have been absent from work for 6 months or more (Wood and Badley, 1980).

TABLE V-1

	Number of subjects
Handicapped/pension	2
General practitioner consultants	20 (58 visits)
Referrals	9
Admissions	1
Operations	0.1
Spinal symptoms	7

The back patients' need for medical and social services, expressed as rates per 1,000 persons at risk (based on Benn and Wood, 1975)

Swedish national health insurance data show that back diagnoses were responsible for an average 12.5 percent of all sickness absence days over a ten-year period (1961-1971) amounting to about 1 percent of all work days (Helander, 1973). The average sickness absence period was 36 days. Forty percent of the periods were shorter than one week, while 9 percent were longer than three months. No other disease group was responsible for a greater number of days off work. The number of sickness absence periods in 1970 was 10 per 100 men, 6 per 100 women (Andersson and Svensson, 1979). The chronicity of back pain is also evident from the Swedish statistics on early retirement and disability pensions. Back pain is the diagnosis in about 25 percent of all new pension cases of this type.

Cross-Sectional Surveys

There are at least seven studies with a cross-sectional design performed over the last 15 year period. Three of these are from the United States, four from Scandinavia, and one from the Netherlands.

The prevalence rate of "persistent back pain" in 18-60 year-old persons living in Columbus (Ohio) was studied in a random sample of 1,135 subjects (Nagi et al., 1973). Eighteen percent had severe frequent low back pain. Four percent of those had had a back operation. Kelsey (1975) performed a study of 20-64 year-old people residing in New Haven, Connecticut. The population was chosen based on radiographs taken over a two year period for suspected herniated discs. No prevalence or incidence data was calculated but a number of risk factors were identified as will be discussed subsequently.

Frymoyer et al. (1980, 1983) studied 1,221 males between the ages of 18-35 who had been enrolled in a family practice facility between 1975-1978. About 70 percent had had low back pain at some time in life, 23.5 percent of considerable severity. Data on the impact of back problems on the health care services were also calculated. Eleven-and-a-half percent of those with moderate low back pain had been to an orthopaedic and/or neurosurgeon, 41.8 percent of those with severe low back pain. The corresponding figures for osteopathic visits were 7.0 percent and 23.8 percent, for chiropractic visits 12.7 percent and 27.5 percent. A back support had been given to 11.3 percent of those with moderate low back pain and 37.4 percent of those with severe, while surgery was performed on 2.0 percent and 10.5 percent respectively.

Hirsch et al. (1969) in a random study of 692, 15-71 year-old women, in the city of Goteborg, Sweden, found the life-time incidence to be 48.8 percent. In the younger years pain was usually mild, and only a small percentage had sciatica. After 35 years of age pain in the back was usually more severe, and sciatica appeared more frequently.

Svensson and Andersson (1982) studied a random sample of 940, 40-47 year-old men in Goteborg, Sweden. Seven hundred and sixteen men were personally interviewed and information about the remaining was obtained from the Swedish National Health Insurance Office. The life-time incidence of low back pain was 61 percent, while the one-month period-prevalence was 31 percent. Forty percent had sciatica. The disability prevented work in 3.6 percent of the participants and 4 percent had been off work more than three months because of low back pain in the three years preceeding the study. Forty percent had consulted a physician, 3.5 percent had been admitted to a hospital, and 0.8 percent had been operated on because of their low back pain. In another study of 1,640 35-60 year-old women quite comparable data were found. The life-time incidence was 67 percent, the one-month prevalence 39 percent. The three-year incidence of sicklisting was 19 percent and 3.5 percent of the women had been off work for three months or more during that period. Thirty-nine percent of the women had consulted a physician, 5.5 percent had been hospitalized, and 1 percent had been operated on because of low back pain.

Biering-Sorensen (1982, 1983) studied 449 men and 479 women in a Copenhagen suburb in Denmark. He found the life-time prevalence to be 62 percent, the one-year incidence 6 percent. Sixty percent of the subjects with low back pain had at some time consulted a physician, and 30 percent had been through an x-ray survey of the lumbar spine. Four-and-a-half percent had been admitted to hospital and 1 percent operated on for low back pain.

Valkenburg and Haanen (1982) studied 3,091 men and 3,493 women in the Netherlands (Table V-2). Fifty-one percent of the men and 57 percent of the women said they had experienced low back pain. In the men, the percentage increased up to above age 65 and then decreased in older age groups, and a similar tendency—although less noticeable—was found in women. Disc prolapse was found in 1.9 percent of the men and 2.2 percent of the women using a clinical definition. Recurrences were reported by 85 percent of those suffering from low back pain, and 30 percent had problems lasting for three months or longer. Nearly half of the men and one-third of the women had been unfit to work at some time and 8 percent (men) and 4 percent (women) had changed occupations because of low back pain. Twenty-eight percent of the men and 42 percent of the women had consulted a doctor for low back pain.

TABLE V-2

	Men (%)	Women (%)
Point-prevalence	22.2	30.2
Life-time incidence	51.4	57.8
> 3 months	11.3	19.6
Unfit for work	24.3	19.5
Work change	4.2	2.4

Low back complaints and work incapacity in the Zoetermeer study (from Valkenburg and Haanen, 1982)

Horal (1969) and Westrin (1970, 1973) studied a random sample of subjects sicklisted in 1964 with low back pain diagnoses, and compared those to a control group (Table V-3). Interestingly, as many as 49 percent of the individuals in the control group who were never sicklisted had had low back pain in the 3-4 years before the study, and 27 percent had pain at the time of the interview.

TABLE V-3

	Probands (%)	Controls (%)
304 year period prevalence	95	49
Of which:		
Duration > 1 week	83	21
Pain medication	73	6
Physiotherapy	47	3
Brace or Corset	18	1
Point-prevalence	53	27

Low back pain in probands and controls (from Westrin, 1973)

Industrial Surveys

There are numerous reports on the frequency of occurrence of back pain in different industries and work situations. (For review see Anderson, 1980; Andersson, 1981; and Snook, 1982).

Anderson (1971) in a British survey of 2,685 men found that 30 percent had backache, 75 percent of whom had low back pain (i.e. 23% of all these men). Twenty-two percent of the low back sufferers were referred to the hospital, 6 percent admitted for treatment, (i.e. 7% and 2% of the total population respectively) (Anderson, 1980). The annual absenteeism from work in Great Britain is calculated to be 70 weeks per 100 men employed (Anderson, 1980).

Magora and Taustein (1969) found prevalence rates from 6.4 to 21.6 per 100 males and females in a survey of 3,316 Israeli workers in eight different jobs, while Ikata (1965) in a study of 1,110 Japanese workers in ten jobs reported on sciatica in between 5.2 percent and 22.4 percent.

The prevalence of back pain in different Scandinavian industries have been reported by several investigators. Hult (1954) found that 60 percent of a sample of Swedish males with different jobs (1,193 persons) had back pain at some time. Four percent had been off work because of these symptoms more than six months, 11 percent between three weeks and six months. Studies from the Swedish building industry (Ostlund, 1975) show that in 1974 22 percent had suffered from work preventing low back pain during the last year and that 33.5 percent had received sickness allowance because of back pain at some time. Corresponding figures from the forest industry show that 37.5 percent had back pain, and about 18 percent had pain at the time of survey (Tufvesson, 1973). A Danish study of back pain among employed males, age 40-59, report

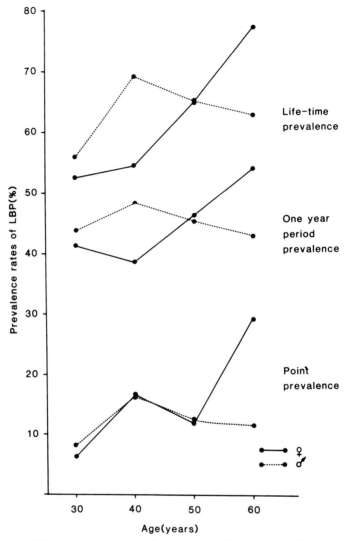

Figure V-1. The prevalence rates of low back pain (from Biering-Sorensen, 1982).

that 25 percent of all had had back pain in the previous year, 8 percent severe enough to warrant bed rest or absenteeism from work (Gyntelberg, 1974).

　　Rowe (1963, 1969) followed the employees at a plant in New York over a ten year period (1956-1965). Low back pain was second to upper respiratory illness in terms of time lost because of illness, and more than four hours were lost per worker each year because of it. From 35 percent to 47 percent of the employees had made visits to the medical department because of low back pain during the study period.

　　Snook (1982) has compiled data from the Liberty Mutual Insurance Company. Annual rates of low back pain in different companies were found to vary from less than 1 percent to over 15 percent. Kelsey (1982) reports that about 20 percent of all employees in the United States have compensable back injury each year.

WORK PLACE FACTORS

Introduction

An increased sickness absence because of low back symptoms has not been found in association with the following six vocational factors: physically heavy work, static work postures, frequent bending and twisting, lifting and forceful movements, repetitive work, and vibrations. These factors are all similar in that they increase the load on the spine. They are often present at the same time, so that the association with any single vocational factor is difficult to establish. Another problem in the evaluation of the relationship between physical work factors and low back pain is the difficulty in defining and measuring the loads on the spine during work. Further, it is known that an increase in mechanical load increases back pain in subjects already suffering such pain. Sickness absence rates and insurance data can therefore be misleading.

In addition to the physical work factors, psychological work factors, as monotony and work dissatisfaction, have also been implicated (see Table V-4).

TABLE V-4

Variable	p-value
Less overtime work	0.01
Diminished work satisfaction	0.01
Decreased potential to influence the work situation	0.01
Less demand on concentration	0.05
More monotonous/boring work	0.001
More physically demanding work	0.001
More lifting	0.001
Less sedentary work	0.05
More walking at work	0.05
More standing at work	0.05

Summary of work-related variables associated with Low Back Pain (Svensson and Andersson, 1983).

Heavy Physical Work

Several investigations indicate an increase in sickness absence due to low back pain, and also an increase in low back symptoms in physically heavy work (Andersson, 1981; Snook, 1982). A few will be discussed here. Most of these studies define heavy physical work as jobs with high energy demand, and contrast those with jobs with a low energy demand. Such an approach can be misleading, since dynamic and static work conditions may both increase the risk of low back pain.

The frequency of low back pain in Hult's study (1954) was 64.4 percent in subjects with "physically heavy work," 52.7 percent in "other types of work." Severe back pain was present in 6.8 percent of those with "light" physical work and 10.6 percent of those with heavy physical work. Differences were more pronounced when work absence was considered; 43.5 (heavy) compared to 25.5 percent (light) had been off work because of back pain. Lawrence (1955) studied 362 workers in four different jobs. Low back pain was found in 41 percent of those working in "physically heavy jobs," in 38-68 percent in miners and in 29 percent in subjects with light physical work. Ikata (1965) reported a point-prevalence of sciatica as high as 22.4 percent in men with heavy jobs, 5.2 percent in men with light, and Magora (1970) found low back pain in 21.6 percent of subjects with heavy industrial work and 10.4 percent in bank employees. Unskilled laborers had the highest prevalence rate for disc prolapse and lumbago in the Dutch study by Valkenburg and Haanen (1982). Svensson and Andersson (1983) found heavy physical work to be strongly associated to the occurrence of low back pain; and the highest prevalence of low back pain in their cross-sectional study was in men with physically heavy professions (Table V-4).

All these studies would seem to support that heavy physical work increases the risk of low back pain. Confounding factors may exist, however, and the level at which physical work load becomes dangerous is not determined.

Static Work Postures

It appears to be important to change one's work posture. Prolonged sitting, and bent over work postures, in particular, seem to carry an increased risk for back pain. But, there is considerable disagreement.

While many studies indicate an increased risk of low back pain in subjects with predominantly sitting work postures (Hult, 1954; Lawrence, 1955; Kroemer and Robinette, 1969; Partridge and Anderson, 1969; Magora, 1972), others do not (Braun, 1969; Westrin, 1963; Bergquist-Ullman and Larsson, 1977; Svensson and Andersson, 1983). Kelsey (1975a,b) and Kelsey and Hardy (1975) found that men who spend more than half their workday in a car have threefold increased risk of disc herniation. This could be due to the combined effect of sitting and vehicle vibration.

Magora (1972) found that those who either sat or stood during most of the workday had an increased risk of low back pain. Frequent changes in posture were also found to be bad for the back, however.

Damkot et al. (1983) recorded body postures required in work situations in subjects with and without low back pain. Forty percent of those with no pain, 36 percent of those with moderate and 59 percent of those with severe low back pain were required to stretch and reach.

Frequent Bending and Twisting

The association between low back symptoms and frequent bending and twisting is difficult to evaluate separately as lifting is usually also involved. Troup, Roantree and Archibald (1970) found the combination mentioned above to be the most frequent cause of back injuries in England. Magora (1973) established a connection between both excessive bending and occasional bending on the one hand and low back pain on the other, and a similar finding was made by Chaffin (1973).

Lifting and Forceful Movements

It has been clearly established that back pain can be triggered by lifting, but the frequency at which back pain occurs after lifting varies from 15 percent to 64 percent in these studies (Bergquist-Ullman and Larsson, 1977; Hult, 1954; Ikata, 1965; Kelsey, 1975; Magora, 1972). Sudden unexpected maximal efforts were found by Magora (1972) to be particularly harmful, and Glover (1960), Tichauer (1965), and Troup et al. (1970) express the same opinion about lifting in combination with lateral bending and twisting.

Chaffin and Park (1973) found that workers involved in heavy manual lifting had about eight times the number of lower back injuries as those with a more sedentary work situation. Svensson and Andersson (1983) found a direct association between occurrence of low back pain and frequent lifting, as did Frymoyer et al. (1980) and Hult (1954).

Snook (1982) found that a worker was three times more susceptible to compensable low back injury if exposed to excessive manual handling tasks.

Kelsey (1975), on the other hand, found no indication that workers with herniated discs did more lifting on the job than workers without such symptoms. Further, there was no indication in that study that jobs requiring pushing, pulling, or carrying either increased or decreased the risk of herniated discs. Herniated discs are a small subset of the total low back pain population, however, perhaps explaining those results.

Repetitive Work

Repetitive work increases, in general, the sickness absence rate. Low back pain seems to be no exception in this respect. This may explain, in part, why assembly line industries have a higher incidence of low back pain among their manual workers than among their office employees (Bergquist-Ullman and Larsson, 1977).

Vibrations

There are several studies suggesting an increasing risk of low back pain in drivers of tractors (Rosegger and Rosegger, 1960; Dupuis and Christ, 1972), of trucks (Kelscy and Hardy, 1975; Gruber, 1976; Wilder et al., 1982), of buses (Gruber and Ziperman, 1974; Kelsey and Hardy, 1975), and of airplanes (Fitzgerald and Crotty, 1972; Schulte-Wintrop and Knosche, 1978). These studies also suggest that low back pain occurs at an earlier age in subjects exposed to vibration.

Kelsey and Hardy (1975) found that truck driving increased the risk of disc herniation by a factor of four, while tractor driving and car commuting (20 miles or more per day) increased the risk by a factor of two. Studies of vibration-exposed populations have also indicated that radiographic changes occur in the spines of these subjects (Rosegger and Rosegger, 1960; Dupuis and Christ, 1972; Gruber, 1976).

Psychological Work Factors

Of different psychological work factors monotony at work and work dissatisfaction have been found to increase the risk of low back pain. Monotony was primarily related to low back pain in the study by Svensson and Andersson (1983); Bergquist-Ullman and Larsson (1977) found the workers with monotonous jobs, requiring less concentration had a longer sickness absence following low back pain than the others. Diminished work satisfaction has also been found to be related to an increased risk of low back pain (Westrin, 1970; Magora, 1973).

INDIVIDUAL FACTORS

Individual factors can, of course, influence the prevalence of low back pain, and also its disabling effects.

Age and Sex

Low back pain usually begins early in life (Bergquist-Ullman and Larsson, 1977; Bierring-Sorensen, 1982; Svensson and Andersson, 1983). The maximal frequency of symptoms appears to be in the age range of 35 to 55, while sickness absence and symptom duration increases with increasing age (as referenced by Andersson, 1981; see Figure V-1). Most cases admitted to hospital and operated on because of herniation are between 35 and 45 years old (as referenced by Spangfort, 1972).

Sex factors seem to be without importance with respect to low back symptoms (Horal, 1969; Valkenburg and Haanen, 1982; Svensson and Andersson,

1982), while operations for disc herniations are performed about twice as often in males as in females (Braun, 1969; Spangfort, 1972; Weber, 1983). The work situation may be quite important in that respect. Swedish insurance statistics indicate a much larger sickness absence in women with heavy physical work than in men doing the same job. A mismatch between the physical strength of the worker and the job requirements can be responsible for these differences. Brown (1973) and Magora (1970) report that females in heavy physical jobs have comparatively more back complaints than men in similar jobs.

Posture

Postural deformities — scoliosis, kyphosis, hypo- or hyper-lordosis and leg length discrepancy — do not seem to predispose to low back pain in general (Hult, 1954; Horal, 1969; Rowe, 1969; Hodgson et al., 1974; Magora, 1975; Sorensen, 1964; Biering-Sorensen, 1983). Scoliosis has been particularly investigated but there is no hard evidence of a true association with low back pain, except in curves of 80 degrees or more (Nilsonne and Lundgren, 1968; Nachemson, 1968; Collis and Ponsetti, 1969; Kostuick et al., 1973; Bradford et al., 1975; Kostuick and Bentivoglio, 1981).

Antropometry

Antropometric data indicate that there is no strong correlation between height, weight, body build and low back pain (Hult, 1954; Horal, 1969; Rowe, 1965, 1969; Chaffin and Park, 1973; Svensson and Andersson, 1983; Biering-Sorensen, 1983; Pope, 1983). However, tallness has been found to be associated with a higher than average risk of back pain in some studies (Kelsey, 1975; Lawrence, 1955; Tauber, 1970) and sciatica is more frequent in the very obese (Ikata, 1965).

Muscle Strength and Physical Fitness

Poor strength in abdominal and back muscles has been found by some investigators in patients with back pain (Alston et al., 1966; McNeill et al., 1980; Rowe, 1963; Addison and Schultz, 1980). Others have found no differences to controls, or differences only in selected groups of strength activities (Berkson et al., 1977; Nachemson and Lindh, 1969; Petersen et al., 1975; Biering-Sorensen, 1983). The question whether a weakness is primary or secondary to back pain remains to be clarified. Kelsey (1975) found insufficient physical exercise, as well as participation in some sports (baseball, golf, and bowling) to be associated with the development of prolapsed lumbar discs.

Cady et al. (1979) concluded from a study of 1,965 Los Angeles firefighters that physical fitness and conditioning have significant preventive effect on the occurrence of back injuries. Chaffin (1974), Chaffin et al. (1978), and Keyserling et al. (1980) have used pre-employment strength testing procedures and found that the risk of a back injury increases threefold when the job requirement exceeds the strength capability on an isometric simulation of the job.

Spine Mobility

Spine motions are reduced in most subjects with back pain. They are usually associated with some pain, particularly at the end of the range of motion. It appears quite unlikely that spine mobility is a factor in the causation of back pain.

Psychological Factors and Psychiatric Problems

Westrin (1970, 1973) when comparing back patients and controls, did not find psychiatric problems to be more common in the back group. Psychological factors, on the other hand, were found to differ significantly. A poorer intellectual capacity, a lesser ability to establish emotional contacts, and a more sociofilic attitude were characteristics of the back patients. Several studies indicate that psychological tests can be used as predictors of treatment and rehabilitation outcome, but this is not always the case.

Social Factors

A high incidence of social problems have been found in back patients. Their general social situation and economy is on an average less good and there is a greater proportion of back patients suffering from drug and alcohol abuse than expected (Magora, 1973; Westrin, 1970). Divorces and family problems are also more frequent, and the education level has been found to be lower in these two studies. Whether social factors are primary or secondary is difficult to assess.

Radiographic and Related Factors

The relationship between the occurrence of *disc degeneration* and low back pain is controversial. It is obvious from many different studies that disc degeneration *per se* is not symptomatic, and is part of a general age process. Back pain appears to be, however, more frequent in subjects with severe degenerative changes, involving several discs (Bistrom, 1954; Caplan et al., 1966; Hult, 1954; Lawrence, 1961; 1969; Magora and Schwartz, 1976; Rowe, 1965; 1969; Torgerson and Dotter, 1976; Wiikeri et al., 1978). In moderate or light degeneration the situation is less clear, and most literature reports that the correlation is negative (Hirsch et al., 1969; Horal, 1969; Hult, 1954; Hussar and Guller, 1956; Magora and Schwartz, 1976; Splithoff, 1953). There seems to be good evidence that disc degeneration is more frequent and occurs earlier in individuals with heavy manual work, although the nature of the stress inducing the degenerative changes is not clear (Hult, 1954; Kellgren and Lawrence, 1958; Lawrence, 1969; Caplan et al., 1966; Kelsey, 1978). Obesity does not appear to be related to degenerative disc disease, nor does generalized osteoarthritis.

Attempts have also been made to relate back pain to the occurrence of *skeletal defects*, congenital or acquired. The prevalence of each defect is so small that studies are difficult to perform. Ninety-eight percent of the defects are located in the L4, L5 and upper sacral segments. As with disc degeneration it has been clearly established that different defects do not necessarily give rise to pain (Horal, 1969; Hult, 1954; LaRocca and MacNab, 1969; Redfield, 1972; Rowe, 1963). Some are associated with an increased risk, however.

Low back pain appears to be more common in subjects with spondylolisthesis (Fisher et al., 1958; Hult, 1954; Kettelkamp and Wright, 1971; Wiltse, 1971), but there are several reports indicating the opposite (LaRocca and MacNab, 1969; Rowe, 1963; 1965). Scheuermann's disease and severe lumbar scoliosis are conditions in which an increased risk has often been claimed, but the association has not been clearly established (Sorensen, 1964). Sacrilization or the presence of a lumbo-sacral transitional vertebra are other abnormalities in association with which an increased prevalence of back pain has sometimes been established (Paillas et al., 1969; Tilley, 1970), but where other studies have failed to confirm a positive correlation. Spina bifida occulta appears not to be more frequent in low back sufferers than in healthy controls.

Osteoarthritis of the intervertebral apophyseal joints may or may not increase the risk of low back pain (Farfan, 1973; Hussar and Guller, 1956; Lewin, 1964). It can cause foraminal narrowing and spinal stenosis symptoms.

Advanced *osteoporosis* with fractures of a macro- or a micro-type is known to be painful. Studies of young or moderately old populations have not indicated that osteoporosis is more common in subjects with low back symptoms than in subjects without (Bistrom, 1954; Horal, 1969; LaRocca and MacNab, 1969).

SUMMARY

Low back pain is one of the most frequent and disabling conditions affecting people in their productive years. Prevention is therefore important, but to be effective we must better identify work place risk factors and individual risk factors. Only then will our preventive efforts be truly successful. It appears clear, however, that mechanical factors play a role, and that therefore work place design and improved work methods are essential. It is also clear that preemployment examinations alone will not suffice in reducing the back problem. Finally all back pain is surely not work related. We must therefore continue in our efforts to find the cause of low back pain and improve our treatment methods.

REFERENCES

Addison, R., Schultz, A. 1980. Trunk strengths in patients seeking hospitalization for chronic low back disorders. *Spine,* 5:539-544

Alston, W.; Carlson, K.E.; Feldman, D.J.; Grimm, Z.; and Gerontinos, E. 1966. A quantitative study of muscle fatigue in the chronic low back syndrome. *Journal of the American Geriatric Society, 14*:1041.

Anderson, J.A.D. 1971. Rheumatism in industry. *British Journal of Industrial Medicine, 28*:103-121.

_____. 1980. Back pain and occupation. In Jayson, M.I.V. (ed.), *The Lumbar Spine and Back Pain.* 2nd Ed., Pitman, London Medical, pp.57-82.

Andersson, G.B.J. 1981. Epidemiologic aspects on low back pain in industry. *Spine* 6(1):53-60.

Andersson, G., Svensson, H.O. 1979. Prevalence of low-back pain. *Social Planerings-och Rationaliserings-institut Rapport 22*:11-23 (in Swedish).

Benn, R.T., Wood, P.H.N. 1975. Pain in the back: An attempt to estimate the size of the problem. *Rheumatology Rehabilitation, 14*(3):121-128.

Bergquist-Ullman, M., Larsson, U. 1977. Acute low back pain in industry. *Acta Orthopaedica Scandinavica, Supplementum 170.*

Berkson, M., Schultz, A., Nachemson, A., Andersson, G.B.J. 1977. Voluntary strengths of male adults with acute low back syndromes. *Clinical Orthopedics, 129*:84-95.

Biering-Sorensen, F. 1982. Low back trouble in a general population of 30-, 40-, 50-, and 60-year old men and women. Study design, representativeness and basic results. *Dan. Med. Bull.* 29(6):289-299.

_____. 1983. A prospective study of low back pain in a general population. I. Occurrence, recurrence and aetiology. *Scandinavian Journal of Rehabilitation Medicine 15*(2):71-79.

Bistrom, O. 1954. Congenital anomalies of the lumbar spine of persons with painless backs. *Ann. Chir. Gynaecol. Fenn. 43*:102-115.

Bradford, D.S., Moe, J.H., Winter, R.B. 1975. Surgical treatment of scoliosis in the adult. *The Spine.* Ed. R.H. Rothman and F.A. Simeone, pp. 347-348, Philadelphia, W.B. Saunders Company.

Braun, W. 1969. Ursachen des lumbalen Bandscheiber-verfalls. *Die Wirbelsaule in Forschung und Praxis 43.*

Brown, J.R. 1973. Lifting as an industrial hazard. *J. Am. Ind. Hyg. Assoc., 34*:292.

Cady, L.D., Bischoff, D.P., O'Connell, E.R., Thomas, P.D., Allan, J.H. 1979. Strengths and fitness and subsequent back injuries in firefighters. *Journal of Occupational Medicine, 21*:269-272.

Caplan, P.S., Freedman, L.M.J., Connelly, T.P. 1966. Degenerative joint disease of the lumbar spine in coal miners—a clinical and x-ray study. *Arthritis Rheum., 9*:693-702.

Chaffin, D.B. 1973. Localized muscle fatigue—definition and measurement. *Journal of Occupational Medicine, 15*:346-354.

_____. 1974. Human strength capability and low back pain. *Journal of Occupational Medicine, 16*:248-254.

Chaffin, D.B., Herrin, G.D., Keyserling, W.M. 1978. Preemployment strength testing. An updated position. *Journal of Occupational Medicine, 20*:403-408.

Chaffin, J.B., Park, K.S. 1973. A longitudinal study of low back pain as associated with occupational lifting factors. *J. Am. Ind. Hyg. Assoc., 34*:513-525.

Collis, D.K., Ponseti, I.V. 1969. Long term follow-up of patients with idiopathic scoliosis not treated surgically. *Journal of Bone and Joint Surgery, 51A*:425-455.

Damkot, D.K., Pope, M.H., Lord, J., Frymoyer, J.W. 1983. The relationship between work history, work environment and low back pain in males. University of Vermont. Manuscript.

Dupuis, H., Christ, W. 1972. Untersuchung der Moglichkeit von Gesundheits-schadigungen im Bereich der Wirbelsaule bei Schlepperfahrern. *Max Plank Inst., Bad Kreuznach.*, Heft A72/2.

Farfan, H.F. 1973. *Mechanical Disorders of the Low Back.* Philadelphia, Lea and Febiger.

Fischer, F.J., Friedman, M.M., Denmark, R.E. Van. 1958. Roentgenographic abnormalities in soldiers with low back pain: A comparative study. *American Journal of Roentgenology, 79*:673-676.

Fitzgerald, J.G., Crotty, J. 1972. The incidence of back-ache among aircrew and ground crew in the RAF. *FPRC/1313.*

Frymoyer, J.W., Pope, M.H., Clements, J.H., Wilder, D.G., MacPherson, B., Ashikaga, T. 1983. Risk factors in low back pain. *Journal of Bone and Joint Surgery, 65A*:213-218.

Frymoyer, J.W., Pope, M.H., Costanza, M.C., Rosen, J.D., Goggin, J.E., Wilder, D.G. 1980. Epidemiologic studies of low-back pain. *Spine, 5*(5):419-423.

Glover, J.R. 1960. Back pain and hyperaesthesia. *Lancet, 1*:1165-1169.

Gruber, J.G. 1976. Relationships between whole-body vibration and morbidity patterns among interstate truck drivers. Nat. Inst. Occ. Safety & Health, Cincinnati. NIOSH Rept. 77-167.

Gruber, G.J., Ziperman, H.H. 1974. Relationship between whole-body vibration and morbidity patterns among motor coach operators. HEW Publication No. (NIOSH) 75-104.

Gyntelberg, F. 1974. One year incidence of low back pain among male residents of Copenhagen aged 40-59 *Dan. Med. Bull, 21*(1):30-36.

Haber, L.D. 1971. Disabling effects of chronic diseases and impairment. *J. Chronic. Dis., 24*:469-487.

Harris, A.I. 1971. *Handicapped and impaired in Great Britain. Part 1. Social Survey Division.* London, Office of Population of Censuses and Surveys, Her Majesty's Stationary Office.

Helander, E. 1973. Back pain and work disability. *Socialmed Tidskr., 50*:398-404. (in Swedish).

Hirsch, C., Jonsson, B., Lewin, T. 1969. Low-back symptoms in a Swedish female population. *Clin. Orthop., 63*:171-176.

Hodgson, S., Shannon, H.S., Troup, J.D.G. 1974. The prevention of spinal disorders in dock workers. *Report to National Dock Labour Board.* (In manuscript).

Horal, J. 1969. The clinical appearance of low back pain disorders in the city of Goteborg, Sweden: Comparisons of incapacitated probands and matched controls. *Acta Orthopaedica Scandinavica, Supplementum 118*:1-109.

Hult, L. 1954. Cervical, dorsal, and lumbar spinal syndromes. *Acta Orthopaedica Scandinavica, Supplementum 17*:1-102.

Hussar, A.E., Guller, E.J. 1956. Correlation of pain and the roentgenographic findings of spondylosis of the cervical and lumbar spine. *American Journal of Medical Science, 232*:518-527.

Ikata, T. 1965. Statistical and dynamic studies of lesions due to overloading on the spine. *Shikoku Acta Med, 40*:262-286.

Kellgren, J.H., Lawrence, J.S. 1958. Osteo-arthrosis and disk degeneration in an urban population. *Ann. of Rheumat. Dis., 17*:388-397.

Kelsey, J.L. 1975. An epidemiological study of acute herniated lumbar intervertebral discs. *Rheumatol. Rehabil., 14*(3):144-159.

————. 1975. An epidemiological study of the relationship between occupations and acute herniated lumbar intervertebral discs. *Int. J. Epidemiol, 4*:197-204.

————. 1978. Epidemiology of radiculopathies. *Adv. Neurol, 19*:385-396.

————. 1982. Idiopathic Low Back Pain: Magnitude of the problem. In *Symposium on Idiopathic Low Back Pain.* A.A. White and S.L. Gordon, Eds., Mosby, St. Louis, pp.5-8.

Kelsey, J.L., Hardy, R.J. 1975. Driving of motor vehicles as a risk factor for acute herniated lumbar intervertebral disc. *Am. J. Epidemiol.,102*:63-73.

Kelsey, J.L., Pastides, H., Bisbee, G.E. Jr. 1978. *Musculo-skeletal disorders: Their frequency of occurrence and their impact on the population of the United States.* New York: Prodist.

Kelsey, J.L., White, A.A. III. 1980. Epidemiology and impact on low back pain. *Spine, 5*(2):133-142.

Kettelkamp, D.B., and Wright, D.G. 1971. Spondylolisthesis in the Alaskan Eskimo. *J. Bone Joint Surg, 53A*:563.

Keyserling, W.M, Herrin, G.D., Chaffin, D.B. 1980. Isometric strength testing as a means of controlling medical incidents on strenuous jobs. *J. Occup. Med., 22*:332-336.

Kostuick, J., Bentivoglio, J. 1981. The incidence of low back pain in adult scoliosis. *Acta Orthop Belgica, 47*:548-559.

Kostuick, J.P., Israel, J., Hall, J.E. 1973. Scoliosis surgery in adults. *Clin. Orthop., 93*:225-234.

Kroemer, K.H.E., Robinette, J.C. 1969. Ergonomics in the design of office furniture. *Industr. Med. Surg., 38*:115-125.

LaRocca, H., Macnab, I. 1969. Value of pre-employment radiographic assessment of the lumbar spine. *Can. Med. Assoc. J., 101*:49-54.

Lawrence, J.S. 1955. Rheumatism in coal miners. Part III. Occupational factors. *Br. J. Ind. Med., 12*:249-261.

————. 1961. Rheumatism in cotton operatives. *Br. J. Ind. Med., 18*:270.

————. 1969. Disc degeneration. Its frequency and relationship to symptoms. *Ann. Rheum. Dis., 28*:121-137.

Lewin, T. 1964. Osteoarthritis in lumbar synovial joints. A morphological study. *Acta Orthop. Scand.* (Suppl.), 73.

Magora, A. 1970. Investigation of the relation between low back pain and occupation. 1. Age, sex, community, education and other factors. *Industr. Med. Surg., 39*:465-471.

————. 1970. Investigation of the relation between low back pain and occupation. 2. Work history. *Industr. Med. Surg., 39*:504-510.

————. 1972. Investigation of the relation between low back pain and occupation. 3. Physical requirements: Sitting, standing and weight lifting. *Industr. Med. Surg., 41*:5-9.

————. 1973. Investigation of the relation between low back pain and occupation. 4. Physical requirements: Bending, rotation, reaching and sudden maximal effort. *Scand. J. Rehabil. Med., 5*:191-196.

————. 1973. Investigation of the relation between low back pain and occupation. 5. Psychological aspects. *Scand. J. Rehabil. Med., 5*:186-190.

————. 1975. Investigation of the relation between low back pain and occupation. 7. Neurologic and orthopaedic conditions. *Scand. J. Rehabil. Med., 7*:146-151.

Magora, A., Schwartz, A. 1976. Relation between the low back syndrome and x-ray findings. 1. Degenerative osteoarthritis. *Scand. J. Rehabil. Med., 8*:115-125.

Magora, A., Taustein, I. 1969. An investigation of the problem of sick-leave in the patient suffering from low back pain. *Industr. Med. Surg., 38*:398-408.

McNeill, T., Warwick, D., Andersson, G., Schultz, A. 1980. Trunk strengths in attempted flexion, extension, and lateral bending in healthy subjects and patients with low back disorders. *Spine, 5*:529-538.

Nachemson, A.L. 1968. Back problems in childhood and adolescence. *Lakartidningen, 65*:2831-2843. (in Swedish).

Nachemson, A.L., Lindh, M., 1969. Measurement of abdominal and back muscle strength with and without low back pain. *Scand J. Rehabil. Med., 1*:60-65.

Nagi, S.Z., Riley, L.E., Newby, L.G. 1973. A social epidemiology of back pain in a general population. *J. Chron. Dis., 26*(12):769-779.

Nilsonne, U., Lundgren, K.D. 1968. Long-term prognosis in idiopathic scoliosis. *Acta Orthop. Scand., 39*:456-465.

Ostlund, E.W. 1975. Personal communication.

Paillas, J.E., Winninger, J., Louis, R. 1969. Role des malformations lombo-sacrees dans les sciatiques et les lombalgies: Etude de 1.500 dossiers radiocliniques dont 500 hernies discales verifiees. *Presse Med., 7*:853.

Partridge, R.E., Anderson, J.A. 1969. Back pain in industrial workers. *Proccedings of the International Rheumatology Congress*, Prague, Czechoslavakia, abstract 284.

Petersen, O.F., Petersen, R., Staffeldt, E.S. 1975. Back pain and isometric back muscle strength of workers in a Danish factory. *Scand. J. Rehabil. Med., 7*:125-128.

Pope, M.H., Rosen, J.D., Wilder, D.G., Frymoyer, J.W. 1983. The relation between biomechanical and psychological factors in patients with low back pain. *Spine, 5*:173-178.

Redfield, J.T. 1972. The low back x-rays as a preemployment screening tool in the forest products industry. *J. Occup. Med., 13*:219-226.

Rosegger, R., Rosegger, S. 1960. Arbeitsmedizinische Erkenntnisse beim Schlepperfahren. *Arch. Landtechn., 2*:3-65.

Rowe, M.L. 1963. Preliminary statistical study of low back pain. *J. Occup. Med., 5*:336-341.

———. 1965. Disc surgery and chronic low back pain. *J. Occup. Med., 7*:196-202.

———. 1969. Low back pain in industry. A position paper. *J. Occup. Med., 11*:161-169.

Schulte-Wintrop, H.C., Knoche, H. 1978. Backache in UHID helicopter crews. *AGARD-CP-255.*

Snook, S.H. 1982. Low back pain in industry. *In Symposium on idiopathic low back pain.* A.A. White and S.L. Gordon, Eds., Mosby, St. Louis, 9-22.

Spangfort, E.V. 1972. The lumbar disc herniation, a computer-aided analysis of 2,504 operations. *Acta Orthop. Scand.* (Suppl.), 142.

Splithoff, C.A. 1953. Lumbosacral junction. Roentgenographic comparison of patients with and without backaches. *JAMA, 152*:1610-1613.

Svensson, H.O.; Andersson, G.B.J. 1982. Low back pain in forty to forty-seven year old men. I. Frequency of occurrence and impact on medical services. *Scand. J. Rehabil. Med. 14*:47-53.

Svensson, H.O.; Andersson, G.B.J. 1983. Low back pain in forty to forty-seven year old men: Work history and work environment factors. *Spine, 8*:272-276.

Sorensen, K.H. 1964. *Scheurmann's juvenile kyphosis.* Copenhagen, Munksgaard (Thesis).

Tauber, J. 1970. An unorthodox look at backaches. *J. Occup. Med., 12*:128-130.

Taylor, D.G. 1976. The costs of arthritis and the benefits of joint replacement surgery. *Proc. R. Soc. Med., 192*:145-155.

Tichauer, E.R. 1965. The biomechanics of the arm-back aggregate under industrial working conditions. *Am. Soc. Mech. Eng.,* 65 WA/HUF-1.

Torgerson, B.R., Dotter, W.E. 1976. Comparative roentgenographic study of the asymptomatic and symptomatic lumbar spine. *J Bone Joint Surg., 58A*:850-853.

Troup, J.D.G., Roantree, W.B., Archibald, R.M. 1970. Survey of cases of lumbar spinal disability. A methodological study. *Med Officers' Broadsheet, National Coal Board.*

Tufvesson, B. 1973. Stockholm, Swedish Work Environment Fund (Unpublished data).

Valkenburg, H.A., Haanen, H.C.M. 1982. The epidemiology of low back pain. *In Symposium on idiopathic low back pain.* eds. A.A. White and S.L. Gordon, Mosby, St. Louis, pp. 9-22.

Weber, H. 1983. Lumbar disc herniation. A controlled, prospective study with ten years of observation. *Spine, 8*:131-140.

Westrin, C.G. 1970. *Sicklisting because of low back pain. A nosologic and medical insurance investigation.* Goteborg. (Thesis, in Swedish).

———. 1973. Low back sicklisting. A nosological and medical insurance investigation. *Scand J. Med.* (Suppl.), 7:1-116.

Wiikeri, M., Nummi, J., Riihimaki, H., Wickstrom, G. 1978. Radiologically detectable lumbar disc degeneration in reinforcement workers. *Scand. J. Work Environ. Health* (Suppl. 1), 4:47-53.

Wilder, D.G., Woodworth, B.B., Frymoyer, J.W., Pope, M.H. 1982. Vibration and the human spine. *Spine, 7*:243-254.

Wiltse, L.L. 1971. The effect of the common anomalies of the lumbar spine upon disc degeneration and low back pain. *Orthop. Clin. North Am., 2*:569-582.

Wood, P.H.N. 1976. Epidemiology of back pain. The lumbar spine and back pain. In *The lumbar spine and back pain*, ed. M. Jayson, pp. 13-17, London: Pitman.

Wood, P.H.N., Badley, E.M. 1980. Epidemiology of back pain. In (eds.) *The lumbar spine and back pain, ed. M.I.V. Jayson, 2nd Ed., pp. 29-55, London: Pitman.*

CHAPTER SIX

AN OVERVIEW OF THE INCIDENCE OF COMPENSABLE OCCUPATIONAL BACK INJURIES IN MICHIGAN: 1970-1981

C. NEWELL AND A. KANNO, Ph.D.

INTRODUCTION

IT is useful for clinicians and those in the public service to be able to exchange information on topics of social significance. Formerly, the different disciplines communicated very little. In spite of the fact that as early as the seventeenth century Bernardino Ramazzini, known as the father of occupational medicine (Lyons and Petricelli, 1978), inquired about the day-to-day problems of the working people in his practice. However, it was not without justification that, even in recent times, members of the learned community spoke of the two cultures. Namely, the exact sciences on the one hand and the social sciences and arts on the other, without a bridge between them (Snow, 1969).

The world of knowledge has come a long way, and the exchange of views and even a certain amount of interdependence has occurred as the social sciences have sharpened their tools of data collection and analysis. It is, therefore, a distinct pleasure to present to concerned clinicians a summary of occupational back injuries in Michigan.

DATA BASE

This paper is based upon information compiled by the Michigan Department of Labor in cooperation with and under the guidelines specified by the U.S. Bureau of Labor Statistics for the supplementary data system. Under the Michigan Workers' Disability Compensation Act, an "Employer's Basic Report

71

of Injury" (Form 100) must be filed for all cases involving a death, a specific loss, or seven or more calendar days of disability beyond the day of injury. The businesses covered by the Workers' Disability Compensation statute and therefore the supplementary data system include all Michigan employers except those specified in the statute. For a sample of the Employer's Basic Report of Injury (Form 100), please contact the authors.

Businesses not covered include the Federal Government, household workers (if employed less than 35 hours/week), maritime employers, merchant seafarers, railroad employers, sole proprietors (without employees), working partners of a partnership (if excluded by an endorsement contained in the Workers' Compensation Insurance Policy for Partnership); and employers covered by the Federal Liability Act, Jones Act, or Longshoremen's and Harbour Workers' Compensation Act.

Each case reported on the Form 100 has been classified and coded by the MIOSHA Information Section, Michigan Department of Labor by the nature of the injury or illness, the part of body affected, the source of the injury or illness, and the type of accident or exposure. Each case is also classified by the age, sex, and occupation of the claimant, the county in which the injury or illness occurred, and the industrial classification of the claimant's employer. All case characteristics for the years 1970-1976 and 1979-1981 were fully encoded for each Form 100 and tabulated.

For the years 1977 and 1978, however, only case characteristics such as age, gender of claimant, county in which injury or illness occurred, and the industrial classification of the affected employee's employer, were fully encoded from each Form 100. For other case characteristics, including nature of injury or illness, part of body affected, source of injury or illness, and type of accident or exposure during 1977 and 1978, a 20 percent sample of all claims were encoded. The sampling procedure was based upon a random sample within each two-digit industrial classification. Estimates for total injuries and illnesses for those two years were derived from sample tabulations. It must also be pointed out that the total numbers given in the tables and figures in this document represent only reported cases and do not include dismissed, denied, or withdrawn cases. Final figures may, therefore, be lower.

The magnitude of occupational safety and health problems deserves public understanding and concern. Michigan has from the early days of its statehood to the present day recognized the need to prevent occupational hazards and improve the workplace environment. The state's continued commitment to occupational safety and health culminated in the enactment of the Michigan Occupational Safety and Health Act, commonly known as MIOSHA, in 1974. MIOSHA, Public Act 154 of 1974, as amended, went into effect on January 1, 1975. This Act outlined employer's and employees' rights and responsibilities in maintaining workplace safety and health and also designated the state agencies to administer the Act. The Bureau of Safety and Regulation of the Michigan Department of Labor, and the Environmental and Occupational Health Service Administration of the Department of Public Health are responsible for administering and enforcing MIOSHA. At the present time, over 135,000 employers and over 3 million workers in Michigan are covered by MIOSHA.

According to a survey report by the Bureau of Labor Statistics of the U.S. Department of Labor, "injuries to the back are one of the more common and costly types of work-related injuries. Based on estimates derived from the Bureau of Labor Statistics' Annual Survey of Injuries and Illnesses and the Supplementary Data System, about 1 million workers suffered back injuries in 1980, accounting for almost 1 out of every 5 injuries and illnesses in the workplace. In eight states which provided information on workers' compensation indemnity payments, almost one-fourth of the expenditures were claims involving back injuries" (U.S. Department of Labor, BLS, 1982).

Furthermore, "about three-tenths of the workers surveyed lost from 1 to 5 workdays and a similar proportion lost from 6 to 15 workdays. Those losing time averaged 14 days away from work. More than two-fifths of the workers who had returned to work were given light duties." These figures clearly underscore the need for concern about occupational injuries and illnesses in general, and back injuries in particular.

An analysis of the reported compensable injuries for 1981 in Michigan showed that the back was the single most affected part of the body; back injuries were 25.2 percent of all cases. This was followed by injuries to fingers: 11.1 percent, knees: 5.8 percent, abdomen: 5.6 percent, hands: 5.1 percent, arms: 5.1 percent, ankles: 4.4 percent, trunk (excluding abdomen, back and shoulders): 4.2 percent and foot: 4.1. the remainder comprised 29.4 percent. Further details are shown on Figure VI-1, and Table VI-1.

The distribution of all reported compensable cases by the nature of injury or illness during 1981 indicates 44.2 percent of the cases as having resulted from sprains and strains. The distribution of reported cases by nature of the injury or illness is given in Figure VI-2. The distribution of the nature of the injury as they relate to the back injuries that occurred from 1970 to 1981 shows that approximately 90 percent of the total were reported as strains and sprains. These conclusions are further elucidated in Table VI-2. In 1981, burns, contusions, cuts, dislocations, fractures, hernias, and inflammation, all together, represented only 7 percent of back injuries, whereas strains and sprains represented almost 89 percent. Verbatim sample descriptions of how occupational back injuries occurred, as reported on the Form 100s, are listed in Appendix VI-1.

The tabulation of reported back injuries by industry groups from 1970-1981 is given in Table VI-3. Throughout the twelve-year period, the manufacturing industry consistently had the largest number of back injuries. In 1981, there were 5,770 reported back injuries in manufacturing: 3,382 in services, 1,825 in retail trade, 1,139 in transportation and public utilities, and 1,114 in

COMPENSABLE CASES BY PART OF BODY AFFECTED
MICHIGAN 1981

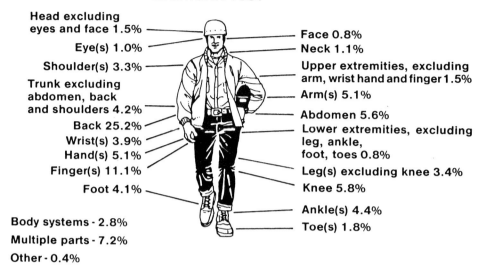

Head excluding
eyes and face 1.5%

Eye(s) 1.0%

Shoulder(s) 3.3%

Trunk excluding
abdomen, back
and shoulders 4.2%

Back 25.2%

Wrist(s) 3.9%

Hand(s) 5.1%

Finger(s) 11.1%

Foot 4.1%

Body systems - 2.8%

Multiple parts - 7.2%

Other - 0.4%

Face 0.8%

Neck 1.1%

Upper extremities, excluding
arm, wrist hand and finger 1.5%

Arm(s) 5.1%

Abdomen 5.6%

Lower extremities, excluding
leg, ankle,
foot, toes 0.8%

Leg(s) excluding knee 3.4%

Knee 5.8%

Ankle(s) 4.4%

Toe(s) 1.8%

Due To Rounding, Sum Of Individual Items May Not Equal 100%.

Source: MIOSHA Information Section, Michigan Department Of Labor

Figure VI-1.

TABLE VI-1

NUMBER AND PERCENTAGE OF COMPENSABLE CASES
BY PARTS OF BODY AFFECTED
MICHIGAN 1974 - 1981

Parts of Body*		1974	1975	1976	1977	1978	1979	1980	1981
Head	#	2,274	2,056	2,143	3,400	3,450	2,861	2,110	1,986
	%	3.9	3.8	0.0	4.7	4.5	3.6	3.3	3.2
Neck	#	520	491	596	530	710	723	629	663
	%	0.9	0.9	1.0	0.7	0.9	0.9	1.0	1.1
Upper Extremities	#	15,065	13,529	15,401	19,865	19,835	22,143	17,206	16,268
	%	25.9	24.9	26.2	27.8	26.0	27.6	26.5	26.7
Trunk (incl. back)	#	21,399	20,798	21,747	25,455	27,375	29,760	24,831	23,325
	%	36.7	38.3	37.0	35.6	35.8	37.1	38.3	38.3
Back**	#	(13,631)	(13,476)	(14,368)	(16,610)	(17,575)	(19,667)	(16,504)	(15,369)
	%	(23.4)	(24.8)	(24.4)	(23.2)	(23.0)	(24.5)	(25.5)	(25.2)
Lower Extremities	#	13,009	11,504	12,461	15,260	16,390	17,011	13,462	12,380
	%	22.3	21.2	21.2	21.3	21.4	21.2	20.8	20.3
Multiple Parts	#	4,812	4,820	5,268	5,005	5,880	5,591	4,738	4,379
	%	8.3	8.9	9.0	7.0	7.7	7.0	7.3	7.2
Body System	#	1,061	1,021	1,107	1,825	2,220	1,804	1,580	1,686
	%	1.8	1.9	1.9	2.6	2.9	2.2	2.4	2.8
Unknown	#	109	120	72	210	590	320	253	242
	%	0.2	0.2	0.1	0.3	0.8	0.4	0.4	0.4
TOTAL NUMBER &	#	58,249	54,339	58,795	71,550	76,450	80,213	64,809	60,929
	%	100.0	100.0	100.0	100.0	100.0	100.0	100.0	100.0

Source: MIOSHA Information Section, Michigan Department of Labor

* Part of Body Affected are classified according to U.S. Bureau of Labor Statistics guidelines for categories. Unknown is the combined
total number and percentage of cases involving body parts but not elsewhere classified and nonclassifiable by body parts.
** The percentage and number of compensable BACK injury and illness cases are also included in the percentage and number of
compensable TRUNK injury and illness cases.

DISTRIBUTION OF COMPENSABLE CASES BY NATURE OF THE INJURY OR ILLNESS - 1981

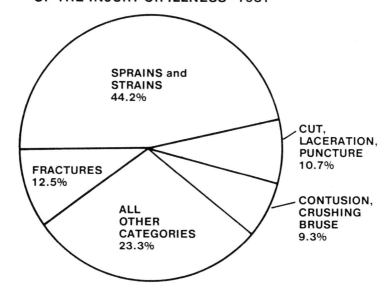

SPRAINS and STRAINS 44.2%

CUT, LACERATION, PUNCTURE 10.7%

FRACTURES 12.5%

CONTUSION, CRUSHING BRUSE 9.3%

ALL OTHER CATEGORIES 23.3%

Source: MIOSHA Information Section, Michigan Department of Labor

Figure VI-2.

TABLE VI - 2
MICHIGAN WORKERS' DISABILITY CLAIMS - BACK INJURIES BY NATURE OF INJURIES 1970 - 1981

Nature of Injury*	1970	1971	1972	1973	1974	1975	1976	1977	1978	1979	1980	1981
Burn	40	30	40	51	10	16	15	10	35	12	11	19
Contusion	661	704	679	711	502	433	510	630	540	601	482	424
Cut	55	53	65	54	40	28	39	55	25	23	15	15
Dislocation	45	61	66	143	300	318	283	380	235	234	119	196
Fracture	252	261	402	524	290	268	259	250	360	250	255	235
Hernia	1	1	1	1	320	326	145	15	10	1	3	1
Inflammation	3	1	4	5	255	272	179	335	215	195	214	135
Strains & Sprains	9,143	9,586	9,869	10,521	11,166	11,611	12,921	14,835	15,370	17,767	14,987	13,648
Injury NEC	--	--	--	--	7	4	2	25	730	469	308	631
Unknown	48	23	50	121	721	168	57	--	--	--	--	--
Other	11	13	12	20	20	32	37	75	55	115	110	65
TOTAL BACK INJURIES	10,259	10,733	11,188	12,151	13,631	13,476	14,466	16,610	17,575	19,667	16,504	15,369

Source: MIOSHA Information Section, Michigan Department of Labor

* Nature of Injuries are classified according to the U.S. Bureau of Labor Statistics guidelines for categories.

NEC = Not Elsewhere Classified

public administration. These five industry groups, together, accounted for 86 percent of the reported back injuries. Throughout the year, agriculture, mining and finance groups reported the least number of back injuries.

In Table VI-4, the employment in industry groups is compared to the number of back injuries for each group to calculate the proportion of back injuries per 10,000 employees for that group. The transportation and public utilities ranks seventh in terms of employment but highest in terms of the percentage of employees suffering back injuries, namely, 84 per ten thousand. This is followed by construction: 82, mining: 81, public administration: 66, and manufacturing: 59 per ten thousand. The industry with the least proportion of back injuries appears to be finance, insurance and real estate with 11 per ten thousand.

TABLE VI - 3

MICHIGAN WORKERS' DISABILITY CLAIMS
BACK INJURIES - BY INDUSTRY GROUPS
1970 - 1981

Industry Groups*	1970	1971	1972	1973	1974	1975	1976	1977	1978	1979	1980	1981
Agriculture, Forestry, Fishing	25	27	24	41	105	98	96	100	90	107	138	125
Mining	122	87	89	114	91	133	159	175	145	134	136	110
Construction	986	1,062	1,081	987	1,038	886	1,093	1,100	1,200	1,489	1,193	883
Manufacturing	5,752	5,808	6,059	7,009	6,717	6,043	6,457	7,705	8,225	8,891	6,543	5,770
Transportation, Public Utilities	794	778	865	837	857	925	975	1,215	1,160	1,424	1,190	1,139
Wholesale Trade	760	790	786	806	696	734	707	790	870	888	891	860
Retail Trade	1,128	1,297	1,361	1,422	1,471	1,479	1,566	1,900	1,815	2,159	2,021	1,825
Finance, Insurance, Real Estate	74	94	80	84	112	126	148	130	105	165	157	161
Services	481	579	592	617	1,563	1,782	2,163	2,515	2,705	3,189	3,181	3,382
Public Administration	137	210	251	234	981	1,270	1,102	980	1,260	1,221	1,054	1,114
Unknown	--	1	--	--	--	--	--	--	--	--	--	--
TOTAL BACK INJURIES	10,259	10,733	11,188	12,151	13,631	13,476	14,466	16,810	17,575	19,667	16,504	15,369

Source: MIOSHA Information Section, Michigan Department of Labor

* 1970-1975 - Industry classification is in accordance with "Standard Industrial Classification Manual of 1967"

* 1976-1981 - Industry classification in accordance with "Standard Industrial Classification Manual of 1972" as amended by the 1977 supplement. U.S. Government Printing Office

TABLE VI - 4

PROPORTION OF EMPLOYMENT COMPARED
TO BACK INJURIES BY INDUSTRY GROUPS
MICHIGAN, 1981

Industry Groups*	Number Employed	Number of Back Injuries	Proportion of Back Injuries per 10,000
Agriculture, Forestry, Fishing	39,793	125	31
Mining	13,583	110	81
Construction	107,848	883	82
Manufacturing	970,447	5,770	59
Transportation and Public Utilities	135,138	1,139	84
Wholesale Trade	161,111	860	53
Retail Trade	555,932	1,825	33
Finance, Insurance, Real Estate	151,955	161	11
Services	880,065	3,382	38
Public Administration	168,717	1,114	66
TOTAL	3,184,589	15,369	48

Source: MIOSHA Information Section, Michigan Department of Labor

* Industry Groups are classified according to U.S. Bureau of Labor Statistics guidelines, which references the Standard Industrial Classification Manual of 1972.

Table VI-5 shows the distribution of reported back injuries by occupational groups. Since 1970, three different occupation encoding systems have been used. The current encoding system, which is shown in Table VI-5, has been in use since 1978. In 1981, four occupations, namely, crafts, operatives, laborers, and service workers accounted for 13,050 or 85 percent of reported back injuries. Operatives (which are defined as occupations having to do with physical work or mechanical action other than transport) accounted for 5,325 back injuries or 35 percent while farmers and farm laborers reported only 62.

TABLE VI - 5

**MICHIGAN WORKERS' DISABILITY CLAIMS
BACK INJURIES BY OCCUPATION GROUPS
1978 - 1981**

Occupation Groups*	1978	1979	1980	1981
Professional, Technical and Kindred	380	394	422	461
Managers and Administrators, Except Farm	365	445	387	374
Sales Workers	170	272	317	308
Clerical and Kindred	750	931	906	885
Crafts and Kindred	3,205	3,714	3,194	2,869
Operatives, Except Transport	6,515	7,616	5,788	5,325
Laborers, Except Farm	2,885	2,950	2,339	1,957
Farmers: Farm Managers, Laborers & Foremen	40	45	68	62
Service Workers, Except Private Household	2,765	2,922	2,826	2,899
Not Reported or Nonclassifiable	500	378	257	229
TOTAL BACK INJURIES	**17,575**	**19,667**	**16,504**	**15,369**

Source: MIOSHA Information Section, Michigan Department of Labor

* Occupation groups are classified according to 1970 U.S. Bureau of the Census Standard Occupational Classification System.

The reported workers' disability cases for back injuries also vary markedly across age groups. As is shown in Table VI-6, the age group of 18-29 consistently accounted for the largest proportion of reported injuries. In 1981, this age group reported 4,957 back injuries, which is 32 percent of the total for that year. During the same year, the age groups of 18-29 and 30-39, together, reported 9,345 back injuries, or 61 percent of the total cases. The age groups of 18-29, 30-39 and 40-49 combined reported 12,420 back injuries, that is 81 percent of total back injury reports for 1981.

Since 1977, an average of about 73 percent of back injury reports filed have been for male employees. This is slightly higher than the proportion of adult male employees in the labor force during those years. The distribution of injuries by gender is given in Table VI-7. In 1981, for instance, 10,882 male employees had reports of work-related back injuries as compared to 4,487 female employees for the same year. The relationship between the proportion of employment and the proportion of reported back injuries by gender is also noteworthy. A positive correlation (r = .93) between the proportion of injuries and employment for both male and female employees is shown in Table VI-8.

Employment breakdowns by gender are currently available for the period

TABLE VI - 6

MICHIGAN WORKERS' DISABILITY CLAIMS
BACK INJURIES BY AGE GROUP
1970 - 1981

Age Group	1970	1971	1972	1973	1974	1975	1976	1977	1978	1979	1980	1981
0 - 17	34	18	36	51	48	38	44	40	85	63	46	49
18 - 29	3,121	3,352	3,481	4,187	4,460	4,316	4,878	5,905	6,490	7,301	5,815	4,957
30 - 39	2,473	2,595	2,676	2,878	3,163	3,245	3,541	4,045	4,450	5,219	4,428	4,388
40 - 49	2,466	2,516	2,604	2,533	2,723	2,730	2,814	2,935	3,075	3,643	3,237	3,075
50 - 59	1,659	1,766	1,846	1,882	2,121	2,169	2,149	2,485	2,390	2,696	2,298	2,259
60 +	458	463	495	499	535	528	566	695	585	623	616	574
Unknown	48	23	50	121	581	450	474	505	500	122	64	67
TOTAL BACK INJURIES	10,259	10,733	11,188	12,151	13,031	13,476	14,466	16,610	17,575	19,667	16,504	15,369

Source: MIOSHA Information Section, Michigan Department of Labor

TABLE VI - 7

MICHIGAN WORKERS' COMPENSATION CLAIMS
BACK INJURIES BY GENDER
1970 - 1981

Gender	1970	1971	1972	1973	1974	1975	1976	1977	1978	1979	1980	1981
Male	8,701	8,866	9,151	9,782	10,152	10,405	11,098	12,400	13,065	14,386	11,946	10,882
Female	1,510	1,844	1,987	2,248	2,841	3,068	3,361	4,210	4,510	5,281	4,558	4,487
Unlisted	48	23	50	121	638	3	7	0	0	0	0	0
TOTAL BACK INJURIES	10,259	10,733	11,188	12,151	13,631	13,476	14,466	16,610	17,575	19,667	16,504	15,369

Source: MIOSHA Information Section, Michigan Department of Labor

from 1970 to 1980. These breakdowns show that the proportion of male employees in the labor force had decreased from 64.5 percent to 58.7 percent in those years. The proportion of reported male injuries also decreased from 85.2 percent to 72.4 percent. In contrast, the proportion of female employees in the labor force increased from 35.5 percent in 1970 to 41.3 percent in 1980. Similarly, the proportion of reports filed for females increased from 14.8 percent in 1970 to 27.6 percent in 1980.

The proportion of compensable back injury reports for males and females during these years decreased or increased in almost direct proportion to their respective employments in the labor force. It appears, however, that male employees suffer a larger proportion of injuries than the proportion in the labor force. (See Figures VI-3, VI-4, and VI-5.) However, since a breakdown of industry employment by gender is not available, it is difficult to explain this difference.

Another important dimension of occupational injuries and illnesses is cost. According to estimates, the cost of work-related injuries in terms of medical expenses and compensation payments is staggering. The National Safety Council estimates that "work accidents" cost $32.5 billion in 1981 in the United States for 12,300 fatalities and 2,100,000 disabling injuries (National Safety Council, 1982). Injuries to the trunk, including the back, were estimated at 610,000 or

TABLE VI - 8
PROPORTION OF EMPLOYMENT AND PROPORTION OF REPORTED BACK INJURIES COMPARED BY GENDER
MICHIGAN, 1970 - 1973, 1975 - 1980

	Male		Female	
Years	% of Employment*	% of Reported Back Injuries**	% of Employment*	% of Reported Back Injuries**
1970	64.5	85.2	35.5	14.8
1971	64.9	82.8	35.1	17.2
1972	64.8	82.2	35.2	17.8
1973	64.3	81.3	35.7	18.7
1975***	62.4	77.2	37.6	22.8
1976	63.0	76.8	37.0	23.2
1977	61.3	74.7	38.7	25.3
1978	61.6	74.3	38.4	25.7
1979	60.2	73.1	39.8	26.9
1980	58.7	72.4	41.3	27.6

$r = .93****$

* Employment figures obtained from the Michigan Statistical Abstract, 1981

** Reported back injury figures obtained from MIOSHA Information Section, Michigan Department of Labor

*** Proportion of employment data for 1974 were not included in the Michigan Statistical Abstract, 1981 edition. However, back injury compensation claims by gender are available for that year. See Table 7

**** $r = .93$ represents the correlation coefficient between percent of employment and percent of reported back injuries during the ten-year period given in the table

29 percent of all work accidents. The National Safety Council also estimates that 38 percent, or $12.35 billion, of the compensation was paid for trunk-related injuries. Other sources estimate an even higher cost of back injuries (Antonakes, 1981; Snook, 1980).

The difficulty in credibly measuring actual costs of work-related injuries must not be overlooked, particularly as they relate to workers' compensation payments. Translating estimated gross national figures to average costs per injury for any particular state would be inaccurate since workers' compensation laws and guidelines vary from state to state. In the case of Michigan, the task is even further complicated because of the difficulty in keeping track of final payments for uncontested cases, and contested closed cases.

A recent survey of Michigan's closed compensation cases indicated that "aside from notifying the worker of the earnings reported by his or her employer (for calculating the weekly benefit level) and checking the accuracy of the benefit calculations, there is little agency involvement in the typical uncontested workers' compensation case in Michigan" (Hunt, 1982).

The cost estimates presented in Table VI-9 for the years 1968 to 1978 are based on Social Security Administration reports. In 1978, the last year for which data was available, compensation payments for Michigan were estimated at $496,987,000. If calculations were made according to proportions of

PROPORTION OF EMPLOYMENT AND PROPORTION OF REPORTED BACK INJURIES COMPARED BY GENDER MICHIGAN 1970-73, 1975-1980

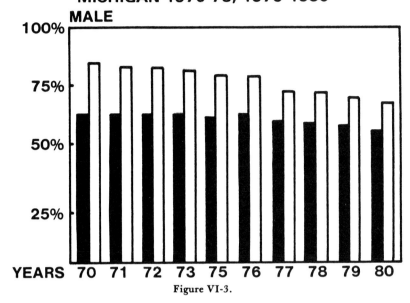

Figure VI-3.

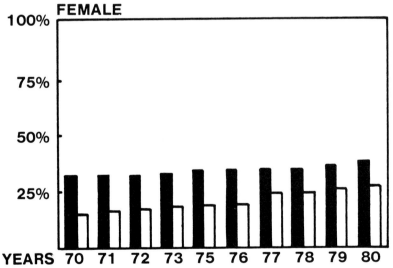

Source: Employment figures obtained from the Michigan Statistical Abstract, 1981. Reported injury figures obtained from MIOSHA Information Section, Michigan Department of Labor.

■ EMPLOYMENT
☐ INJURIES

Figure VI-4.

injuries, the payments for back injuries in Michigan in 1978 would amount to over $125,000,000. There are very strong indications, however, that the actual final figures may be significantly lower for those years. But even so, the figures confirm the extreme social significance of occupational injury problems.

As a concluding remark, it is encouraging to note that the overall number of comparable back injury reports filed in Michigan reached a peak of 19,667 in 1979 and started declining in 1980 and 1981 to 15,369. Unfortunately, thousands of deaths on the job, and millions of disabling injuries still occur in the United States every year. In 1981, according to a report from the U.S. Department of Labor, 4,370 work-related deaths and 5.3 million occupational injuries, as well as about 126,100 recognized job-related illnesses, occurred nationwide. These occurrences resulted in over 39 million lost workdays by our nation's employees.

It is, therefore, important to continue our efforts to understand why and how occupational injuries occur. It is hoped that this description of how work-related back injuries occur in Michigan will help place in socio-environmental perspective the clinical trials of manipulation. Through the dedication and concern of professional groups significant progress can undoubtedly be made toward improving safety and health in the workplace.

In addition to the efforts of clinicians in treating back pain after it occurs, there are also other approaches worthy of attention. Biomechanical problems are being studied and major design principles are becoming understood. This field is called ergonomics, which is a scientific attempt to make the job fit the person, instead of making the person fit the job. Such efforts will most certainly make the preventative approach more effective. There is also increasing evidence that suggests the need for this approach (MacLeod, 1982; Greenberg, and Chaffin, 1976; Tichener, 1978; NIOSH, 1981; McCormick, 1982).

For example, in the survey of back injuries associated with lifting, the U.S. Bureau of Labor Statistics noted that, "Material handling equipment to lift and transport the objects was, reportedly, not available in 61 percent of the cases studied. Even where workers had access to such equipment, 58 percent found it impractical to use" (U.S. Department of Labor, BSL, 1982).

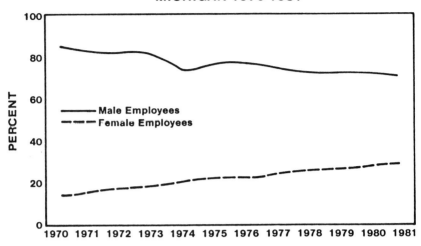

Source: MIOSHA Information Section, Michigan Department of Labor

Figure VI-5.

TABLE VI - 9

ESTIMATES OF WORKERS' COMPENSATION PAYMENTS IN MICHIGAN BY TYPE OF INSURANCE: 1968 - 1978

(As reported in the Michigan Statistical Abstract, 16th Ed., 1981)

(In thousands of dollars)

Year	Insurance losses paid by private insurance carriers	State and federal fund disbursements	Self-insurance payments	Total
1968	80,602	5,691	51,345	137,638
1969	94,226	6,420	59,885	160,531
1970	105,090	6,646	66,485	178,221
1971	119,700	8,033	76,000	203,733
1972	140,677	8,362	93,745	242,784
1973	158,141	9,759	105,620	273,530
1974	180,536	10,845	120,400	311,781
1975	193,410	11,500	128,800	333,710
1976	222,754	16,975	151,000	390,729
1977	252,569	14,116	168,000	434,685
1978	270,700	20,437	205,850	496,987

SOURCE: Social Security Administration, Social Security Bulletin, January 1966 through January 1977 (Washington, D.C.: Monthly), vol. 40, no. 1 (January 1977): 35, vol. 41, no. 3 (March 1978): 33, and vol. 42, no. 10 (October 1979): 20 (October 1980: 8.)

REFERENCES

Antonakes, J.A.: *Claims Costs of Back Pain*, in the Proceedings of the Liberty Mutual Back Pain Symposium, Boston, Massachusetts, March 22-24, 1981.

Greenberg, L., Chaffin, D.: *Workers and Their Tools*. Pendell Press Publishers, 1976.

Hunt, H.A.: *Workers' Compensation System in Michigan*. Kalamazoo, W.E. Upjohn Institute for Employment Research, 1982.

Lyons, A.A., Petrucelli, R.J.: *Medicine: An Illustrated History*, New York, Harry N. Abrams, Inc., 1978. p. 463.

MacLeod, D.: *Strains & Sprains: A Worker's Guide to Job Design*. Detroit, UAW, 1982.

McCormick, E.J., Sanders, M.F.: *Human Factors in Engineering and Design* (5th ed.), New York, McGraw-Hill, 1982.

Michigan Statistical Abstract, 16th ed., Detroit, Wayne State University, 1981.

National Safety Council, *Accident Facts*, 1982 ed.

NIOSH Technical Report, *Work Practices Guide for Manual Lifting* (DHHS) (NIOSH) Publication No. 81-122, Washington, D.C., U.S. Government Printing Office, 1981.

Snook, S.H.: Low back pain in industry, in White, A.A. and Gordon, S.E. (ed.) *Symposium on Idiopathic Low Back Pain*, St. Louis, C.V. Mosby, 1982, pp. 23-39.

Snow, C.P.: *The Two Cultures*, Cambridge, England, Cambridge University Press, 1969.

Tichaner, E.R.: *The Biomechanical Basis of Ergonomics*. New York, John Wiley and Sons, 1978.

U.S. Department of Labor, Bureau of Labor Statistics (BLS), *Back Injuries Associated with Lifting*, Bulletin 2144, August 1982.

Appendix VI-1

SAMPLE DESCRIPTIONS OF HOW OCCUPATIONAL BACK INJURIES OCCURRED AS REPORTED ON FORM 100s

1. Picked up a bag of heavy wet grass.
2. Spraying donuts—bent over while carrying screen of donuts.
3. Helping patient from the commode to the bed.
4. Slipped on steps.
5. Pushing scrap cart when front wheel hit a guard in floor.
6. Climbing over boxes 7 ft. high. When climbing down, something pulled in back.
7. Picking up wood skid, moving it over.
8. Stepped back on embankment, slipped, twisted body trying to regain balance.
9. Trying to lift and tie down a job.
10. Lifting panels off jig to put in pile.
11. Doing patient care.
12. Transporting files from one room to another and from one drawer to another.
13. Putting back bag of potatoes that fell.
14. Fell in parking lot over a piece of wood that was over a puddle.
15. Unknown—While employed at the Detroit Plaza.
16. Bent over and felt a sprain in back.
17. Using a shovel to clean walls of sand hopper, lost balance and footing and started to fall in, grabbed a rail going across bin to catch himself.
18. Lifting a steel door,
19. Taking 70 lb. parts from machine and stacking them.
20. Pulling a patient up in bed.
21. Folding hoist on truck.
22. Moving furniture.
23. Tightening large bolt with wrench.
24. Bending over to pick up piece of iron.
25. Unknown—possible aggravation of pre-existing injury.
26. Bent over to change the liner in waste basket.
27. Bending over to pick up steel.
28. Pulling a water pump.
29. Greasing lawn equipment.
30. Lifting cores.

Section 3

INTRODUCTION — SOME CHARACTERISTICS OF SPINAL MANIPULATION

THE quantification of the characteristics of manipulable patients and of the effects of manipulation is a largely unknown and unproven area. One approach is the randomized clinical trial upon a relatively ill-defined patient population. Another is the painstaking examination and characterization of manipulable populations. The following three papers exemplify the latter approach and are very important. One can only give the authors credit for attempting one giant step forward in a very difficult area.

CHAPTER SEVEN

DIFFERENTIAL DIAGNOSIS OF BACK PAIN

PHILIP E. GREENMAN, D.O., F.A.A.O.

INTRODUCTION

THE musculoskeletal system comprises 60% of the body. It is the site where patients experience a large number of painful syndromes. Back pain is the most common presenting complaint within the musculoskeletal system (e.g. Newell and Kanno, this volume). It is usually localized in the cervical or lumbar regions. Evaluation of patients presenting with back pain must be comprehensive. The physical examination of the back should be extensive, and will be described, but must be accomplished within the context of examination of the total patient. In this paper, I will discuss the problems in arriving at an accurate diagnosis of low back pain patients in order to decide upon appropriate therapeutic intervention.

Back pain is a multi-factorial problem with many etiologies. As a result, a number of therapeutic approaches are utilized, each with its advocates and detractors. Primary care physicians, orthopaedic surgeons, neurosurgeons, neurologists, rheumatologists, rehabilitation medicine specialists, general surgeons, and manual medicine specialists all treat patients with back pain, each with their own approaches, and based upon their experience and expertise. Other health care practitioners including chiropractors, acupuncturists, psychologists, and social workers all contribute their expertise in the management of patients with back pain. A team approach, utilizing the expertise of many disciplines in order to obtain the best results for the back pain patient may be especially valuable (O'Brien, 1980). Any therapeutic intervention, whether through an individual practitioner or a team approach, should be based upon the recognition of the natural course of a patient's back pain. Approximately 70% of back pain patients will be better in three weeks; 90% are self limiting; 99% recover without hospitalization; and 99.5% do not require surgery. What is necessary before therapeutic intervention of any kind is the most accurate diagnosis that is possible (Snook, 1982).

Farfan, (1980, page 159) has said:

> "I believe that the aetiological factor in back pain is mechanical in nature."

If that statement is true (and I support this hypothesis in most cases) then what is necessary is a simple, comprehensive approach to searching for the mechanical fault(s). Unfortunately, our present taxonomy of illness is oriented toward disease rather than mechanical functional analysis. Perhaps we should focus more attention on identifying the mechanical fault and less on the disease process. To emphasize this point one only has to look at the lack of correlation between the incidence of back pain and the incidence of spondylosis of the spine. It is easy to make a diagnosis of spondylosis by x-ray examination but its relationship to back pain is in serious question. To have diagnosed the presence of vertebral spondylosis may have little or nothing to do with the mechanical fault causing the back ache. Farfan (1980, page 159) states that:

> ". . . there are many side effects of excessive mechanical stress in a tissue, which may be involved singly or severally in exciting the central nervous system."

Therefore our investigation should lead us toward those structures which, when subjected to mechanical stress, may cause abnormal excitation of neural structures and which might result in the perception of pain. (See Neumann, this volume.) The lumbar vertebral motion unit consists of two lumbar vertebra, each with a body, pedicles, transverse processes, articular processes and facet joints and spinous process, together with the intervening intervertebral disk. Each vertebral motion unit forms the intervertebral foramen through which exit the spinal nerves. Sometimes this intervertebral foramen is actually a canal within which the spinal nerve divides into the anterior and posterior primary divisions. There are several structures which can mechanically influence the nerve root. They include the posterior longitudinal ligament, intervertebral disk, ligamentum flavum, and facet joint. Wyke (1980) has studied extensively the nociceptive receptor system throughout the vertebral column. He describes the distribution of lumbosacral nociceptive receptor systems as:

(1) skin, subcutaneous and adipose tissue.
(2) fibrous capsules of the apophyseal facet and sacroiliac joints.
(3) longitudinal spinal, interspinous, flavum and sacroiliac ligaments.
(4) periosteal covering of vertebral bodies and arches (and attached fascia, tendons and aponeuroses).
(5) dura mater, epidural fibro adipose tissue.
(6) walls of blood vessels supplying the spinal and sacroiliac joints, and intervertebral cancellous bone.
(7) walls of epidural and paravertebral veins.
(8) walls of intramuscular arteries and lumbosacral muscles.

Of particular importance is the sino-vertebral nerve, a branch of the anterior primary division which returns through the intervertebral foramina to innervate the posterior longitudinal ligament and the annulus fibrosis of the intervertebral disk. There is an extensive anastomosis of the spinal vertebral nerve system, crossing over the midline, and traveling both cephalically and caudally. Also important is the medial branch of the posterior primary ramus which extensively innervates the articular processes and facet joints on each side (Fisk, 1977; Riley et al., 1978).

The intervertebral disk is a major component of the vertebral motion unit (see Pope, this volume). It is a structure which is much discussed, much maligned, and receives a lot of therapeutic attention. There appears to be a natural history of degenerative change within the disk. Kirkaldy-Willis (1982) has described the degenerative process in which the disk progresses from a structure well delineated between its nucleus and annulus to a phase wherein the demarcation between the nucleus and annulus is lost, and culminating in the fibrotic disk in which there is marked internal disruption. Since the classical report of Mixter and Barr (1934), the so-called "herniated" disk has received much attention. We now recognize three types of intervertebral disk disease:

(1) The "prolapsed" intervertebral disk describes the condition which some of the nucleus pulposus passes through fissures in the annulus fibrosis or vertebral end plate resulting in narrowing of the intervertebral disk space and bulging of its lateral aspects.

(2) The "extruded" intervertebral disk occurs when nuclear material extrudes through and creates bulging at the disk periphery.

(3) The "sequestrated" intervertebral disk is the condition wherein nuclear material is found within the spinal canal.

While the intervertebral disk receives a great deal of attention, a diagnosis of prolapse or displacement is made only about 15 percent of the time in patients presenting to a general practitioner (Wood and Badley, 1980). When present it does account for a large percentage of those disabled by back pain, that is probably greater than 80 percent.

The symptoms of low-back disk disease are primarily those of the effect upon lumbar and sacral nerve roots. The pathophysiology of the nerve root includes those of compression, inflammation (Murphy, 1977), and potentially an immune response (Marshall et al., 1977). When there is involvement of the nerve roots, there may be changes in the deep tendon reflexes, strength of muscle groups, bowel and bladder function, sensory change, nerve stretch signs (e.g. straight leg raising and femoral stretch) and the distribution of pain. Frequently accompanying the back pain and these root signs is the finding of sciatic scoliosis with distortion of the spinal complex to the ipsilateral side of the sciatica. Examples are the loss of the Achilles reflex with an S-1 radiculopathy commonly associated with herniation of the L-5 disk. Another classic finding is weakness of the extensor hallucis longus muscle due to an L-5 radiculopathy which is frequently associated with herniation of the L-4 disc. There are many such classic findings in discogenic radiculopathy, but the examiner must be aware that there are many overlaps of nerve roots, both due to their development and their level of exit from the spinal canal (Cailliet, 1962).

HISTORY

The history may well be the most important aspect of the evaluation of a patient presenting with back pain (see Finneson, 1980a; Mennell, 1960). It is essential that a total patient history be made. The familial and past personal history are obtained as well as an intensive historical review of organ systems. One important purpose is to rule out the presence of referred back pain from visceral pathology.

A detailed history of the back pain starts with the history of the present episode. One must ask such questions as:

(1) Where is the pain located?
(2) Is it in the lumbar, lumbosacral or sacroiliac region?
(3) Is it unilateral or bilateral?
(4) Is there radiation of the pain?
(5) If it radiates into the leg, where in the leg is the pain?
(6) Is it all on the posterior, lateral, anterior, or medial side?
(7) Does it radiate only to the knee or below the knee?
(8) Is there numbness or tingling or weakness associated with the pain?
(9) What was the position of the patient at the time of onset?
(10) Was there trauma of a fall, lift, or other injury?
(11) What positions of the body make the pain better and worse?
(12) Is the pain worse with coughing, sneezing, or straining for a bowel movement? In addition to the history of the present episode, it is most important to obtain a history of previous episodes of back pain.
(13) At what age was the first episode?
(14) Was the original onset insidious or following some trauma?
(15) How frequently have recurrences occurred?
(16) How much disability was related to both the present episode and to all previous attacks? It is also important to ascertain what previous therapies have been utilized and their effectiveness. We are interested in treatment for all conditions and not just that for back pain.
(17) What previous surgeries have occurred.
(18) What medications has the patient received?
(19) Have there been previous fractures, particularly of the lower extremities, which might alter the gait or pelvic declination?

It is beyond the scope of this paper to discuss all the permutations of symptoms which lead the skilled clinician through the problem solving process. Perhaps a synopsis of one typical case will be helpful in understanding the subtleties of understanding the history; unilateral lumbosacral pain radiating to the buttock and posterior leg is a common presenting complaint among people with acute and recurrent back pain. If the pain radiates below the knee, the index of suspicion of radicular irritation is higher than if the radiation of the pain stops at the knee or above. Frequently pain radiates to the posterior hip and thigh with biomechanical faults at the posterior facets in the lower lumbar spine and also in the presence of a sacroiliac syndrome. Obviously, radiculopathies with radiation of pain below the knee and in typical distributions to the calf and foot, have an even more guarded prognosis.

In summary, the history is well worth the time that it takes to acquire. Recurrent probing with questions during the examination can clarify the circumstances and nature of the patient's back pain.

PHYSICAL EXAMINATION

The physical examination is the second most important element in the differential diagnosis of back pain (See Finneson, 1980b). The objective is to elicit information about local and distant pathology which might account for the presenting complaint. The physical examination of the musculoskeletal system must be conducted in the context of a complete physical examination of the patient. This presentation will focus upon the musculoskeletal system, but a complete physical examination is essential to rule out pathologics which might cause back pain. The examination should attempt to identify, or rule out, neurological and orthopedic pathologies. While accomplishing this objective, the physical examination should also attempt to determine the functional capacity of the musculoskeletal system as well as the presence of organic path ology.

The examination (Eaton, 1965) begins with the initial observation of the patient in the act of disrobing, *moving* around the examining room, and assuming examining chairs or tables.

The screening examination (Mitchell et al., 1979) of the musculoskeletal system begins with the observation of the patient *walking* from the side, from the front, and from the rear. Observation of the stride, the foot, ankle, knee, and pelvis while participating in the stride, looking for symmetry and ease of movement. One observes the swing of the arms and the participation of the torso in a walking function.

The patient is then asked to *heel-walk* in order to evaluate strength or the level of function of the tibialis anterior and extensor muscle group.

Then the patient is asked to *toe-walk,* evaluating the gastrocnemius and soleus mechanism.

Tandem walking is used to evaluate neurological function of fine motor performance.

Static posture is then evaluated from the front, rear, and both lateral directions. Evaluation of body symmetry or asymmetry, weight distribution, levels of shoulders and hips, head carriage, are all made. In the lateral position, one looks for the posture against a plumb line dropped from the tragus of the ear: Is there good antero-posterior (AP) symmetry to the plumb line? Is there an increase or decrease in the lumbar lordosis? Is the abdomen protuberant or flat?

What is the weight distribution in the lateral projection? Asymmetries of spinal curvatures both in the anterior-posterior and coronal planes are of particular interest.

One then examines the bony parts at the *acromioclavicular* joint, the iliac crests, the greater *trochanters* of the femurs for relative symmetry. *Unleveling* of these anatomical landmarks suggests postural imbalance as a factor in the genesis of the patient's complaint. To test the *sidebending* capacity *of the trunk*, one observes the posterior aspect of the patient and instructs the patient to reach to the knee on the left side with the left hand, and then to the right knee with the right hand while maintaining the body erect so that the motion occurs in the coronal plane. One can observe the range of movement to each side as well as the participation of the thoracic spine, lumbar spine, and pelvis in this sidebending movement. Normally there should be a smooth convexity to the opposite side during sidebending. Straightened or flattened areas within the lateral curvature are usually indicative of restricted vertebral mobility in that region.

The *posterior superior iliac spines* are *palpated* with the thumbs while the index finger lies along the posterior aspect of the iliac crest. This gives additional evaluation of pelvic obliquity or the normal leveling. From this position, the *standing flexion test* is initiated. The relative movement of the posterior superior iliac spines on each side is evaluated. If one posterior superior iliac spine appears to move more in a cephalic and anterior direction than the opposite side, the standing flexion test is termed positive on that side; a positive test is presumptive evidence of restricted pelvic mobility on that side. During this same forward bending procedure, one observes the lumbar and lower thoracic spine looking for the normal response of progressive segmental participation in the forward bending arc, or the abnormal response of dysrhythmia, blocked movement, and the introduction of lateral curvatures.

While the patient remains in the standing position, instructions are given to *stand on one foot and lift the weight of the body* up on the toes repetitively; this is a second test for the strength of the gastrocnemius/soleus muscle group; early fatigue of one side versus the other is frequently found in pathologies involving the S-1 nerve root.

The functional capacity of the joints of the lower extremity are screened by the squat test with the feet flat on the floor. If there is loss of motion of the feet,

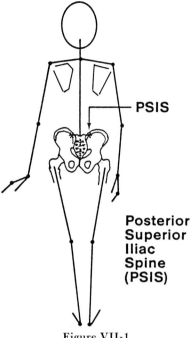

PSIS

**Posterior
Superior
Iliac
Spine
(PSIS)**

Figure VII-1.

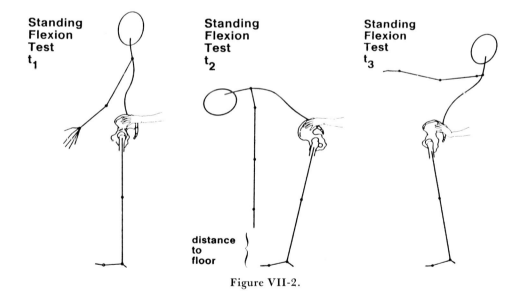

**Standing
Flexion
Test
t_1**

**Standing
Flexion
Test
t_2**

**Standing
Flexion
Test
t_3**

**distance
to
floor**

Figure VII-2.

ankles, knee, hip joints, the patient is unable to perform this task. While not definitely diagnostic, it calls attention to loss of functional capacity of the lower extremities.

A modified Schober test (Moll and Wright, 1980) is used to evaluate mobil-

Modified Schober's Test

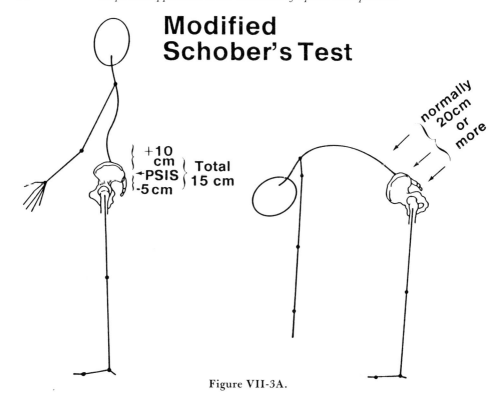

Figure VII-3A.

Modified Schober's Test

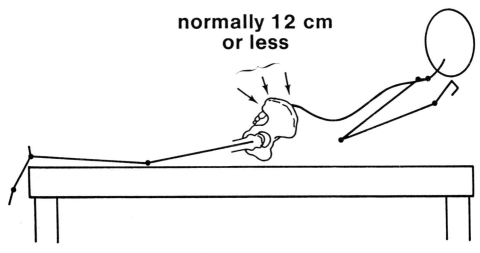

Figure VII-3B.

ity within the lumbar and lumbosacral regions of the back. Three marks are made on the back. The first is at the mid-point of the posterior superior iliac spines, the second ten centimeters above and the third five centimeters below the first point. The patient is asked to forward bend completely and the excursion from the superior to inferior mark is identified. Normally in flexion the distance should be greater than twenty centimeters, that is it should increase more than five centimeters. This test can be done in conjunction with measurements of distance between the patient's extended fingers and the floor. With the patient in the prone position and asked to extend the spine, measurement is again made between the superior and inferior marks. Reduction of the distance by at least three centimeters is considered normal. It must be emphasized that the modified Schober test must be interpreted cautiously since normal variations occur. Its value is two-fold. First, it is useful in screening for restricted mobility in both the forward and backward bending movements; and second, it is valuable for following the progress of a patient over time and especially in evaluating the response to therapeutic intervention.

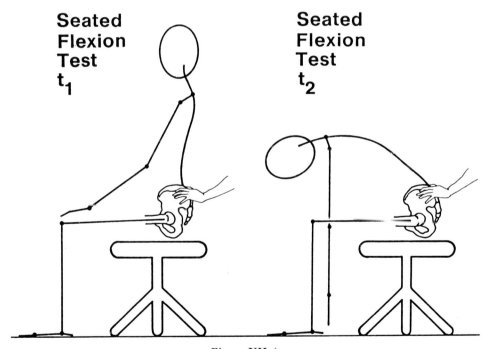

Seated Flexion Test t_1

Seated Flexion Test t_2

Figure VII-4.

With the patient seated on a firm stool, the posterior superior iliac spines are again palpated and the patient is instructed to forward bend with the arms between the knees and with the feet flat on the floor. This procedure is called the *seated flexion test*; one observes the relative motion of both posterior superior iliac spines (PSIS) during the forward bending movement. Excursion of one posterior superior iliac spine in a more cephalic and anterior direction than the opposite PSIS, is interpreted as a positive seated flexion test and is presumptive evidence of restricted pelvic mobility on the ipsilateral side without the influence of the lower extremities upon pelvic mechanics. Again the response of the vertebral column for dysrhythmia, flattening, or introduction of lateral curvatures is made. Comparison of the findings of the standing flexion test and the seated flexion test, and the lumbar responses thereto, are helpful in differentiating difficulties introduced due to pathology in the lower extremities versus dysfunctions due to pathology in or above the pelvis without the involvement of the lower extremities.

With the patient seated on an examining table, the *patellar reflex* is tested bilaterally. Absence of a patellar reflex is frequently found in the presence of pathology of the L-4 nerve root.

With the patient kneeling on the table or a chair, the *Achilles reflex* is tested. Absence of the Achilles reflex is frequently due to disturbance of function of the S-1 root.

With the patient seated on the table the knee is extended passively to test the nerve stretch on that side. In effect this is the same as a *straight leg raising test* in the *supine* position and is useful in determining a psychological overlay: patients may fake a positive straight leg raising test while in the supine position, but are unaware that this *seated* test provides the same information

Passive trunk movements are made with the patient seated in the erect and not the slouched position. Rotation right and left are passively introduced to determine the range and quality of motion during this movement and to feel the end point of the range of motion. This is also done in the sidebending direction. Evaluation is made of symmetry or asymmetry of participation of the thoracic and lumbar spines in these rotational and sidebending movements. The sidebending test is compared with the findings when the patient was standing.

Evaluation is then made of the relationship of a number of osseous landmarks of the pelvis against the three planes of the body. Palpation of anatomical landmarks in the pelvis is fraught with potential danger because of the developmental asymmetries which are so frequently present within the osseous pelvic ring. However, presumptive evidence of functional derangement of both sacroiliac joints and the symphysis pubis can be made when there are asymmetries in a number of the parts palpated. The landmarks palpated are:

1) *anterior superior iliac spine* (ASIS).
2) *pubic tubercles*.
3) *medial malleoli in the supine position*.

With the patient in the supine position the *Patrick or Fabere Test* is made bilaterally to test for hip joint pathology. Place the foot of his involved leg on his opposite knee. The hip joint is then flexed, abducted, and externally rotated.

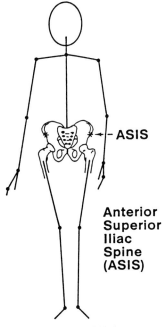

ASIS

**Anterior
Superior
Iliac
Spine
(ASIS)**

Figure VII-5.

**The Patrick
or
Fabere Test**

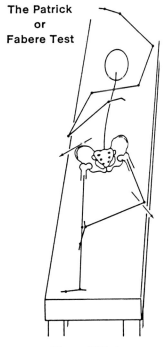

Figure VII-6.

In this position, inguinal pain is an indication of pathology in the hip joint or the surrounding muscles. When the end point of flexion, abduction, and external rotation has been reached, fixation of the femur in relation to the pelvis occurs. To stress the sacroiliac joint, extend the range of motion by placing one hand on the flexed knee joint and the other hand on the anterior superior iliac spine of the opposite side. Press down on each of these points. If the patient complains of increased pain, there may be pathology in the sacroiliac joint.

The *straight leg raising test* is then carried out in several *variations*. First the straight leg is raised *passively* while the movement of the opposite anterior superior iliac spine is monitored for movement. The first motion felt by the monitoring hand is the end point of the capacity of straight leg raising due to the length of the hamstrings. The equality of hamstring muscles can then be identified; abnormal hamstring equality is a common finding in chronic back pain syndromes. Straight leg raising is then carried on to the point of the initiation of *nerve stretch pain* and the angle is noted. Increased pain due to dorsi-flexion of the foot at this level *(Bragard's sign)* is further evidence of nerve root irritation. Plantar flexion at this level should not exacerbate pain as does dorsi-flexion and is a useful test in differentiating the patient with psychological overlay. With the knee and hip flexed, the classical *Lasegue's sign* is tested by straightening the knee and determining if pain is exacerbated by that movement. It is confirmatory evidence of nerve root irritation.

Dermatomal patterns are then identified for abnormalities of sensation. These are carried out across the thigh, calf, and foot with both the rolling pinwheel, single pin prick, and light superficial brush testing. Of particular value is the observation of sensory perception across the dorsum of the foot wherein the medial side is innervated by L-4, the dorsum by L-5 and the lateral side by S-1 nerve roots. Sensory testing is difficult and requires concentration by both the physician and the patient. One looks for variations in sensation bilaterally. Is it dermatomal? Sensory changes which do not follow typical neurologic patterns are of particular interest.

Strength testing is made *of the great toe* as well as the other dorsi flexors of the foot. If the patient is unable to resist the physician's effort to plantar flex the great toe, a weakness of the extensor hallucis longus is presumed and this is frequently related to root irritation at L-5. The *Babinski test* is elicited bilaterally. Plantar flexion is normal while dorsi-flexion of the great toe and splaying of the remaining toes is positive. Of course, a positive Babinski is frequently associated with upper motor neuron lesions.

The *dorsalis pedis and posterior tibial pulses* are palpated bilaterally to identify presence or absence. Vascular deficiencies are common in the elderly age groups with arteriosclerosis, and at any age in patients with diabetes. Vascular changes and a neuropathy are commonly associated with diabetes mellitus.

Range of motion, length and strength of muscle groups of the hips and thighs are then identified by taking the extended leg into abduction bilaterally, and internal and external rotation with the hip and knee at 90/90 degree flexion. Internal rotation in this 90/90 position stretches the piriformis muscle; and exacerbation of leg pain in the *"piriformis syndrome."*

As described earlier, the length of the hamstrings is tested by passive straight leg raising while monitoring the opposite anterior superior iliac spine. An increased frequency of shortening of the hamstrings on the left leg has been reported by Fisk (1978), the reason for which is unknown. Fisk (1978) has also reported changes in hamstring length following manipulation of the lumbar spine.

Assessment is then made of the *relative lengths of the two psoas muscles* by having the patient bring both knees to the chest, holding one knee in that position and attempting to extend the opposite hip. If the posterior thigh is unable to strike the table, psoas muscle shortening is a common cause. Both sides are tested. However, *note with caution* that this test puts strain upon the facet joints of the lower lumbar spine, particularly at the lumbosacral level.

The patient is placed in the prone position and observation of the *relative lengths of the lower extremities* are made again by palpating and comparing the inferior slopes of each medial malleolus. Is there a difference from that found in the supine position? If so, and it frequently is, the probability of functional alteration in pelvic mechanics is high.

The *inferior slope of the posterior superior iliac spines* are palpated and evaluated against the horizontal plane. The *base of the sacrum*, just medial to each posterior superior iliac spine, is palpated and evaluated against the coronal plane. The *inferior lateral angle of the sacrum* is then palpated in the neutral position and is utilized as an indicator of symmetrical or asymmetrical position of the sacrum.

Since asymmetry of the sacrum is so common, dynamic testing of the anatomical landmarks is made to ascertain if it is a structural or functional asymmetry. This is done by *evaluating the inferior lateral angle* in the forward bent position (similar to the position used for the *seated flexion test*) and in the *hyperextended position with the patient prone* on the table. Change in the relationship of the inferior lateral angles on both sides in these three positions is indicative of functional disturbance within the pelvis while maintenance of the same asymmetry in all three positions is usually found in patients with structural asymmetry of this osseous part. The *sacro-tuberous ligaments* are palpated bilaterally as well as the tension within the sciatic notch. Tenderness and tension in this area is frequently related to sciatic irritation with or without piriformis hypertonicity. The relative levels of the *ischial tuberosities* are palpated against the horizontal plane, again looking for asymmetry of form of function. The *lumbar spring test* is then accomplished. This is done by downward pressure on the lumbar spine while the patient is in the prone position, evaluating both the presence or absence of the lumbar lordosis and its ability to respond to backward bending movement as the physician presses anteriorly. Flattening of the lumbar lordosis and resistance to springing are common in acute lumbar disk disease. The knees are then flexed and relative lengths and strengths of the quadriceps muscles are identified. Flexion of the knee in this position also stretches the femoral nerve and aggravation of pain might be due to femoral nerve irritation. With the knees at 90 degrees internal and external hip rotation is accomplished. These tests are paired with the internal and external rotation that was accomplished with the patient in the supine position and the knees and hips at 90/90 degrees of flexion.

Evaluation of vertebral mobility has been classically described as an observation during the forward bent position with the patient standing. This procedure both in the standing and the seated postures has already been described above. In addition to these, observation of the segmental relationship of the tips of the transverse processes of each vertebral segment is accomplished in the neutral position and in the backward bent position. It is possible to segmentally identify the transverse processes in these three positions from approximately T-6 or T-7 to the sacrum. By following the excursion of the transverse processes in all three positions, one gets information as to segmental vertebral hypermobility or hypomobility as well as that of asymmetrical movement. *Individual vertebral segmental motion* testing is a finite art but hypomobility of vertebral segments is highly correlated to patients with acute and chronic back pain. *Hypomobility* of vertebral segments is readily amenable to appropriate manipulative therapeutic intervention. *Hypermobility* of a vertebral segment is a contraindication to manipulative therapeutic intervention.

As described, the physical examinationof the musculoskeletal system, with particular reference to the lower back and lower extremities, can be accomplished rapidly and thoroughly in the sequence described herein. Please note that the patient is examined both passively and actively in the standing, seated, supine, and prone positions. Several tests are done to elicit the same information for corroboration of findings. This sequence of examination techniques requires minimal movement of a patient who is uncomfortable. Orthopedic and neurologic pathologies can be identified. Anatomical and functional asymmetries of the osseous parts of the vertebral column and pelvis can be identified. Specific segmental vertebral motion characteristics can also be identified and structural and functional asymmetries ascertained.

LABORATORY TESTING

For a more complete discussion of these tests, consider the excellent symposium edited by Wagner and Galen (1977); the chapter by Ward (1977) may be of special interest.

In evaluating the back pain patient, laboratory testing is primarily useful to rule out other distinct pathologies rather than being diagnostic for the cause of the back pain. The patient should have the benefit of a baseline laboratory evaluation. A complete blood count, erythrocyte sedimentation rate (ESR), rheumatoid factor test, uric acid, fasting blood sugar, proteins with albumin-globulin (A/G) ratio, and if indicated, a B-27 human leukocyte antigen test (HLA-B27) should be included. In most instances, rheumatoid disease does not present a problem in differential diagnosis. For example, an elevated sedimentation rate and a positive HLA-B27 in a young, otherwise healthy, patient, usually a male, with bilateral low-back pain would be consistent with ankylosing spondylitis. A commonly overlooked condition is gout which can present itself as back pain and can easily be identified by an elevation in uric acid. Abnormalities of the blood sugar level would raise the suspicion of a diabetic neuropathy. Abnormalities of proteins and A/G ratio together with an elevated sedimentation rate would suggest the possibility of a myeloma as the etiology of the back pain.

ELECTROMYOGRAPHY (EMG)

Electromyography and nerve conduction studies are particularly useful in localizing the nerves involved in a radiculopathy (DeLisa et al., 1978). The study also is useful in monitoring the deterioration of a neurologic deficit. It should be pointed out that a positive EMG is not present early in the pathology and only becomes positive two to three weeks following nerve injury. Electromyography is a most useful tool in differentiating a wide variety of neurologic and muscle diseases, when performed by a well trained and experienced clinician.

RADIOLOGY

All patients presenting with acute or recurrent back pain should have a routine radiographic study. A *"six film study"* (Greenman, 1979) is a minimum and should include: a transverse film of the pelvis, hip joints, sacroiliac joints, symphysis pubis, and an angle study made with a 30 degree cephalic angle for both sacroiliac and the lumbosacral joints. Some people prefer a "spot lateral" of the lumbosacral junction, but in my experience the angle study is more valuable in discerning pathologic change at the lumbosacral level and gives a second film for evaluation of the sacroiliac joints. The left and right obliques are made for evaluation of the posterior elements and the facet joints. The oblique studies give evaluation of the pars intra-articularis for disruption (spondylolysis) and separation (spondylolisthesis). An anterior-posterior projection of the lumbar spine including all five vertebra allows one to look at vertebral architecture. Of particular importance is the observation of each pedicle at each vertebral level. Absence of a demonstrable pedicle is a common finding in early metastatic disease of lumbar vertebrae. If this film is made in the erect position, it is also possible to identify the level of the sacral base plane and the presence of a weight bearing lumbar scoliosis. Sacral base unleveling as a factor in back pain remains controversial. In my experience, it is one of the more common findings in patients who have chronic recurrent low back pain. The lateral projection provides opportunities to look at the vertebral bodies and posterior arches. Particular evaluation should be made of the *intervertebral disk heights.* It should be pointed out that the lumbosacral disk is normally more narrow than the others. Caution must be exercised before stating that narrowing of the intervertebral disk is the cause of the back pain. Evaluation of the normality, flattening and increase of lumbar lordosis is easily made. Three measurements are useful on a lateral erect film. They are the lumbosacral angle measured between the posterior aspect of the sacrum and the fifth lumbar body; the sacral base angle of Ferguson (1949), the angulation of the sacrum against the horizontal plane; and the mid-third lumbar perpendicular plumb line to see if it strikes within the confines of the sacral base.

Evaluation of the routine "six film study" can also provide information on congenital and developmental variations such as spina bifida occulta, sacralization, lumbarization, and facet tropism. Degenerative spondylosis and spondylarthrosis are common findings in routine radiographic examination of the lower back. One must be very cautious before stating that degenerative changes are a cause of a painful back syndrome since these changes frequently occur in patients without back pain. Alterations in the trabecular pattern of the osseous parts should alert one to metabolic or pathologic bony pathology. Haziness, irregularity, narrowing, and erosion of the sacroiliac joints are common early findings in ankylosing spondylitis, which in later stages can be readily identified by the classical "bamboo spine."

Routine radiographic studies can be supplemented by *stress films* of flexion-extension and films in the lateral projection and in right and left lateral flexion films both in the anterior-posterior projection. These studies provide some information on the functional capacity of the lumbar spine. The use of the erect films in the anterior-posterior and lateral projections for postural analysis can be most helpful.

SPECIAL RADIOLOGY STUDIES

There are a number of both invasive and non-invasive special radiographic techniques which can be used in both localizing and identifying the causes of pain in the lower back (Park, 1980). These studies include:

(1) myelography,
(2) epidural venography,
(3) epidurography,
(4) discography,

(5) radionucleid bone scan,
(6) computerized tomographic scanning (CT-scan), and
(7) nuclear magnetic resonance.

Myelography is an invasive procedure which carries a certain risk. It can be most useful in localizing pathologies within the dura as well as extradural lesions. The new aqueous medium, metrizamide, appears to have improved diagnostic results because of its superior filling of the lateral recesses and nerve sleeves, and because it is less dense than Pantopaque. In addition, being water soluble, metrizamide is absorbed and excreted by the body and is not retained as a potential long-term irritant. Myelography should only be utilized to identify a specific level prior to surgery or to rule out intra-dural pathology.

CT-scan (Glenn et al., 1980) has rapidly become a valuable diagnostic tool in the differential diagnosis of back pain. Its accuracy rate is at least equal to or superior to that of myelography in localizing intervertebral disk lesions. It is also a useful tool in the diagnosis of central and lateral recess stenosis. It is also helpful in evaluating inflammatory, neoplastic, and other organic pathologies of the region.

Epidural venography and epidurography have fallen into disuse with the advent of CT-scan and with improved myelography with metrizamide. Both of these procedures can still be useful but should be reserved for individuals who have experience with the technique.

Discography calls for the introduction with a needle of contrast material directly into the nucleus pulposus of the disk. This procedure is done at multiple levels and is useful in the diagnosis of intervertebral disk disease. Not only does the procedure provide for the radiographic study of the integrity of the disk, but it is also a provocative test which in the presence of symptomatic disk disease can cause exacerbation of the patient's back and referred leg pain. This procedure has become more popular recently because its use in combination with chemonuclcolysis may yield improved results in intervertebral disk disease.

As useful as many of these imaging techniques are, they should not be viewed as substitutes for an accurate history and physical examination of the patient and should be used for corroboration and specific localization of the etiology of the back pain.

PSYCHOLOGICAL EVALUATION

Because pain is a subjective experience, and because many patients with back pain have sustained injuries, from compensable occupational or personal liability injuries, psychological evaluation can be most useful. The *Minnesota Multiphasic Personality Inventory (MMPI)* test has been the instrument most frequently utilized in research in the field (Wiltse and Rocchio, 1975). Abnormal

MMPI, particularly with elevations of the hypochondrical, hysterical, and depressive scales, are frequently found in patients with a poor response to therapy, particularly in surgical cases.

The pain drawing is another instrument which has been of value in differentiating the organic from non-organic pain patterns. Despite the value of these instruments, they are no substitute for an in-depth psychological interview with a psychiatrist or psychologist experienced with pain patients and especially chronic pain. However, one must be cautious when identifying a patient's pain as being psychological in origin unless an intensive and concerted effort has been made to rule out all possible organic causes of the painful syndrome presented by the patient.

CONCLUSION

The differential diagnosis of the patient with back pain can be a tremendous challenge to the clinician as well as the patient. An accurate diagnosis must be made before any intervention is contemplated. A comprehensive approach including an extensive history, physical examination, psychological evaluation, radiographic examination, laboratory studies, and electromyography may all be necessary to arrive at a conclusion. It may well be that the most important analysis is that of functional capacity of the musculoskeletal system. The goal of any therapeutic intervention should be the restoration of the maximum possible pain free function. In the large number of patients with back pain in whom no specific etiology is found, and are therefore termed idiopathic, perhaps we should focus more attention upon the analysis of mechanical functional rather than upon the continued search for a disease process. It is in those back pain cases which demonstrate mechanical functional loss of motion that are usually most amenable to manipulative therapeutic intervention.

REFERENCES

Cailliet, R.: *Low Back Pain Syndrome*, Philadelphia, PA, F.A. Davis Company, 1962.

DeLisa, J.A., Kraft, G.H., Gans, B.M.: Clinical electromyography and nerve conduction studies. *Orthopedic Review, 7*(10):75-84, 1978.

Eaton, J.M.: The differential diagnosis of the low back syndrome, 1965 Yearbook, *Academy of Applied Osteopathy Yearbook, 2*:122-128, 1965.

Farfan, H.F.: The scientific basis of manipulative procedures. *Clinics in Rheumatologic Diseases, 6*(1):159, 1980.

Ferguson, A.B.: *Roentgen Diagnosis of Extremities and Spine*. New York, Paul B. Hoeber, Inc., 1949, pp. 382-387.

Finneson, B.E.: *Low Back Pain* (2nd ed.), Philadelphia-Toronto, J.B. Lippincott Co., 1980a, pp. 45-48.

Finneson, B.E.: *Low Back Pain* (2nd ed.), Philadelphia-Toronto, J.B. Lippincott Co., 1980b, pp. 48-57.

Fisk, J.B.: *The Painful Neck and Back*, Springfield, IL, Charles C Thomas, 1977, pp.15-19.

Fisk, J.W.: *The Significance of Disordered Muscle Activity in the Perpetuation and Treatment of Low Back Pain, with Particular Reference to the Effect of Manipulation.* M.D. Thesis, University of Edinburgh, 1978.

Glenn, W.V., Brown, B.M., Rhodes, M.L., Lancourt, J.E.: Computerized body tomography and evaluation of lumbosacral spinal disease in Finneson, B.E. (ed.) Low Back Pain, 2nd ed. Philadelphia-Toronto, J.B. Lippincott, 1980, pp.115-178.

Greenman, P.E.: Lift therapy: Use and abuse. *Journal of American Osteopathic Association, 79*:238-250, 1979.

Kirkaldy-Willis, W.H.: Pathogenesis of lumbar spondylosis and stenosis. North American Academy of Manipulative Medicine Annual Meeting, 1982.

Marshall, L.L., Trethewie, E.R., Curtain, C.C.: Chemical radiculitis. *Clinical Orthopedics, 129*:61-67, 1977.

Mennell, J.McM.: *Back Pain*. Boston, Little Brown and Co., 1960, pp.39-46.

Mitchell, F.L., Moran, P.S., Pruzzo, N.T.: *An Evaluation and Treatment Manual of Osteopathic Muscle Energy Procedures*, P.O. Box 371, Valley Park, MO, Mitchell, Moran and Pruzzo Associates, 1979.

Mixter, W.J., Barr, J.S.: Rupture of the intervertebral disc with involvement of the spinal canal. *New England Journal of Medicine, 211*:210-215, 1934.

Moll, J., Wright, V.: Measurement of spinal mobility. In Jayson, M. (ed.) *The Lumbar Spine and Back Pain* (2nd ed.), Tunbridge Wells, Kent, England, Pittman Medical Publishing Co., 1980.

Murphy, R.W.: Nerve roots and spinal nerves in degenerative disc disease. *Clinical Orthopedics and Related Research, 129*:46-60, 1977.

O'Brien, J.P.: The multidisciplinary approach to back pain disorders. *Clinics in Rheumatologic Diseases, 6*:133-142, 1980.

Park, W.M.: Radiographic investigation of the intervertebral disc. In Jayson, M. (ed.) *The Lumbar Spine and Back Pain* (2nd ed.) Tunbridge Wells, Kent, England, Pittman Medical Publishing Co., 1980, pp.185-230.

Riley, J., Yong-Hing, K., MacKay, R.W., Kirkaldy-Willis, W.H.: Pathological anatomy of the lumbar spine. In Helfet and Gruebel Lee, *Disorders of the Lumbar Spine*, Philadelphia-Toronto, J.B. Lippincott, 1978, pp.26-50.

Snook, Stover H.: *Epidemiology*, Low Back Pain Course, Harvard Medical School, November 29, 1982.

Wagner, B.M., Galen, R.S. (eds.): Symposium on the role of the laboratory in orthopedic practice. *Orthopedic Clinics of North America, 10(2)*:1-500, 1979.

Ward, P.C.J.: Chemical profiles of disease, pp.405-436, in Wagner and Galen, 1979, cited immediately above.

Wiltse, L.L., Rocchio, P.D.: Preoperative psychological tests as predictors of success of chemonucleolysis in the treatment of the low-back syndrome. *Journal of Bone and Joint Surgery, 57A*:478-483, 1975.

Wood, P.H.N., Badley, E.M.: Epidemiology of Back Pain. In Jayson, M. (ed.) *The Lumbar Spine and Back Pain* (2nd ed.) Tunbridge Wells, Kent, England, Pittman Medical Publishing Co., 1980, pp.29-55.

Wyke, B.: The neurology of low back pain. In Jayson, M. (ed.). *The Lumbar Spine and Back Pain* (2nd ed.) Tunbridge Wells, Kent, England, Pittman Medical Publishing Co., 1980, pp.265-339.

CHAPTER EIGHT

INTER-RATER RELIABILITY IN THE SELECTION
OF MANIPULABLE PATIENTS

WILLIAM L. JOHNSTON, D.O., F.A.A.O.

IN discussing the selection of manipulable patients, I will address several questions relating to design of clinical investigations that involve manipulation, and especially, the manner in which design may be influenced by inter-rater reliability studies of palpation. The purpose of inter-rater reliability studies is to observe the reliability of subjective judgement in trained examiners (Koran, 1975). Reliability in examiners' use of a clinical test is an essential component for clinical research — as important as standardization of the instruments used for biomechanical measurement. It is understandable that the degree of accuracy may not seem comparable to many bioengineers — still, between our related fields, with a similar goal of knowledge in human biomechanics, some degree of reliability may become a basis for future communication. For a clinical research setting, inter-examiner studies can contribute a confidence not only in the use of diagnostic palpatory tests for somatic system function, but also in the reproducibility of findings of *disturbance* in that system's function. Both of these diagnostic features are essential to a clinical trial of manipulation, and, in principle, they direct the application of appropriate treatment in manipulable patients. My emphasis will be that considerations of diagnosis of musculoskeletal problems have been seriously lacking in studies of patients with back pain.

The title of this conference, "Empirical Approaches to the Validation of Manipulation", suggests a bias that has, until now, been rather widely accepted by us all. That bias is: it is the clinician's role to test the efficacy of manipulative treatment by conducting controlled studies of manipulation for back pain. I want to challenge that bias, and offer an alternative direction in clinical research, one that involves the use of manipulation, but first tests concepts of somatic system function and of somatic pain. This direction places emphasis on

106

testing *diagnostic* hypotheses rather than alternative forms of treatment. Studies that compare the results of different methods of treatment, however, have already pre-empted the investigation of diagnostic signs. Until criteria for diagnostic findings are clearly established, and patients are selected on the basis of presence or absence of those findings, we have little basis for comparing results of treatment.

Let me use the field of surgery as an example. The *initial* question is not whether surgery is an effective form of medical treatment. The question is: Is the diagnosis a confined pathology, one that can be removed, repaired, or replaced, and still maintain life? Stated simply, these are the major categories that surgery can address, and the accent is on diagnosis. If the diagnosed pathology is not confined, if essential function cannot be maintained in the face of removal, repair, or replacement, then surgery is not a natural choice. How we perceive the diagnosis is critical to the decision on choice of treatment. A primary stage in medical investigation must involve diagnosis; approaches to treatment are, relatively, a secondary question.

One does not, therefore, test surgery as an appropriate treatment unless one asks the reason for surgery. Likewise, one does not investigate manipulation unless one asks the reason for manipulation. Is the answer to be "idiopathic or non-idiopathic low back pain"? Pain is subjective, a complaint rather than a diagnosis and, in my opinion, to make a diagnosis of chronic pain is, in many instances, to set aside palpatory testing for more objective somatic findings that not only describe the patient's condition, but also establish a diagnostic category. It is only when these somatic findings are established, and not until then, that legitimate questions about approaches to treatment can be tested in a research setting.

The patient complaining of back pain shows physical signs of a problem evident on a somatic system examination (Schwab, 1933; Allen and Stinson, 1941a and b; Denslow, 1964; Dinnar et al., 1980; 1982). One of these signs is palpable muscle tension; a second sign involves structural or positional irregularity, and (almost always) there is altered mobility. Together, these three make up the cardinal signs of musculoskeletal dysfunction sometimes referred to as a biomechanical fault. As a diagnostic category, this triad of signs is termed somatic dysfunction (Siehl, 1970). Palpatory procedures (Johnston, 1982c) initially test for the presence of somatic dysfunction and secondarily for the specific location of the dysfunction; once this location is defined, there is also a third level of tests to detail major characteristics of the disturbed function that may be focused at a particular mobile unit (Figure VIII-1). The term mobile unit, as applied here to the vertebral column, refers to the bony segment and its adnexal tissues. Each vertebra has articular surfaces for movement; its adnexal tissues can move it, can allow it to be moved from one position to another, and can stabilize it in one position. Especially, the elements of local muscular tension and motion limitation characterize the disturbance in segmental function

(Johnston, 1962, 1966, 1972, 1975): there is an asymmetry to the limited response to motion at the segment. Besides tissue tests for local increased tension
in muscle, other tissue tests provide palpable signs of alteration in fluid content
and thermal properties; these can be important qualifiers of the disturbed function in the mobile unit.

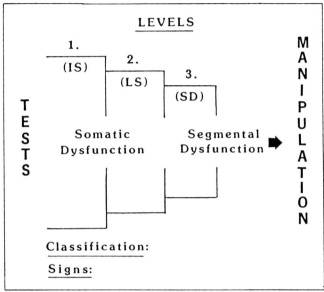

Figure VIII-1: A diagnostic process for dysfunction in the somatic system. IS is the initial
screen; LS is the local scan; and SD is the segmental definition (after Johnston [1982c], reproduced with permission of the author and editors).

Several items emerge from this emphasis on palpatory diagnosis. 1) There
may be a possible relation between the patient's somatic pain and the presence
of diagnosed somatic dysfunction. 2) Major signs of somatic dysfunction do relate to limited mobility, that is, increased tension of muscle and increased resistance to motion at bony segments. 3) Manipulation addresses these biomechanical faults that serve as impediments to motion function. 4) Manipulation
may then be a medium for testing a hypothesis; that is, we might use manipulation as one experimental variable to test the hypothesis that the presence of
somatic pain bears a relation to the presence of the limited mobility of somatic
dysfunction.

Selecting manipulable patients requires first of all ruling out other pathological causes of pain, but equally important, carefully establishing diagnosis of
the presence of somatic dysfunction. We have recently completed several case
studies (Kelso, 1982; Johnston, 1983) using manipulative treatment as an experimental variable. Let me use one of these studies (Johnston, 1983) as an example to explain the role that inter-examiner reliability studies have played,
not only in selecting a manipulable patient, but also in developing instrumental

measures of the palpable signs of somatic dysfunction present on physical examination.

Acute pain was not a *current* complaint of the patient to be described. A 27-year-old male medical student volunteered to participate in a clinical study of somatic dysfunction involving manipulative treatment. His health history was relatively negative for major illness and major surgery. A sports injury 12 years previously had resulted in acute neck sprain, involving a 3-month recovery period; he had four or five subsequent attacks of acute neck pain and limited mobility, each lasting one to two weeks. There had also been a moderate degree of chronic intermittent discomfort in the neck region, but he was relatively pain-free at the time of the study.

He was selected for study because a finding of asymmetry in response to a passive gross motion test of the cervical region of the spine was reproducible by independent examiners during repeated examinations. Examiners used a single motion test for response to passive gross cervical sidebending as the basis for his selection. We were able to use this test with some confidence because in previous inter-rater reliability studies with passive gross motion tests (Johnston, 1982b) we had achieved a significant level of agreement on findings from tests for both cervical rotation and cervical sidebending. In our case study we based the tentative diagnosis of somatic dysfunction on this level 1 test for cervical asymmetry, eliciting greater palpable resistance in response to sidebending to the right than left. The diagnosis was supported by other palpable findings of muscular and structural asymmetries in the region.

For this case study, we also had available to us two instrumental measurements that could provide additional descriptors of the disturbance present in this patient's cervical region, measurements of head-and-neck motion range and of myoelectric activity in cervical muscle. These measures had become appropriate for investigating group differences once we had a reliable test to separate prospective subjects into symmetric and asymmetric groups. Let me outline briefly this preliminary study of instrumental measurement of symmetric and asymmetric groups, involving a total of 16 subjects. A kinematic measure of motion range, recorded during active and passive motion tests, was synchronized with the myoelectric activity recorded from 12 surface electrodes at six selected bilateral muscle sites in the neck region. Groups were made up of male volunteers, matched for age, and relatively asymptomatic. Procedures have been detailed in previous reports (Vorro et al., 1982; Becthold et al., 1983). Kinematic differences between groups were significant; Figure VIII-2 indicates the grand mean total ranges of motion for all members of respective groups for all directions of motion tested, that is, head-and-neck sidebending, axial rotation, and flexions in the sagittal plane; all ranges were introduced both actively by the subject and passively by the examiner. The symmetric group, as indicated in the center, shows a mean total range of motion significantly greater than either the right or left asymmetric groups. Mean ranges for individual motions, in each of the three planes, were also significantly greater in the symmetric group. Detailed analysis of the EMG data from the six muscle sites, during these movements, provided the following information. In the symmetric group, muscles began their activity sooner, they reached peak electrical output sooner, and their strength of contraction was greater than the asymmetric group. These data provide models of performance in response to regional motion tests; they further describe characteristics related to a diagnosis of somatic dysfunction in the cervical spine.

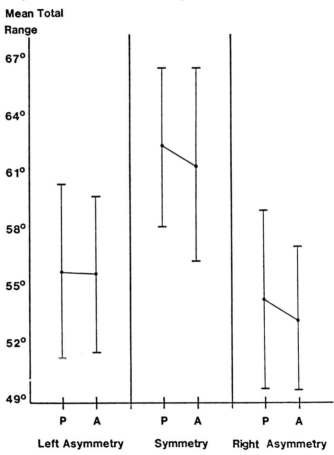

Figure VIII-2: The passive (P) and active (A) grand mean total range of motion for symmetric and asymmetric groups of asymptomatic individuals. Note that the range of motion is greater in symmetric individuals.

In this essential area of diagnostic signs, the inter-examiner reliability studies of passive gross motion tests (Johnston, 1982b) had already played a very significant role in making our case study feasible. By establishing greater confidence in subjective decisions by trained examiners on palpable signs of somatic dysfunction, these studies had led to instrumental measurements for evaluating

the patient's condition, measures that were more objective than the patient's report of pain or lack of pain.

At this point, our case-study patient is confirmed to have a positive finding
on a single palpatory test for asymmetry in response to passive gross sidebending in the cervical region, a decreased total range of motion in the cervical
region, and myoelectric indication of disturbed regional muscular activity.
I am very purposefully repeating the term "region" here in each of these findings to emphasize the initial diagnostic level of these tests, and the relation of
this level of definition to the term "somatic dysfunction." These are level 1 tests,
significant in defining tentative signs of the *presence* of a problem in the somatic
structure, but not yet defining the problem. Palpable findings from a number
of level 1 tests performed on this patient are detailed in Figures VIII-3 and
VIII-4.

We still do not have diagnostic findings sufficient to establish our patient
specifically as a manipulable patient for study. Once ruling out the presence of
other relevant pathology, there is still a need to localize the *site* and the *characteristics* of the musculoskeletal problem. These features are addressed with the following questions. How carefully can findings of increased muscular tension be
localized within the region indicated? What *tissue* tests elicit information about
the intensity of the tissue reaction? What *motion* tests elicit motion characteristics that are manipulable — or — what motion characteristics provide a diagnostic basis supporting the use of manipulation? The next level of testing in the
diagnostic sequence is level 2, defining the location of the problem within the
region.

In order to utilize this second level of palpatory diagnostic tests with confidence, we had investigated the reliability of a number of level 2 test procedures
before finally reaching significant agreement in a study of a percussion type of
palpatory test in the thoracic spinal region (Johnston, 1983). Using this test,
multiple examiners had identified the location of bony segments with palpable
signs of increased resistance/decreased rebound and then had used response to
a shearing type of deep pressure to rate intensity of the deep muscular tension
present at the segment identified. Results of the study of 30 subjects indicated
80% to 86% agreement among independent examiners in distinguishing between a significantly lesioned thoracic spinal segment and an unlesioned segment, as shown in Table VIII-1. And with 4 examiners and 15 subjects, on the
basis of Chi square, calculated 91.2 vs. 3.54, we could totally reject the hypothesis that the distribution of agreements on location of even moderately lesioned segments could be reached by chance (see Table VIII-2).

In our case study, we used this same test sequence of palpatory tests (percussion and deep pressure shearing) to define the segmental location of a major
area of deep muscular tension and limited mobility at T1, and modified the
procedures for application in the cervical region to localize upper cervical dysfunctions at C2 and occiput; segmental findings are illustrated in Figure VIII-5

Somatic Findings **Level I : Initial Screen**

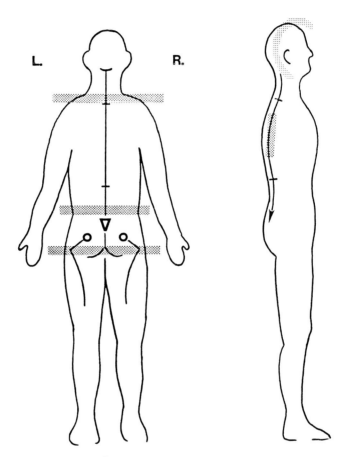

Gross Visual Symmetry

Figure VIII-3: Gross Visual
— symmetry of levels at shoulders, trochanters and crests
— anterior carriage of head
— reduction in normal mid-thoracic kyphosis

(to include costal dysfunctions, 2 and 7 left, and 6 right).

During osteopathic management in patient care, when manipulation is selected as a specific part of the treatment regimen for an identified problem, the physician localizes manual forces at major areas of diagnosed segmental dysfunction. In consideration now of the segmental dysfunctions diagnosed at T1, C2 and occiput, we can qualify our case study patient as a potentially manipulable patient.

At the point when specific manipulation becomes a consideration in osteopathic care, the critical question is not with regard to what manipulative

Somatic Findings   Level I : Initial Screen

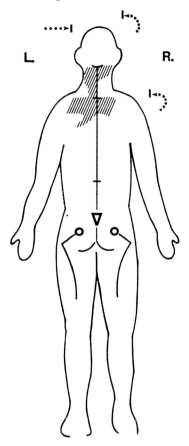

Gross Palpatory

Figure VIII-4: Gross Palpatory
- paravertebral muscle tension, superficial and deep in upper thoracic and upper cervical regions bilaterally, especially left.
- passive gross motion asymmetries at shoulders, limited in rotation left, and at head and neck, limited in sidebending right and rotation left.

procedure is to be applied. Instead, the major issue is still one of diagnosis, because the tissue and motion characteristics at the lesioned/dysfunctional segment form the basis of information on which principles of a manipulative approach are applied. The manipulative procedure itself is then designed to effectively address the particular pattern of segmental motion asymmetry presented, and adapted according to body region and other clinical concerns. Obviously, this is not the routine application of a procedure, like massage, or a poultice for example, nor is manipulation a procedure that one applies to pain

TABLE VIII-1

EXAMINER AGREEMENT ON AREAS MARKED
(LESIONED VS UNLESIONED)

Student examiners	Number of examinations	Agreements	Percentage agreement
1	7	6	86
2	29	23	79
3	28	23	82
4	16	13	81
5	7	6	86

(after Johnston et al. [1983], reproduced with permission of the authors and editors)

TABLE VIII-2

DISTRIBUTION OF AGREEMENTS BY 4 EXAMINERS,
ON 15 SUBJECTS, IN 10 AREAS

	Observed	Expected
Total agree (4-0, 0-4)	61	20.75
Slight agree/disagree (3-1, 1-3)	56	75
Total disagree (2-2)	33	54.25

(after Johnston et al. [1983], reproduced with permission of the authors and editors)

as one applies aspirin—for relief of pain. The technique of manipulation, in a given instance, emerges in direct relation to the diagnosed asymmetry at the lesioned segment.

Previously, in our professional history, palpable findings on many tests for vertebral bony position have been interpreted as reflecting a diagnosis of asymmetry of the mobile unit; even when segmental motion was tested, findings were often interpreted in relation to a basic concept of asymmetry in bony position. Within these positional concepts, manipulative forces were then used to

Segmental Findings   Level 2 : Regional Scan

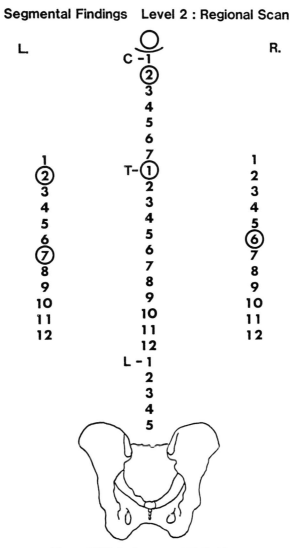

Figure VIII-5. Segmental Definition
- cervical dysfunctions at C_2 and occiput
- thoracic dysfunction at T_1
- costal dysfunctions at ribs 2 and 7 left, and 6 right

encourage a realignment of bony positional relations. In recent years additional emphasis has been placed on segmental motion tests as a reliable means of providing specific information about the dysfunction occurring at a vertebral segment. Results of several initial studies (Johnston, 1980; 1982a) have shown significant agreement among examiners when responses to opposing directions of selected passive movements were monitored by palpation for symmetry at specific thoracic spinal segments. Palpatory cues about motion asymmetries form the basis on which direct and indirect principles of specific manipulation are applied. Research involving manipulation requires a design that will make use of diagnostic palpatory cues to direct the specifics of the procedure, monitor response to the procedure, and assess therapeutic change following the procedure.

Our case-study protocol required examination of our subject at 3-week intervals for 6 weeks in order to establish reliable palpatory, kinematic, and myoelectric findings. Each examination procedure was repeated again following a 3-month interval of 10 manipulative treatments addressing the dysfunctions identified in the cervical and thoracic spinal regions and thoracic cage. The strategy of manipulative approach to treatment utilized functional techniques that apply an indirect principle in manipulation (Bowles, 1955; 1956; 1957; Johnston, 1966; Bowles, 1981). Frequency of treatment visits, choice of treatment procedures, and selection of areas to be treated were all clinical decisions based on assessment of the patient's condition at each visit. On completion of the 3-month treatment period, symmetry in response to the test for gross cervical sidebending had been stable for one month; areas of segmental dysfunction were reduced to the point where no further treatment was indicated.

The initial pre-treatment mean total motion range showed active motions $55.2°$ and passive $55.2°$, within the ranges of the model for right asymmetrics in Figure VIII-2. Post-treatment motion ranges were active $66.9°$, passive $66.3°$, reflecting a significant increase in regional mobility. Vorro used Fourier analysis to determine the power density spectrum of each myoelectric signal in order to examine the median frequency of discharge of motor units during active and passive movements. An asymmetry, reliably present in active sidebending during pre-treatment EMG examinations, showed a significant trend away from distortion and toward greater uniformity when reexamined following the treatment interval. Table VIII-3 illustrates this trend in one aspect of the median frequency data, recorded at the C3 paravertebral muscle site during active sidebending left.

This example of a case study has been used to discuss the relevance of interrater reliability studies to research investigations of manipulation. We don't predict that the findings of this case study are necessarily reproducible in every case of spinal asymmetry or following all instances of manipulation. In order to achieve the instrumental measurements, however, it has been essential to establish confidence in palpatory procedures, palpable findings, and the presence of somatic dysfunction. The emphasis has been shifted from the question of whether manipulation is an effective approach to treatment of pain; instead, the study has looked at reliable findings of somatic and segmental dysfunction, reliable measures of muscular and motion properties, using manipulation as the experimental variable. The interaction of these signs offers more objective criteria for clinical research than the patient's complaint of pain, especially when

Table VIII-3

Case Study

During Active Side Bending		Frequencies Recorded At C3	
		On Right	On Left
I.	To Right	70.3 Hz	101.6 Hz
	To Left	**64.5**	**107.5**
II.	To Right	98.7	80.1
	To Left	**54.7**	**109.4**
III.	To Right	76.2	85.9
	To Left	**68.4**	**95.7**
Pretreatment Means (I, II, III)			
	To Right	81.7	89.2
	To Left	**62.5**	**104.2**
Post Treatment			
IV.	To Right	82.0	87.9
	To Left	**72.3** ↑	**91.8** ↓

the cause of pain is without diagnostic confirmation. Diagnostic signs of the presence of somatic and segmental dysfunction are absolutely essential if research of any value is to be carried out with regard to the use of manipulation.

REFERENCES

Allen, P.V.B. and Stinson, J.A.: The development of palpation: Part I; *Journal of the American Osteopathic Association, 40*:207-10, 1941a; Part II: *Journal of the American Osteopathic Association, 40*:276-8, 1941b.

Becthold, J.E., Ridl, P., Hubbard, R.P., and Vorro, J.: Head orientation measured with a video system. *Journal of Biomechanical Engineering, 105*:404-6, 1983.

Bowles, C.H.: A functional orientation for technique. *Academy of Applied Osteopathy Year Book*, Part I: 177-191, 1955; Part II: 107-114, 1956; Part III: 53-58, 1957.

Denslow, J.S.: Palpation of the musculoskeletal system. *Journal of the American Osteopathic Association, 63*:1107-15, 1964.

Dinnar, U.; Beal, M.C.; Goodridge, J.P.; Johnston, W.L.; Mitchell, Jr., F.L.; Upledger, J.E. and McConnell, D.G.: Classification of diagnostic tests used with osteopathic manipulation. *Journal of the American Osteopathic Association, 79*:451-5, 1980.

Dinnar, U.; Beal, M.C.; Goodridge, J.P.; Johnston, W.L.; Karni, Z.; Mitchell, Jr., F.L.; Upledger, J.E. and McConnell, D.G.: Description of fifty diagnostic tests used with osteopathic manipulation. *Journal of the American Osteopathic Association, 81*:314-21, 1982.

Johnston, W.L.: Manipulative specifics. *Journal of the American Osteopathic Association, 61*:535-9, 1962.

Johnston, W.L.: Manipulative skills. *Journal of the American Osteopathic Association, 66*:389-407, 1966.

Johnston, W.L.: Segmental behavior during motion. I. A palpatory study of somatic relations. *Journal of the American Osteopathic Association, 72*:352-61, 1972.

Johnston, W.L.: The role of static and motion palpation in structural diagnosis, in NINCDS Monograph #15, *The Research Status of Spinal Manipulative Therapy*, DHEW Publication No. (NIH), 76-998, 1975, pp. 249-53.

Johnston, W.L.; Hill, J.L.; Sealey, J.W.; and Sucher, B.M.: Palpatory findings in the cervicothoracic region: variations in normotensive and hypertensive subjects. A preliminary report. *Journal of the American Osteopathic Association, 79*:300-308, 1980.

Johnston, W.L.; Hill, J.L.; Elkiss, M.L.; and Marino, R.V.: Identification of stable somatic findings in hypertensive subjects by trained examiners using palpatory examination. *Journal of the American Osteopathic Association, 81*:830-836, 1982a.

Johnston, W.L.; Elkiss, M.L.; Marino, R.V.; and Blum, G.A.: Passive gross motion testing: Part II. A study of inter-examiner agreement. *Journal of the American Osteopathic Association, 81*:304-308, 1982b.

Johnston, W.L.: Inter-examiner reliability studies. Spanning a gap in medical research. *Journal of the American Osteopathic Association, 81*:819-29, 1982c.

Johnston, W.L.; Allan, B.R.; Hendra, J.L.; Neff, D.R.; Rosen, M.E.; Sills, L.D.; and Thomas, S.C.: Inter-examiner study of palpation in detecting location of spinal segmental dysfunction. *Journal of the American Osteopathic Association, 82*:839-845, 1983.

Johnston, W.L. and Vorro, J.: Biomechanical measurements of changes in cervical muscle function following manipulation. Presented at the 27th Annual Research Conference, American Osteopathic Association/National Osteopathic Foundation, Chicago, IL, 1983.

Kelso, A.F.; Grant, R.G.; and Johnston, W.L.: Use of thermograms to support assessment of somatic dysfunction or effects of osteopathic manipulative treatment. *Journal of the American Osteopathic Association, 82*:182-188, 1982.

Koran, L.M.: The reliability of clinical methods, data and judgments. (First of two parts.) *New England Journal of Medicine, 293*:642-6, 1975.

Schwab, W.A.: Principles of manipulative treatment. The low back problem. *Journal of the American Osteopathic Association, 32*:436-40, 1933.

Siehl, D.: Chairman, Hospital Assistance Committee of the Academy of Applied Osteopathy Recording of osteopathic diagnostic and therapeutic terms for office and hospital. *The DO, 11*:209-10, 1970.

Vorro, J.; Johnston, W.L.; and Hubbard, R.P.: Biomechanical analysis of symmetric and asymmetric cervical function. Presented at the 26th Annual Research Conference, American Osteopathic Association/National Osteopathic Foundation, Chicago, IL, 1982.

CHAPTER NINE

SPINAL MANIPULATION FOR THE TREATMENT OF CHRONIC LOW-BACK AND LEG PAIN: AN OBSERVATIONAL STUDY

J.D. CASSIDY, D.C., B.Sc., F.C.C.S.(C), W.H. KIRKALDY-WILLIS, M.A., M.D., F.R.C.S. (E and C), AND M. McGREGOR, B.Sc., D.C.

INTRODUCTION

THERE is little doubt that low-back pain affects the quality of life for just about everyone in contemporary Western society (Kelsey and White, 1980). Despite the resultant medical, economic, and social burden created by this disorder, only recently has there been an escalation of scientific effort to study the problem. At present, there are two equally important and related issues. The first, and most obvious, concerns the cause or causes of low-back pain, and the second concerns its treatment.

With the exception of some cases of nerve root entrapment from herniation of the nucleus pulposus and degenerative lateral and central spinal stenosis, the exact cause of low-back pain remains a mystery in a large number of cases. It has been estimated that between 20 and 90 percent of low-back pain is idiopathic (Kelsey, 1982). Since the cause is often unknown, there are enormous difficulties encountered in the assessment of various forms of treatment for the low back. This is particularly true for therapies such as spinal manipulation where the treatment is directed towards specific structures such as the lumbar posterior joints and the sacroiliac joints.

Practitioners of manipulation, along with most other clinicians, have developed various diagnostic categories based mostly on subjective criteria. The objections raised to this approach include the lack of objective distinguishing tests and the implication of an unproven pathogenesis. The posterior facet and sacroiliac syndromes are two good examples of controversial diagnoses. In neither case are there truly objective tests to demonstrate these syndromes, nor is the pathogenesis scientifically proven. Yet many clinicians accept the existence of these syndromes and direct their treatment towards these structures. In fact, most practitioners of manipulation direct their treatment to specific levels of the spine contingent on palpatory findings and other highly subjective criteria (Gitelman, 1980; Maigne, 1972; Maitland, 1973; Mennel, 1960; Stoddard, 1959). As a result, the scientific community has had difficulty in assessing the efficacy of this form of therapy.

Many of the past studies of spinal manipulation have avoided the diagnosis controversy by studying undiagnosed low-back pain (Coxhead et al., 1981; Doran and Newell, 1975; Evans et al., 1978; Glover et al., 1974; Hoehler et al., 1981; Jayson et al., 1981). The treatment is applied to the symptom of back pain with little or no mention made of the criteria used to select the level and direction of the manipulative treatments. In some cases, there is no attempt to identify a manipulable lesion, and the maneuvers are applied nonspecifically throughout the painful region of the spine. In such cases, it is possible that the direction and level of the manipulation is wrong. Furthermore, this general approach ignores the large empirical data base which forms the foundation of the various schools of manipulative therapy. Future studies should include parallel investigations into the criteria used to direct the manipulative treatments.

Finally, there appears to be considerable disagreement on what actually constitutes a manipulation. In fact, many of the past clinical trials on manipulation fail to define exactly what sort of manipulations were studied. In some instances, the term mobilization is used interchangeably with manipulation—even though the two terms describe different maneuvers. Other studies include both manipulation and mobilization, but do not differentiate between their frequency of use (Jayson et al., 1981; Sims-Williams et al., 1978, 1979) Most of the clinical trials of manipulation don't even define the treatment studied. Even the best designed study becomes clinically insignificant without a clear definition of the type of treatment tested.

METHODS

A. Definition of Joint Manipulation

Early research into the phenomenon of joint manipulation was done in 1947 by two British anatomists, Roston and Haines (1947). They utilized x-rays to study the behavior of the metacarpophalangeal joint under traction. Their results are shown in Figure IX-1 as modified by Sandoz (1981). On the abscissa is the applied tension in kilograms, and on the ordinate is joint separation in millimeters. The initial separation of 1.8 mm represents the thickness of the two radiolucent articular cartilages. Under preliminary tension, the joint behaves in an elastic manner, until at 8.3 kg the joint surfaces suddenly jump apart from 2 to 4.7 mm with a cracking noise. Further separation, up to the tolerance of the subject, results in an additional separation to 5.6 mm. This additional separation can only be achieved after cracking the joint, and has been labeled the paraphysiological zone.

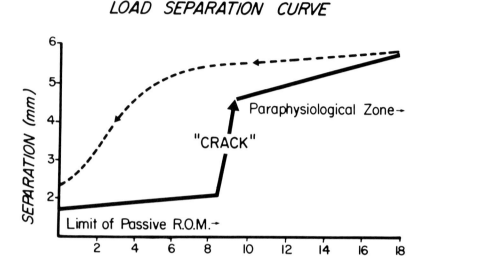

Figure IX-1.

When the tension is reduced, the joint separation is still 5 mm at 5 kg of tension. After the tension is entirely released, the joint remains slightly more separated than its original position. This added separation slowly decreases over 15 to 30 minutes. A mobilization involves taking the joint to its limit of the passive range of motion, while a manipulation involves movement into the paraphysiological zone with an associated cracking noise. At the end of the paraphysiological zone, the limit of anatomical integrity is encountered, beyond which there is damage to the articular ligaments.

Normally, at rest, there exists a slight negative or subatmospheric pressure in a joint space which is a factor in coaptation of the joint surfaces (Sandoz, 1976; See Figure IX-2). Under axial traction, the soft tissues tend to become invaginated or aspirated centripetally because the joint cavity is airtight. When the limit of possible invagination is reached, at the limit of the passive range of motion, an elastic barrier of resistance is encountered. If the separation is forced beyond this barrier of resistance, gases are suddenly liberated from the synovial fluid, and form a radiolucent cavity visible on the radiograph. This extraction of gases from the synovial fluid is a complex phenomenon known to physicists as cavitation. The energy released by this phenomenon is thought to be responsible for the cracking noise. After manipulation, the gas bubble breaks up and slowly redissolves into the synovial fluid, and the joint space returns to its original position. Therefore, a joint manipulation involves a sudden separation of articular surfaces with an associated cracking noise, and the appearance of a radiolucent cavity within the joint space.

Joint Manipulation

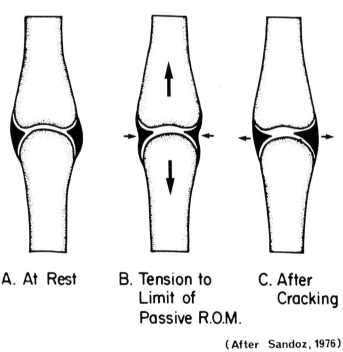

A. At Rest   B. Tension to   C. After
                       Limit of   Cracking
                    Passive R.O.M.

(After Sandoz, 1976)

Figure IX-2.

B. Spinal Mobilization and Manipulation

During spinal mobilization and manipulation, a combination of rotation, lateral flexion and traction is utilized to move the posterior facet joints. The two maneuvers are contrasted in Figure IX-3 (Sandoz, 1976). The lightly-colored central arc on the diagram represents the active range of motion of a joint in one plane. When the joint is passively mobilized, the range of motion is slightly increased. At the end of this passive range of motion, a resistance is encountered due to tensing of the joint capsule. During *mobilization*, the joint is passively moved, back and forth in both directions, up to this barrier of resistance. If the movement is forced beyond this initial barrier, a sudden give is felt, a crack is heard, and the range of motion is increased beyond the usual physiological limit into the paraphysiological space. At the end of this space is the limit of anatomical integrity for the joint. A spinal *manipulation* involves a carefully graded and directed thrust applied at the end of the passive range of motion. The force must be great enough to overcome coaptation of the joint surfaces and separate them into the paraphysiological space without taking them beyond their limit of anatomical integrity. At present there is no clear evidence that "cracking" or "popping" a joint is essential to a clinically effective manipulation.

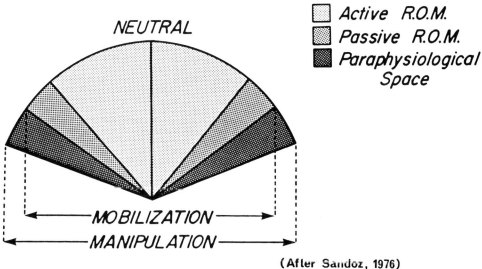

Figure IX-3.

C. Technique of Manipulation

Lumbar spine manipulation can be performed with the patient sitting, lying prone or supine, but is most often done with the patient in the side posture (Figure IX-4). In this position, the upper knee and hip are flexed on the lower leg, so that the upper thigh can be used as a lever. At this point, the spine is relatively straight.

To begin the process of manipulation, the patient's upper body is twisted which introduces an element of rotation and lateral flexion into the lumbar spine (Figure IX-5). At this point, there is a counter-rotation of the upper torso on the pelvis, and the patient's spine is at, or near, its limit of the active range of

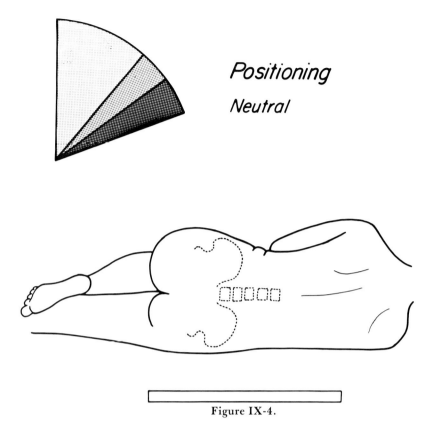

Positioning

Neutral

Figure IX-4.

motion (R.O.M.). During the next step, the manipulator must localize the point of counter-rotation to the desired spinal motion segment (Figure IX-6). This is achieved by varying the amount of flexion in the upper knee and hip. This, in turn, varies the degree of tension placed on the posterior elements of the lumbar spine and the point of counter-rotation of the levers. By increasing this tension, the force of the manipulation can be localized to higher levels of the lumbar spine. With experience, the manipulator can be very specific in selection of the spinal level to be manipulated.

Once the level to be manipulated has been selected, the process of manipulation can begin. The patient has already been positioned to the limit of the active range of motion in the lumbar spine. The next step is to increase slowly the counter-rotation in the spine up to the capsular barrier of resistance at the limit of the passive range of motion (Figure IX-7). At this point, the motion segment at the point of counter-rotation between the two levers has been mobilized in one direction. To manipulate that level, a carefully-applied, high-velocity, short-amplitude thrust is applied with the contact hand and forearm which is hooked over the patient's buttock (Figure IX-8). This thrust must be sufficient to overcome the capsular barrier of resistance, yet not exceed the paraphysio-

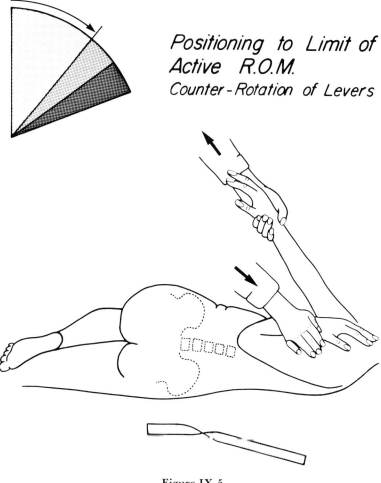

Figure IX-5.

logical space and the limit of anatomical integrity. This requires considerable control and coordination.

D. **The Manipulable Lesion**

Since manipulative therapy introduces motion into the spine, it would seem logical that it should be applied to the spinal levels where motion is restricted or lacking. Painful stiffness or lack of lumbar mobility is a common feature of low-back pain, and has often been described by the terms joint dysfunction and fixation (Gillet, 1960; Liekens, 1960; Mennell, 1960). This condition includes the painful loss of mobility due to muscle spasm, soft tissue contracture, articular adhesion, and degenerative joint disease. In the acute stage, there may be paravertebral muscle spasm. In more chronic cases, there may be early degenerative changes and fibrous adhesion formation in the posterior

Segmental Localization of Force

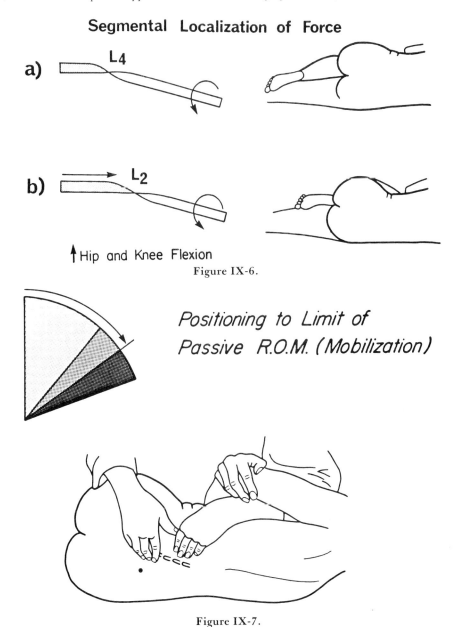

a) L4

b) L2

↑Hip and Knee Flexion

Figure IX-6.

Positioning to Limit of Passive R.O.M. (Mobilization)

Figure IX-7.

facet joints (Cassidy, 1979). A similar process can occur in the sacroiliac joints, where degenerative changes and fibrous adhesions can be seen as early as the third decade of life (Bowen and Cassidy, 1981).

The diagnosis of joint dysfunction or fixation relies heavily on subjective palpatory findings, but can be confirmed by a dynamic radiographic examination. Each motion segment of the spine is examined to determine the level and direction of reduced mobility. This is accomplished by manually stressing each

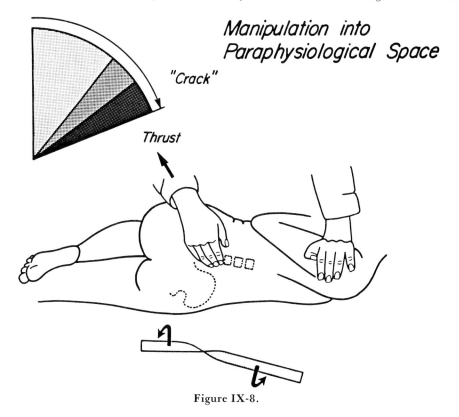

Figure IX-8.

spinal level in extension, rotation and lateral bending while the patient is seated, or if necessary, lying down. In extension, the examiner uses the back of his hand or fist to force the spine into and out of more lordosis (Figure IX-9). With this test, the examiner gains a general impression of muscle tone and anteroposterior mobility in the lumbar spine. A more detailed segmental examination is then performed at each spinal level, utilizing the spinous process as a lever. Each level is stressed in rotation and lateral bending, taking great care to compare the degree of mobility and tenderness on each side of the spine (Figures IX-10 and IX-11).

The radiographic examination includes anteroposterior views in lateral bending and lateral views in flexion and extension. The anteroposterior views in lateral bending are more useful in determining areas of reduced mobility of dysfunction (Cassidy, 1976; Sandoz, 1965). Lateral bending is a composite of rotation and lateral tilt in the lumbar spine, and one or both motions may be blocked or fixed. Figure IX-12 shows a rotational fixation which is reduced on bending to the left and aggravated on bending to the right. Figure IX-13 shows a lateral tilt fixation at L4-5 on right lateral bending with hypermobility at the same level on left lateral bending. In both cases, the manipulation must be directed into the fixation at the proper level while avoiding the hypermobile

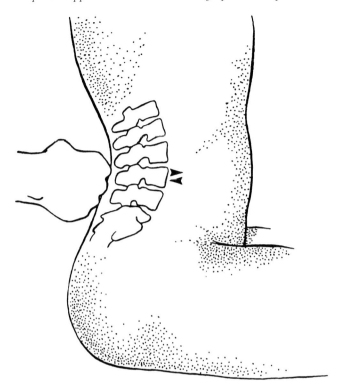

Motion Palpation
Extension

Figure IX-9.

side. The lateral x-ray views in flexion and extension are most useful in diagnosing gross segmental instability which constitutes a contraindication for manipulation at that particular level (Cassidy et al., 1983; Kirkaldy-Willis and Farfan, 1982; see Figure IX-14). However, the radiographic picture must be viewed as supplemental and confirmatory information to the clinical examination findings.

Once the level of joint dysfunction and the direction of fixation has been determined, the involved segments should be manipulated in a manner which will increase their mobility. The manipulation should be as specific as possible in order to avoid areas of normal mobility and instability. The motion examination should be performed prior to and after each treatment, in order to assess any changes in mobility. Since the level and direction of each manipulation is decided by this examination, it is a very important factor in the study of spinal manipulation.

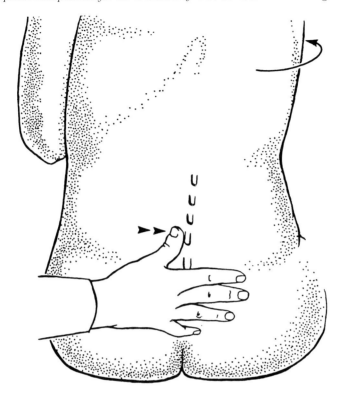

Motion Palpation
Rotation

Figure IX-10.

E. Patient Population

Over a five-year period, 463 patients from the Low-Back Clinic at the University of Saskatchewan were considered eligible for this study. Patients were not eligible if they presented with severe or progressive neurological deficit requiring surgical intervention, bone and joint pathologies including cancer, infection, inflammatory arthritis, demyelinating disease, etc., or if they, or the referring doctor, were unwilling to agree to their inclusion in this study. All eligible patients had to have a minimum of six months of pain and fit into one of the four main diagnostic categories (posterior joint syndrome, sacroiliac syndrome, lateral nerve root entrapment syndrome, and central spinal stenosis syndrome). Patients with herniation of the nucleus pulposus were not included.

Of the 463 eligible patients, this study reports on the results of treatment in 285. The remaining 178 patients were excluded because of:

(1) poor psychological profile—based on a pain drawing, an M.M.P.I.

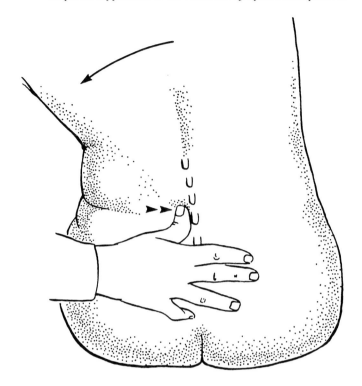

Motion Palpation
Lateral Bending
Figure IX-11.

and an interview with a clinical psychologist — 65 patients.

    (2) less than a grade IV low-back disability on our rating scale at the onset of therapy — 75 patients.

    (3) too obese to manipulate — 8 patients.

    (4) undiagnosed bone and joint pathologies which became evident during or immediately after treatment — 10 patients.

Twenty patients did not return for the initial follow-up after completing their course of treatment.

    Of our sample of 285 patients, 154 were males and 131 were females. The mean age was 42 with a wide range from 16 to 79 years. The duration of symptoms varied from 6 months to 40 years with an average of 8.2 years. Twenty-four percent had undergone previous lumbar surgery and all had undergone previous conservative treatment. This treatment included:

    (1) non-manipulative physiotherapy — 86 percent

    (2) two weeks of bed rest — 72 percent

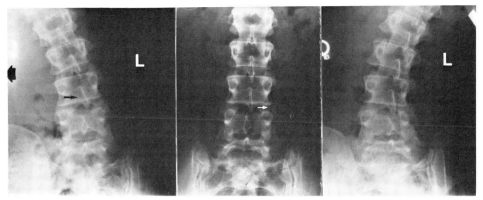

Figure IX-12. Anteroposterior lateral bending series of the lumbar spine. The small white arrow shows a rotation malalignment of L3 on L4 on the straight anteroposterior view in the center. On left lateral flexion, the spinous processes are aligned with good rotation and lateral tilt coupling. On right lateral flexion, there is a blockage (fixation) of rotation at L3-4 (black arrow).

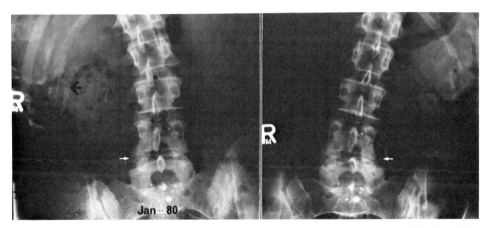

Figure IX-13. Anteroposterior views of the lumbar spine in right and left lateral flexion. The small white arrows point to a lateral tilt blockage (fixation) of L4 on L5 on right lateral flexion, and hypermobility at L4-5 on left lateral flexion.

    (3) various medications—66 percent
    (4) previous manipulative therapy—47 percent
    (5) lumbar support—35 percent
    (6) low-back school—26 percent
    (7) lumbar injections—18 percent
    (8) lumbar traction—5 percent

F. Study Design

    The results of the treatment were graded by the patient during an interview with an orthopaedic surgeon or resident. The emphasis of the grading

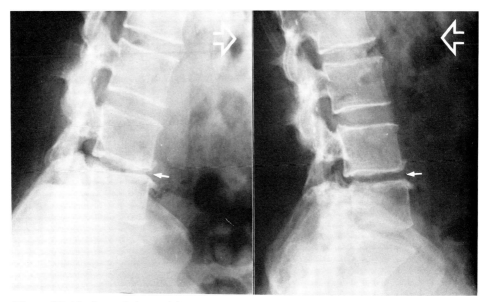

Figure IX-14. Lateral views of the lumbar spine in flexion and extension. These views show evidence of segmental instability at the L4-5 motion segment. There is narrowing of the disc space with anterior osteophyte formation, and retrolisthesis of L4 on L5 on extension.

method was on pain and activity levels. All patients began at the grade IV level. These patients had shown no lasting improvement with any previous treatment. Their pain was described as constant and severe, and they were unable to work or go about their normal daily activities.

In order to be upgraded to grade III, there had to be improvement with treatment. Grade III patients did, however, still have constant pain. They also had some restriction in their work and daily activities, but were not totally disabled. They often required periodic manipulations to maintain this improvement.

Grade II patients were considerably improved following their treatment. They all complained of mild intermittent symptoms, but were able to resume their work and daily activities without restriction. They occasionally required re-manipulation, but responded quickly to this treatment.

Grade I patients were very much improved after manipulative treatment. They were symptom-free and unrestricted in their work and daily activities. Some of them complained of occasional pain, but it always settled quickly without treatment.

Our method of study is diagrammed in Figure IX-15. During the initial assessment, the patient underwent a complete history and physical, psychological and radiographic examinations. Special notice was made of the patient's past history (duration of symptoms, past treatment), neurological status (reflexes, motor power and sensation), extent of sciatic radiation of pain (proximal to the knee or distal to the knee), and degree of spondylosis seen on the lumbar radiographs (1 — none, 2 — mild, 3 — moderate, and 4 — severe). With the aid of this information, the patients were placed within a diagnostic category. Some patients required specialized examination procedures before the diagnosis could be made (myelography, EMG, CT scan, etc.).

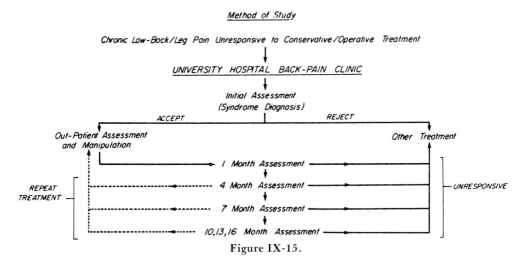

Figure IX-15.

Once the syndrome diagnosis had been established, those patients with sacroiliac, posterior joint, nerve root entrapment and central spinal stenosis syndromes were considered for this study. If the patient satisfied our other inclusion criteria, they were sent to an outpatient clinic for a lumbosacral motion assessment and a two-week course of manipulative treatment. Only fixed or dysfunctional levels of the spine and sacroiliac joints were manipulated.

At one month, the results of treatment were recorded at the Low-Back Pain Clinic, and the patients were followed at three month intervals thereafter. If their condition was unchanged, they were given a grade IV rating and removed from the study. If their condition initially improved and then deteriorated, they were given two choices — either repeat the therapy or be graded at their present level and removed from the study. Those that repeated the therapy were assessed again at one month, and then followed at three month intervals thereafter. With this method of study, grade II and III patients were able to have more treatment if they so please. If, in our opinion, they were overusing this option with little benefit, they were graded and removed from the study.

RESULTS

Table IX-1 shows the distribution by diagnosis of the patients studied. Four basic syndromes were studied, two referred pain syndromes — posterior joint syndrome (P.J.S.), and sacroiliac syndrome (S-I.S.), and two nerve compression syndromes — nerve root entrapment syndrome (N.R.E.S.) and central spinal stenosis syndrome (C.S.S.S). The mobility of the pain-producing lesion is designed as fixed (hypomobile) or unstable (hypermobile) according to the motion assessment made before manipulative treatment. There were no patients with unstable segments in the central spinal stenosis group, and only fixed segments were manipulated in all groups. Therefore, in the case of the unstable posterior joint syndrome and the unstable nerve root entrapment syndrome, manipulations were directed to adjacent dysfunctional levels, and not the primary pain producing lesion. This choice was made on the basis of past clinical experience (Cassidy et al.,1978).

TABLE IX-1

DISTRIBUTION OF PATIENTS BY DIAGNOSIS AND SEX

DIAGNOSIS	M:F	TOTAL
Fixed posterior joint syndrome (F.P.J.S.)	34:21	55
Unstable posterior joint syndrome (U.P.J.S.)	22:9	31
Fixed sacroiliac syndrome (F.S-I.S.)	30:39	69
Fixed posterior joint and sacroiliac syndrome (F.P.J. & S-I.S)	18:30	48
Fixed nerve root entrapment syndrome (F.N.R.E.S.)	36:25	61
Unstable nerve root entrapment syndrome (U.N.R.E.S.)	5:5	10
Central spinal stenosis syndrome (C.S.S.S)	9:2	11
		285

A. The Posterior Joint Syndrome

This syndrome has been well described in the past (Kirkaldy-Willis and Hill, 1979; Mooney and Robertson, 1976). The pain is thought to emanate from mechanical derangement of the posterior facet joints. It begins as a midline low backache which may be referred into the buttock, thigh or leg. The referred pain is non-dermatomal and difficult to localize. Although straight-leg raising may be somewhat restricted, it is on the basis of hamstring spasm, and there are no signs of nerve root tension. There may be altered sensation, reflexes and motor power in the lower extremities, but no major neurological deficit is present. There is increased pain with pressure over the lumbar spine, and often a reduced range of motion with muscle spasm and segmental joint dysfunction. In the majority of cases, there are radiographic signs of reduced lumbar mobility or fixation (Kirkaldy-Willis and Hill, 1979). In some instances, posterior joint syndrome can be caused by lumbar instability.

Sixty-two percent of patients with a fixed posterior joint syndrome achieved a grade I result while only 26 percent achieved the same result in the unstable group (Figures IX-16 and IX-17). If we consider significant clinical improvement to be the attainment of at least a grade II rating, patients with a

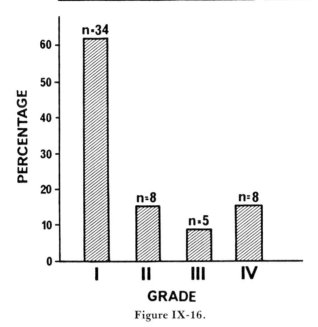

Figure IX-16.

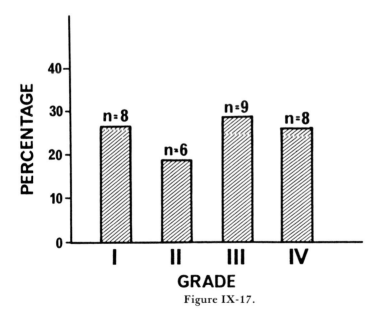

Figure IX-17.

fixed posterior joint syndrome responded to spinal manipulation significantly better than those with an unstable form of this syndrome (Table IX-2). The two groups were similar in age, duration of pain, follow-up and degenerative

TABLE IX-2

IMPROVEMENT IN FIXED AND UNSTABLE POSTERIOR JOINT SYNDROMES

	IMPROVED	NOT IMPROVED
FIXED	42 (76%)	13 (24%)
UNSTABLE	14 (45%)	17 (55%)

Corrected X^2 = 7.83, df = 1, p<0.01

TABLE IX-3

CHARACTERISTICS OF PATIENTS WITH FIXED AND UNSTABLE
POSTERIOR JOINT SYNDROMES

	FIXED		UNSTABLE			
	$\overline{X}$	S.D.	$\overline{X}$	S.D.	t	P
Age (yrs.)	38.6	± 13.9	41.8	± 14.3	1.02	N.S.
Duration of pain (yrs.)	5.9	± 6.0	8.5	± 8.8	1.61	N.S.
Follow-up (mos.)	9.0	± 9.2	8.0	± 7.9	0.51	N.S.
Degenerative score	2.2	± 1.0	2.6	± 0.9	1.90	N.S.
Number of treatments	6.9	± 3.4	8.9	± 4.8	2.27	< 0.05

score. However, the unstable posterior joint syndrome patients received significantly more treatments (Table IX-3). The unstable group also had a greater percentage of previous lumbar operation and neurological deficit (Table IX-4).

B. The Sacroiliac Syndrome

The sacroiliac joint is an atypical synovial joint with a well innervated joint capsule, and a small range of motion (Frigerio et al., 1974; McGregor and Cassidy, 1983). Like the lumbar posterior joints, this joint is susceptible to mechanical derangement which results in painful stiffness in one or both joints (McGregor and Cassidy, 1983). Since the sacroiliac joint lies deep to the body surface, it has been difficult to study in vivo. As such, the exact function of this joint is not presently known.

The sacroiliac syndrome is characterized by lateral sacral and buttock pain which may radiate in a non-dermatomal distribution into the thigh and leg (Cavienzel, 1973). Like the posterior joint syndrome, straight-leg raising may

TABLE IX-4

FIXED VS. UNSTABLE POSTERIOR JOINT SYNDROME

	FIXED % (n)	UNSTABLE % (n)
Previous operation	15 (8)	26 (8)
Proximal sciatica	35 (19)	32 (10)
Distal sciatica	22 (12)	32 (10)
Reflex deficit	9 (5)	19 (6)
Sensory deficit	15 (8)	39 (12)
Motor deficit	9 (5)	10 (3)

be diminished, but there are no signs of nerve root tension or major neurological deficit. There is tenderness over the dorsal aspect of the sacroiliac joint, but no mid-line tenderness over the lumbar spine. Several different methods of diagnosing fixation or dysfunction of the sacroiliac joint have appeared in the literature (Gillet, 1976; Grice and Fligg, 1980; Wiles, 1980).

Seventy-one percent of patients with a fixed sacroiliac syndrome achieved a grade I improvement with manipulation of this joint (Figure IX-18). A further 22 percent achieved a grade II improvement for a total of 93 percent improved overall. Similarly, 88 percent of patients with a combination of fixed posterior joint and sacroiliac syndrome achieved a grade I and II improvement (Figure IX-19). Characteristics of the two patient groups are presented in Tables IX-5 and IX 6. It would seem that when a diagnosis of sacroiliac or posterior joint syndrome is made, the results of manipulative treatment are promising.

C. **The Nerve Root Entrapment Syndrome**

The nerve root entrapment syndrome results from compression of the nerve root in the lateral recess. It is most often due to narrowing of the recess by degenerative enlargement of the superior articular process of the vertebra below and posterior osteophytes from the adjacent vertebral body (Kirkaldy-Willis et al., 1978).

This syndrome produces predominately distal leg pain in a corresponding dermatomal distribution. There may also be some backache, since this syndrome rarely appears without associated neurological deficit, including diminution of sensation, reflex loss and muscle weakness and wasting. The sciatic nerve is usually tender at the sciatic notch and behind the knee at the level of

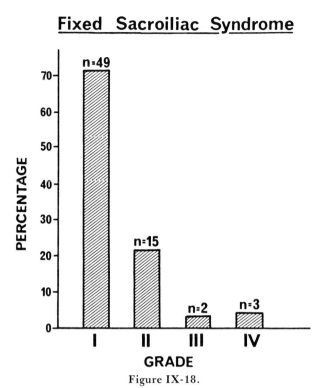

Figure IX-18.

the posterior tibial and lateral popliteal nerves. Diagnostic EMG and high resolution C-T scanning can often help to confirm the level of compression.

Within this category, there were 61 patients with a fixed nerve root entrapment syndrome and only 10 patients with an unstable nerve root entrapment syndrome. In both groups, 50 percent achieved a grade I or II improvement, and there was significant difference in the results of treatment (Figure IX-20 and IX-21 and Table IX-7). The two groups were similar in age, duration of pain, follow-up, degenerative score and number of treatments (Table IX-8). Fifty percent of the unstable group had undergone a previous spinal operation (Table IX-9). Perhaps there were too few patients with the unstable form of this syndrome for any significant differences to become apparent. Considering the chronicity and disability with this group, it is surprising that as many as 50 percent achieved significant clinical improvement with manipulation.

D. Central Spinal Stenosis Syndrome

The central spinal stenosis syndrome results from narrowing of the spinal canal secondary to degenerative enlargement of the posterior part of the vertebral bodies and the posterior facet joints. This results in the impairment of nerve function, either by direct pressure, traction or irritation to the nerves, or as a result of interference with the vascular supply to the nerves (Bowen et al.,

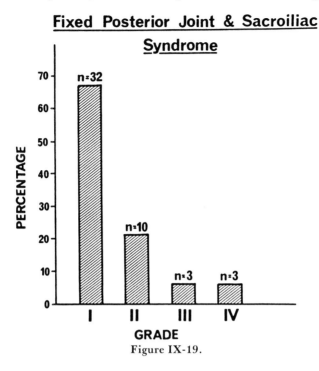

Fixed Posterior Joint & Sacroiliac Syndrome

Figure IX-19.

TABLE IX-5

CHARACTERISTICS OF PATIENTS WITH FIXED SACROILIAC SYNDROME ALONE AND THOSE WITH FIXED POSTERIOR JOINT AND SACROILIAC SYNDROME COMBINED.

| | FIXED S-I.S. | | FIXED P.J. & S-I.S. | |
	$\bar{X}$	S.D.	$\bar{X}$	S.D.
Age (yrs.)	41.1	± 13.9	41.9	± 12.3
Duration of pain (yrs.)	7.9	± 8.4	8.9	± 9.1
Follow-up (mos.)	10.8	± 11.9	13.9	± 15.0
Degenerative score	2.3	± 1.0	2.3	± 0.9
Number of treatments	6.7	± 3.4	7.6	± 3.6

1978).

This syndrome produces predominately multidermatomal and often bilateral leg pain which is made worse by walking. These patients complain of restless legs at night, and may have to get up and walk for relief. However, too much walking can make the leg pain worse. Their neurological deficit may involve several roots, and is often bilateral. In order to detect this deficit, it may

TABLE IX-6

FIXED SACROILIAC SYNDROME ALONE AND
FIXED POSTERIOR JOINT SYNDROME WITH SACROILIAC SYNDROME

	FIXED S-I.S. % (n)	FIXED P.J.S. & S-I.S. % (n)
Previous operation	23 (16)	15 (7)
Proximal sciatica	38 (26)	29 (14)
Distal sciatica	41 (28)	42 (20)
Reflex deficit	17 (12)	10 (5)
Sensory deficit	23 (16)	15 (7)
Motor deficit	20 (14)	2 (1)

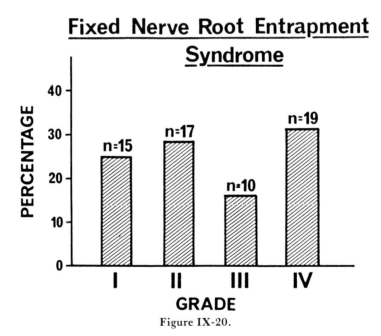

Figure IX-20.

be necessary to have the patient walk in the corridor prior to the examination. Narrowing of the central canal can be confirmed by myelography or by the C-T scan.

The results of manipulative treatment of 11 patients with a central spinal stenosis syndrome are illustrated in Figure IX-22. Only 36 percent of these patients achieved significant clinical improvement after manipulative treatment.

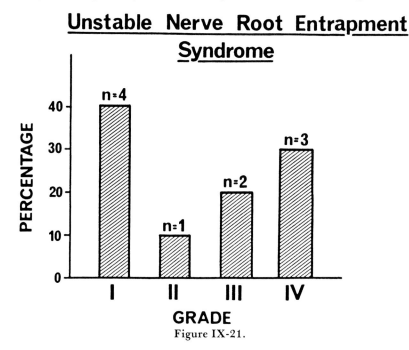

Figure IX-21.

TABLE IX-7

IMPROVEMENT IN FIXED AND UNSTABLE NERVE-ROOT ENTRAPMENT SYNDROMES

	IMPROVED	NOT IMPROVED
FIXED	32 (53%)	29 (48%)
UNSTABLE	5 (50%)	5 (50%)

Corrected X^2 = N.S.

This outcome is not surprising in such a chronic and disabled group of patients (Table IX-10).

The overall results are summarized in Figure IX-23. If significant clinical improvement is considered the attainment of at least a grade II outcome, the patients with the referred pain syndromes (posterior joint and sacroiliac syndromes) responded significantly better to manipulation than those with the nerve compression syndromes (nerve root entrapment and central spinal stenosis syndromes) (Table IX-11). The one exception to this rule was the patients with an unstable posterior joint syndrome.

The extent of sciatic radiation of pain into the lower extremities had a significant effect on the treatment outcome (Table IX-12). Patients with pain radiating past the knee (distal sciatica) didn't respond to manipulation as well as

TABLE IX-8

CHARACTERISTICS OF PATIENTS WITH FIXED AND UNSTABLE
NERVE ROOT ENTRAPMENT SYNDROMES

	FIXED		UNSTABLE			
	$\overline{X}$ ± S.D.		$\overline{X}$ ± S.D.		t	P
Age (yrs.)	43.8	± 12.4	43.6	± 13.9	0.05	N.S.
Duration of pain (yrs.)	7.7	± 8.6	11.1	± 13.9	1.06	N.S.
Follow-up (mos.)	13.9	± 12.8	12.6	± 13.6	0.30	N.S.
Degenerative score	2.8	± 0.9	3.1	± 1.0	0.94	N.S.
Number of treatments	11.2	± 5.5	12.2	± 13.6	1.31	N.S.

TABLE IX-9

FIXED VERSUS UNSTABLE NERVE ROOT ENTRAPMENT SYNDROME

	FIXED % (n)	UNSTABLE % (n)
Previous operation	33 (20)	50 (5)
Proximal sciatica	20 (12)	0
Distal sciatica	72 (44)	90 (9)
Reflex deficit	49 (30)	70 (7)
Sensory deficit	44 (27)	30 (3)
Motor deficit	34 (21)	10 (1)

those with proximal or no sciatica. We also studied the effect of degenerative changes (radiographic), previous lumbar surgery, duration of symptoms and age, and found no significant effect on the treatment outcome. There was, however, a tendency for older patients to do less well than younger patients, and for the results to decrease with increasing duration of pain.

DISCUSSION

This paper raises several issues regarding the assessment of spinal manipu-

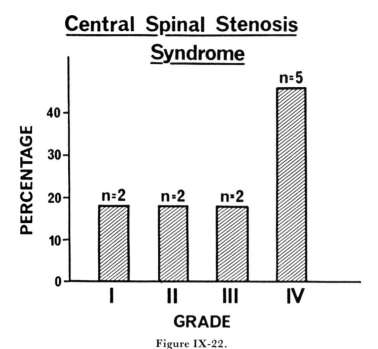

Figure IX-22.

TABLE IX-10

CHARACTERISTICS OF PATIENTS WITH CENTRAL SPINAL STENOSIS SYNDROME

	$\bar{X}$	± S.D.		%	(n)
Age (yrs.)	52.6	± 19.6	Previous operation	46	(5)
Duration of pain (yrs.)	16.9	± 13.4	Proximal sciatica	27	(3)
Follow-up (mos.)	7.0	± 6.6	Distal sciatica	73	(8)
Degenerative score	3.3	± 1.0	Reflex deficit	9	(1)
Number of treatments	9.3	± 4.6	Sensory deficit	55	(6)
			Motor deficit	27	(3)

lation in the treatment of low-back pain. First and foremost, investigators should define more precisely what sort of manipulative techniques they have used in their studies. At present, there are many different techniques of manipulation and mobilization, and it is wrong to assume that they are all equally effective. Moreover, if the technique is not adequately described, it is not possible to draw any meaningful conclusions from that particular study. Sec-

TABLE IX-11

REFERRED PAIN SYNDROMES VS. NERVE COMPRESSION SYNDROMES

	IMPROVED	NOT IMPROVED
REFERRED PAIN SYNDROMES	162 (80%)	41 (20%)
NERVE COMPRESSION SYNDROMES	41 (50%)	41 (50%)

Corrected X^2 = 23.9, df = 1, p<0.005

TABLE IX-12

EFFECT OF SCIATICA

	IMPROVED	NOT IMPROVED
NO LEG PAIN	54 (77%)	16 (23%)
PROXIMAL SCIATICA	70 (82%)	15 (18%)
DISTAL SCIATICA	77 (60%)	51 (40%)

Corrected X^2 = 13.9, df = 2, p<0.001

ondly, the criteria used to direct the level and direction of the manipulation must be clearly stated. Some investigators have applied their manipulations nonspecifically — without regard to level and direction. Others have tried to localize their manipulations to dysfunctional segments only (Cassidy and Potter, 1979). In the former case, it is possible that the manipulations were not directed to the dysfunctional or fixed spinal segments. In the latter case, the diagnosis of spinal joint dysfunction becomes a very important variable in the assessment of spinal manipulative therapy.

Although the exact cause of low-back pain is often not apparent, on the basis of this study, it would seem reasonable to make a syndrome diagnosis prior to manipulative treatment. At the very least, there should be some differentiation between the referred pain and the nerve compression syndromes. Our results indicate that the former group will respond significantly better than the

Percentage of Patients Improved Vs. Syndrome Diagnosis

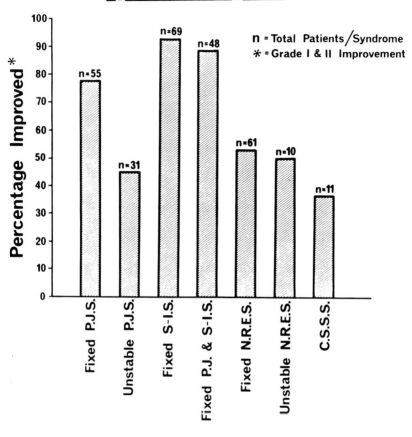

Syndromes

Figure IX-23.

latter group to specific manipulative therapy. Furthermore, we recommend that a motion assessment be completed on each patient prior to manipulative treatment, and that only the dysfunctional or fixed spinal segments be manipulated. In this study, patients with a fixed posterior joint syndrome responded significantly better to spinal manipulation than those with an unstable posterior joint syndrome. Further studies of manipulation should include investigations into the phenomenon of joint dysfunction, as well as the indications for the direction and level of the manipulation. Ultimately, a better understanding of the manipulable lesion will result in more accurate clinical trials.

The treatment of back pain by spinal manipulation is not a simple matter. It is an art that requires considerable experience and dexterity. Like other spinal treatments, it is not a panacea, but when applied skillfully to the appropriate spinal level, the results are often rewarding.

CONCLUSIONS

The conclusions from this observational study are:

1. Referred pain syndromes respond significantly better to specific spinal manipulative therapy than nerve compression syndromes.
2. Patients with no leg pain or proximal leg pain respond significantly better to specific spinal manipulative therapy than those with distal leg pain.
3. Patients with a fixed posterior joint syndrome respond significantly better to specific spinal manipulative therapy than those with an unstable posterior joint syndrome.

ACKNOWLEDGEMENTS

The authors would like to acknowledge the financial assistance of the Canadian Memorial Chiropractic College and the Foundation for Chiropractic Education and Research. We would also like to acknowledge the assistance of Dr. G. E. Potter, Dr. J. H. Wedge, Dr. A. Grice, Dr. R. Gitelman, Mr. D. Manderville, Ms. S. Stacey, and Ms. K. Frydenlund.

Figures 9, 10, 11 and 14 appear by courtesy of the editors of the *Journal of Manipulative and Physiological Therapeutics*, reprinted from Cassidy, J.D and Potter, G.E.: Motion examination of the lumbar spine. 2:151-158, 1979.

REFERENCES

Bowen, V., Shannon, R., Kirkaldy-Willis, W.H.: Lumbar spinal stenosis. *Child's Brain, 4*:257-277, 1978.

Bowen, V., Cassidy, J.D.: Macroscopic and microscopic anatomy of the sacroiliac joint from embryonic life until the eighth decade. *Spine, 6*:620-628, 1981.

Cassidy, J.D.: Roentgenological examination of the functional mechanics of the lumbar spine in lateral flexion. *Journal of the Canadian Chiropractic Association, 10*:13-16, 1976.

Cassidy, J.D., Potter, G.E., Kirkaldy-Willis, W.H.: Manipulative management of low-back pain in patients with spondylolisthesis. *Journal of the Canadian Chiropractic Association, 22*:15-20, 1978.

Cassidy, J.D., Potter, G.E.: Motion examination of the lumbar spine. *Journal of Manipulative and Physiological Therapeutics, 2*:151-158, 1979.

Cassidy, J.D., Dupuis, P., Yong-Hing, K.: Radiological diagnosis of lumbar instability. In Proceedings of the 10th meeting of the International Society for the Study of the Lumbar Spine. Cambridge, England, April 5-9, 1983.

Cavienzel, V.H.: Beitrag zur kenntnis des iliosakralsyndroms. *Manuelle Medizin, 11*:102-108, 1973.

Coxhead, C.E., Inskip, H., Meade, T.W., North, W.R.S., Troup, J.D.G.: A multicentre trial of physiotherapy in the management of sciatic symptoms. *Lancet, 1*:1065-1068, May 16, 1981.

Doran, D.M.L., Newell, D.J.: Manipulation in treatment of low-back pain: a multicentre study. *British Medical Journal,, 2*:161-164, 1975.

Evans, D.P., Burke, M.S., Lloyd, K.N., Roberts, E.E., Roberts, G.M.: Lumbar spinal manipulation on trial: Part 1 — Clinical assessment. *Rheumatology and Rehabilitation, 17*:46-53, 1978.

Frigerio, N.A., Stowe, R.R., Howe, J.W.: Movement of the sacroiliac joint. *Clinical Orthopaedics, 100*:370-377, 1974.

Gillet, H.: Vertebral fixations: An introduction to movement palpation. *Annals of the Swiss Chiropractic Association, 1*:30-33, 1960.

Gillet, H.: Clinical measurements of sacro-iliac mobility. *Annals of the Swiss Chiropractic Association, 6*:59-70, 1976.

Gitelman, R.: A chiropractic approach to biomechanical disorders of the lumbar spine and pelvis. In Haldeman, S. (ed.): *Modern Developments in the Principles and Practice of Chiropractic.* New York, Appleton-Century-Crofts, 1980, pp.297-330.

Glover, J.R., Morris, J.G., Khosla, T.: Back pain: a randomized clinical trial of rotational manipulation of the trunk. *British Journal of Industrial Medicine, 31*:59-64, 1974.

Grice, A., Fligg, D.B.: Biomechanics of the pelvis. *A Collection of Monographs on the Biomechanics of the Pelvis from the Denver Conference of the ACA Council on Technic,* held June 17-20, 1980, pp.96-111.

Hoehler,F.K., Tobis, J.S., Buerger, A.A.: Spinal manipulation for low-back pain. *Journal of the American Medical Association, 245*:1835-1838, 1981.

Jayson, M.I.V., Sims-Williams, H., Young, S., Baddeley, H., Collins, E.: Mobilization and manipulation for low back pain. *Spine, 6*:409-416, 1981.

Kelsey, J.L., White, A.A.: Epidemiology and impact of low-back pain. *Spine, 5*:133-142, 1980.

Kelsey, J.L.: Idiopathic low-back pain: magnitude of the problem. In White, A.A. and Gordon, S.I. (eds.): *Idiopathic Low-Back Pain.* St. Louis and Toronto, C.V. Mosby, 1982, pp. 5-8.

Kirkaldy-Willis, W.H., Wedge, J.H., Yong-Hing, K., Reilly, J.: Pathology and pathogenesis of lumbar spondylosis and stenosis. *Spine, 3*:319-328, 1978.

Kirkaldy-Willis, W.H., Hill, R.J.: A more precise diagnosis for low-back pain. *Spine, 4*:102-109, 1979.

Kirkaldy-Willis, W.H., Farfan, H.F.: Instability of the lumbar spine. *Clinical Orthopaedics and Related Research, 165*:110-123, 1982.

Liekens, M.: Movement palpation. *Annals of the Swiss Chiropractic Association, 1*:34-42, 1960.

Maigne, R.: *Orthopaedic Medicine: A New Approach to Vertebral Manipulations.* Springfield, IL, Charles C Thomas, 1972.

Maitland, G.D.: *Vertebral Manipulation.* London, Butterworths, 1973.

McGregor, M., Cassidy, J.D.: Post-operative sacroiliac syndrome. *Journal of Manipulative Physiological Therapeutics, 6*:1-11, 1983.

Mennell, J. McM.: *Back Pain.* Boston and Toronto, Little, Brown and Co., 1960.

Mooney, V., Robertson, J.: The facet syndrome. *Clinical Orthopaedics, 115*:149-156, 1976.

Roston, J.B., Hains, R.W.: Cracking in the metacarpo-phalangeal joint. *Journal of Anatomy, 81*:165-173, 1947.

Sandoz, R.: Technique and interpretation of functional radiography of the lumbar spine. *Annals of the Swiss Chiropractic Association, 3*:66-106, 1965.

Sandoz, R.: Some physical mechanisms and effects of spinal adjustments. *Annals of the Swiss Chiropractic Association, 6*:91-141, 1976.

Sandoz, R.: Technique and interpretation of functional radiography of the lumbar spine. *Annals of the Swiss Chiropractic Association, 3*:66-106, 1965.

Sandoz, R.: Some physical mechanisms and effects of spinal adjustments. *Annals of the Swiss Chiropractic Association, 6*:91-141, 1976.

Sandoz, R.: Some reflex phenomena associated with spinal derangements and adjustments. *Annals of the Swiss Chiropractic Association, 7*:45-66, 1981.

Sims-Williams, H., Jayson, M.I., Young, S.M., Baddeley, H., Collins, E.: Controlled trial of mobilization and manipulation for patients with low-back pain in general practice. *British Medical Journal, 2*:1338-1340, 1978.

Sims-Williams, H., Jayson, M.I., Young, S.M., Baddeley, H., Collins, E.: Controlled trial of mobilization and manipulation for low-back pain: Hospital patients. *British Medical Journal, 2*:1318-1320, 1979.

Stoddard, A.: *Manual of Osteopathic Technique.* London, Hutchinson, 1959.

Wiles, M.R.: Reproducibility and interexaminer correlation of motion palpation findings of the sacroiliac joints. *Journal of the Canadian Chiropractic Association, 24*:59-69, 1980.

Section 4

RANDOMIZED CLINICAL TRIALS OF MANIPULATION FOR LOW BACK PAIN

As is repeatedly pointed out in this volume, there are few *objective* quantifiable measures describing a manipulable patient and/or describing the effects of manipulation. This is a very important point; however some hope in this regard can be gained from the work of G.G. Rasmussen (1979, and this volume) using a modified *Schober's test* and the work of S.M.S. Young and others (Sims-Williams et al., 1978, 1979; and Young in this volume) using such measures as patients' reports of time elapsed until *return of specific physical abilities* (e.g., Jayson et al., 1981; and Young in this volume). In addition, the reports of J.W. Fisk (1978) and possibly Jayson et al., (1981) and Hoehler and Tobis (1982) and others concerning *straight leg raising tests* offer additional hope of objective measures of the susceptibility to and the effects of manipulation.

In addition, reproducible *subjective* measures are possible, as shown in the results of the randomized clinical trials reported in this section and elsewhere. Perhaps some interaction with psychologists or sociologists might yield useful ways of characterizing and improving the reproducibility of these results. The characteristics of reproducible objective and subjective measures are further discussed in the conclusion to this book.

As was pointed out by Newell and Kanno of Michigan Department of Labor in this volume, modification of the work place may play a significant role in reducing low back pain among workers with this common problem, but these modifications are seldom implemented and when they are implemented they are sometimes so impractical that they are not used. For example, in the study by Bergquist-Ullman and Larsson (1977), one wonders about the proportion of the Low Back School patients who reported relief of back pain who also had their work place successfully altered and also about the distribution within the Low Back School group between those with and without successful work place alteration in relation to "successful" treatment.

We have not included in this volume reviews of the early papers of Glover *et al.* (1974) and Doran and Newell (1975), primarily because these works have been reviewed by their authors in a previous work (Buerger and Tobis, 1977).

Unfortunately, one excellent clinical trial comparing (1) mobilization and manipulation with (2) diathermy, isometric abdominal exercises and ergonomic instruction was not known to us when this volume was organized (Farrell and Tohmey, 1982). Both the duration of symptoms and the number of treatments required to achieve a pain free state were less for the mobilized and manipulated group. This study was well designed and implemented and is of special interest because its results are not entirely compatible with those of Bergquist-Ullman and Larsson (1977).

An additional paper of great importance appeared while this volume was going to press; Deyo (1983) reviewed over 50 clinical trials of various types of conservative therapies for low back pain, including 14 randomized or unrandomized trials of manual medicine, and suggested some possible solutions to problems in the design of rigorous studies of low back pain. Both of these papers are essential reading for those interested in clinical trials of manipulative techniques.

REFERENCES

Bergquist-Ullman, M., Larsson, U.: Acute low back pain in industry: A controlled prospective study with special reference to therapy and confounding factors. *Acta Orthopaedica Scandinavica, Supplementum 170*:1-117, 1977.

Buerger, A.A., Tobis, J.S. (eds.): *Approaches to the Validation of Manipulation Therapy*, Springfield, IL, Charles C Thomas, 1977.

Deyo, R.A., Conservative therapy for low back pain: Distinguishing useful from useless therapy. *Journal of the American Medical Association (JAMA), 250*:1057-1062, 1983.

Doran, D.M.L. and Newell, D.J.: Manipulation in treatment of low-back pain: a multicentre study. *British Medical Journal, 2*:161-164, 1975.

Farrell, J P., Twomey, L.T.: Acute low back pain. Comparison of two conservative treatment approaches. *Medical Journal of Australia, 1*:160-164, 1982.

Fisk, J.W.: *The Significance of Disorders of Muscles' Activity in the Perpetuation and Treatment of Low Back Pain, with Particular Reference to Manipulation.* M.D. Thesis, University of Edinburgh, 1978.

Glover, J.R., Morris, J.G., Khosla, T.: Back pain: A randomized clinical trial of rotational manipulation of the trunk. *British Journal of Industrial Medicine, 31*:59-64, 1974.

Hoehler, F.K. and Tobis, J.S.: Low back pain and its treatment by spinal manipulation: Measures of flexibility and asymmetry. *Rheumatology and Rehabilitation, 21*:21-26, 1982.

Jayson, M.I.V., Sims-Williams, H., Young, S., Baddeley, H., Collins, E.: Mobilization and manipulation for low-back pain, *Spine, 6*:409-416, 1981.

Rasmussen, G.G.: Manipulation in treatment of low back pain — A randomized clinical trial. *Manuelle Medizin , 1*:8-10, 1979.

Sims-Williams, H.L., Jayson, M.I.V., Young, S.M.S., Baddeley, H., Collins, E.: Controlled trial of mobilization and manipulation for patients with low back pain in general practice. *British Medical Journal, 2*:1338-1340, 1978.

Sims-Williams, H.L., Jayson, M.I.V., Young, S.M.S., Baddeley, H., Collins, E.: Controlled trial of mobilization and manipulation for low back pain: Hospital patients. *British Medical Journal, 2*:1318-1320, 1979.

CHAPTER TEN

THE RANDOMIZED CONTROLLED TRIAL
AND LOW BACK PAIN:
AN INTRODUCTION

VICTOR M. HAWTHORNE, M.D.

WIDESPREAD recognition of the value of the randomized controlled trial as a means of determining the efficacy of treatment in medical practice seems to have taken place shortly after World War II with the publication of the early trials of chemotherapy in the treatment of tuberculosis in Great Britain (Brockington, 1969). However, the technique of treating one set of patients and not treating another and then comparing the results is not new. One of the earliest documented clinical trials and one with a commendable preventive emphasis, was that of James Lind's experiment at sea on May 20, 1747 (Daniels and Hill, 1952). His twelve seamen suffering from scurvy diagnosed by putrid gums, spots, lassitude and weakness of the knees, were put into the fore-hold of the H.M.S. Salisbury and onto the standard seaman's diet of that day: watery gruel and sugar, fresh mutton broth, light pudding, boiled biscuit with sugar and a supper of barley, raisins, rice currants, sago and wine. The patients were then allocated, two by two, to six different regimens of daily care ranging from a quart of cider through a half pint of sea water to two teaspoons of vinegar three times. The regimen "of most sudden and good effect" was two oranges and one lemon a day. Efficacy was measured by the simple criterion of being fit for duty. Lind notes "one was fit for duty at the end of six days and was quite healthy by the time the ship reached Plymouth on June 16th." The other was apparently well enough to be appointed sick nurse to the others during the month at sea.

Lind's classical experiment had all the elements, if not the precise plan, of any randomized clinical trial of treatment; and the principles are as applicable today as they were then.

151

THE HYPOTHESIS

A National Institutes of Health Study Section today would probably have criticized Lind for not enunciating a hypothesis. However, if none is stated, one can quite readily be inferred from his report. Lind's hunch was that a deficiency of acid in the diet was associated with scurvy; and this inference seems to emerge fairly clearly from the nature of the treatments to which the seamen were allocated: cider, elixir of vitriol on an empty stomach after a strongly acidulated gargle, vinegar, acidulated barley water, and oranges and lemons.

A review of the low back pain literature would suggest the need to restate the hypothesis of manipulation as a treatment of choice. Lind's range of interventions might also suggest the need to describe a detailed range of different manipulations as well as alternative modalities of intervention in low back pain. It would also be helpful to support that hypothesis by suggesting that manipulation can affect low back pain, at least in the short term, by attempting to describe a biologically plausible mechanism as the rationale for this type of intervention.

THE STUDY POPULATION

Review of the low back pain literature suggests need for much more detailed description of the types of population being studied. Clinical trials in general, because they are dealing with sick as opposed to apparently well people, tend to describe in adequate detail the entry and exclusion criteria to the trial, largely upon clinical terms, but all too often with insufficient regard to demographic factors like age and sex, marital status and occupation. Although generalizability is more the concern of the epidemiologist than the clinician, the widespread nature of low back pain in the general population suggests that generalizability should not be completely overlooked. A more serious problem is the exent to which insufficient regard to age, sex and socio-economic status can produce major bias in drawing inferences from results. Education, income and socioeconomic class are now widely recognized as having a major influence on the distribution of disease and disability across such disparate indices as coronary heart disease and low birth weight babies. In low back pain a higher socio-economic group may well have freer access to treatment, obtain earlier treatment and secure a more favorable outcome, and again, examples range from the efficacy of single dose therapy for urinary infections to perinatal mortality.

Low back pain presents its own special problems in respect of the criteria used to select patients. This is a problem inherent in the subjective nature of pain itself. Here it would seem that research must continue among the newer technologies to instill more objectivity into diagnoses, and in this the problems

of classifying chronic rheumatoid arthritis and in particular, the three digit rubrics used to describe disorders of the spine, need careful attention (World
Health Organization, 1970).

The Lind sample was highly selective but highly generalizable to seamen of
all nations. The spots and putrid gums no doubt excluded the possibility of ma-
lingerers among his sample. But the problem of deciding when a patient is a
patient and perhaps, even more cogently, when a patient is no longer a patient,
still calls for the special awareness of all investigators, particularly those working in such a highly subjective area of assessment as low back pain.

ETHICS

In recent years, Human Subjects' Committees working in close collaboration with investigators, have helped to ensure that, fairly universally, all
participants in trials are kept fully informed of the purpose of the study, the
nature of the intervention to be used and of any risks attaching to the procedure. Assurances to the patient which must not be overlooked are for confidentiality and probably also a commitment on the part of the investigator to
inform the patient of the results of any examinations performed in the trial
and the outcomes of any interventions. In a chronic condition like low back
pain it may also be advantageous to keep patients informed of group as well
as personal results in the interests of maintaining high response in long term
follow-up.

There are a number of ethical considerations which must exercise the
judgement of the investigator. An important issue is the efficacy of the new
treatment compared with the old. If the new treatment is obviously better, the
experiment may not be justified. Is it safe to use placebos — what about treatments involving, say, injections? Is it safe to make the trial "double-blind"? In
the case of an emergency the investigator must be able to "break the code" and
discover which treatment the patient is receiving. Again, should intermediate
results be examined? If in a trial of predetermined size, there is an early,
marked difference between treatment and control, is it ethical to continue the
trial in order to satisfy criteria for statistical significance? Finally, there is the
difficult area experienced by most investigators, of explaining to the patient
that he may be placed on a placebo, if one is to be used; and that, irrespective
of whether he is on treatment or a control, he must abide by the decision,
otherwise he is not acceptable for inclusion in the trial.

The low back pain literature seems deficient in brief descriptions of how
patients are recruited and informed. Reports also frequently lack information
regarding the proportion of those who consent and who are entered in the trial,
factors which can produce bias and diminish generalizability (Mosteller,
Gilbert and McPeek, 1980).

RANDOMIZATION

One would hope that the two seamen allocated to oranges and lemons were not selected because they had friends in high places. All participants must have an equal opportunity of being allocated either to control or treatment. The method of randomization must be described in any report not just to satisfy skeptics, but mainly as a means of checking the actual procedure retrospectively. If selection bias has occurred, perhaps it can still be adjusted.

There are many methods of randomization. In the Scottish trials of smoking cessation (Hawthorne, 1983), the top decile of smokers at risk of coronary artery disease were allocated to treatment or control by "odd" or "even" last digit of a unique seven digit personal identification number. That number itself was randomly allocated in advance of determining eligibility for entry into the trial. In the large British Medical Research Council (MRC) randomized control trial of treatment of mild to moderate hypertension now entering its eighth year (MRC, 1977), the patients were randomly allocated to one of four regimens by a program of randomization run by the central computer for the country situated at Northwick Park near London. There are many other methods. Flipping coins or drawing cards expose investigators to the temptation to intervene in the allocation process if there is a long run of heads or tails, and this method provides no record afterwards of what actually happened. Another common method is to prepare the necessary number of cards labelled "T" for treatment and "C" for controls. These can then be shuffled and placed in opaque envelopes, and opened when the next eligible patient appears. Perhaps the systematic use of random numbers best serves the needs of convenience, security and reproducibility.

The main purpose of randomization is to ensure that the treatment and control groups are similar in respect of all possible "confounding" factors (i.e. factors other than treatment which might influence outcome, e.g., occupation). A further refinement of randomization is stratification. This is used to ensure that equal numbers of patients with certain characteristics (e.g., "mild" and "severe" low back pain) fall into equal groups for treatment or control. In this case, patients might be classified at entry into "mild" or "severe" and distributed thus:

PATIENT	MILD	SEVERE
1	T	C
2	T	T
3	C	C
4	T	C
5	C	T
6	C	T
-	-	-
-	-	-

It is worth remembering that randomization without regard to major risk factors can bias results. If concomitant risk factors like obesity are suspected as having an influence on outcome, some form of prognostic stratification should be considered to ensure equal distribution of that risk between the two groups. Finally in randomized clinical trials, scientific reports should always give a brief description of how randomization was done.

MATCHING

Although the matching of treated with control patients is a major concern in epidemiologic studies, the issues which arise cannot be altogether overlooked in randomized control trials. As a general rule, subjects may be matched by characteristics related to the outcome of the trial provided these characteristics exist in comparable numbers in both the treated and control groups. In a study of bronchitis, for example, it would be important to ensure equal numbers of smokers in both groups.

Some designs enter patients into the trial in matched pairs, each pair being as alike as possible for factors influencing outcome: age, sex, severity of disease are common examples. One of each pair may be randomly allocated to treatment, the other to placebo or existing treatment. Both participants are followed at the same time, and outcomes are compared in each pair. Gehlbach (1980) provides a useful summary of subject selection. It includes consideration of the origin of the study population: are they from hospital outpatient departments or primary care? Does their back pain represent the whole spectrum of symptomatology or just part of the distribution? Do patients all have the disability they are supposed to have and are the criteria reasonable? Are the techniques used for classifying subjects practical and reproducible?

ASSESSMENT

Similar standards of patient assessment must be applied at the beginning, throughout and at the end of the trial. In Lind's study, remission of putrid gums and spots would be preferred to recovery from lassitude and weakness of the knees, and both outcomes would certainly have been preferred to transition from "unfit" to "fit."

Review of the back pain literature would suggest that a growing number of specific procedures providing enhanced objectivity in diagnosis and in degree of back pain are available; examples are the passive hamstring stretch test (Fisk, 1979a, 1979b) and skin hyperesthesia, deep tenderness, etc., used to assess change "before" and "after" intervention by Glover and his colleagues (Glover, Morris and Khosla, 1974). If new diagnostic methods are to be developed or existing ones adopted, each must be validated, i.e., tested to ensure that the procedure is measuring what it purports to measure. The general principles are probably governed by those for tests of work capacity and physiological response to work (Rose and Blackburn, 1968). The test should be a simple procedure requiring no special skills and lasting a relatively short time, should be safe and within the capacity of all ambulatory subjects whether patients or healthy persons, involve relevant muscle masses and skeletal structures rather than isolated tissues, provide steady state periods for recording comparative quantitative measures, give reproducible results, be related to body mass, provide estimates of maximum responses and work capacity, and serve investigatory interest in both diagnosis and function. The literature suggests the probability that there is not yet available for low back pain any single test of adequate sensitivity, specificity, predictive value and reproducibility. Again, the deficiency hints at present need for review of more recent technology for procedures which might be used in new clinical trials.

In low back pain trials, the literature suggests general need to exercise care in standardizing the conditions under which tests are made. An extreme example, in cardiovascular epidemiology, is the measurement of blood pressure. The patient must not have eaten, smoked, or exercised a half-hour before examination. The width of the cuff, position of the cuff on the arm, position of the arm, speed of cuff inflation and deflation, are all necessary requisites of a standardized examination to avoid intra- and inter-observer error. Precautions are needed to prevent confusion between aural and visual signals of blood pressure level. The number and duration of the intervals between examinations must be adequate to exclude the phenomenon of regression to the mean, in order to estimate the true biological level of blood pressure. It is conceivable that similar needs for standardization may have to be considered for low back pain.

Assessment also involves the problem of bias on the past of the assessor. This can be countered by keeping the assessor ignorant of the participant's classification as a treated or control patient or by using a completely "masked" or "blind" independent assessor. In general, "blindness" means that the nature of the intervention used has been concealed from investigator and patient alike. "Single blind" is the term used when the investigator is unaware of who is the patient and who the control; "double blind" is used when both investigator and patient are unaware; and "triple blind" is employed when the independent evaluator or assessor is also "blind." The MRC Trial of Mild Hypertension (MRC, 1977) probably exemplifies use of the last approach. As mentioned above, the measures taken to achieve blindness must be described in scientific reports (Mosteller, Gilbert and McPeek, 1980).

SAMPLE SIZE

Trials of Fixed Size

Most trials are of fixed size. The number of patients to be treated and the number of controls to participate are determined beforehand. The factors which govern the numbers needed to test a hypothesis depend on four considerations:

(1) The first is the *size of the difference* to be detected between the treated and control groups. Fewer patients for example would be needed to detect a three-fold than a two-fold difference.

(2) Next, *statistical significance* sought. Two significance levels are considered:

    (a) The *alpha significance*, for which a probability value is usually quoted. This is a statement that, if there is really no difference between treatments, the results obtained could have been due to chance with a probability of P=alpha. The alpha level is usually 5% or 1%.

    (b) *Beta significance* is the probability that if there really is a difference between treatments, it will fail to show up. The probability of this happening is usually regarded as less serious than an alpha error. The level often chosen is 10% or 20%.

(3) The fourth factor is the *variance of the outcome measurement*. Where this is considerable, for example, when there is a large standard deviation, more patients will be needed.

Standard tables are available providing sample sizes for all four factors but a statistician should always be consulted.

Sequential Trials

Sequential trials differ from fixed size trials because results are examined and statistical significance tested after each result is obtained. Repeated significance testing requires special statistical techniques, and a sequential design must be decided on before the trial commences. An advantage of a sequential design is that no more patients than are needed to attain statistical significance, are exposed to whatever risks may be inherent in the treatment. Sequential trials are suitable for paired designs or cross-over designs in which the problems of differences between treatment and control groups are eliminated because each patient receives all the treatments being tested. The comparison between treatments is made between each patient who acts as his or her own control. The sequential cross-over design is particularly suitable for chronic diseases and for those conditions which do not vary greatly in severity over time, but in which the condition can undergo spontaneous remission without treatment like arthritis and low back pain.

Sequential methods in clinical trials are described with statistical detail by Armitage (1971) whose trial of two hypertensive agents is used here to suggest a possible model for a study of intervention in low back pain (See Figure X-1).

The figure describes a plan for sequential analysis for two drugs designed to lower blood pressure during anesthesia. A paired design was used; and the outcome measured by blood pressure recovery after anesthesia. The outcome was expressed as a preference for one or the other drug for each pair of sub-

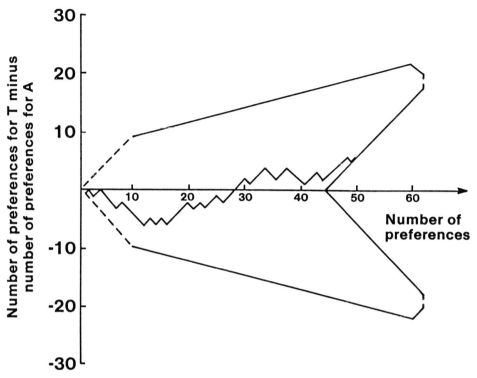

Figure X-1. Trial of two hypotensive agents — restricted pain with $2\alpha=0.05$, $1-\beta=0.95$, $\theta=0.75$, and $N=62$. (Robertson and Armitage, 1959).

jects. The design chosen in this illustration was closed: the maximum number of pairs that were to be used was restricted to 62. The significance levels employed were alpha $=0.05$ and beta $=0.05$. In regard to the outcome (theta, the probability of one drug being preferable to the other) was set at 0.75. After each pair was assessed, a preference for drug A would move the trace line one square toward the top and right of the chart. A preference for drug B would move the trace line one square to the right and toward the bottom of the chart.

The trial would conclude when the trace line coincided with the upper limiting line giving the result that drug A was preferable at the prescribed significance levels. If the lower limit was reached by the trace line, the advantage would go to drug B at the prescribed significance level. An equivocal result would be indicated by the absence of a significant, cumulative move to the upper or lower limit by the completion of entry of the final results for the 62 pairs. An equivocal outcome is shown in Figure X-1.

SIGNIFICANCE OF THE NON-SIGNIFICANT RESULT

A caveat suggested by review of the low back pain literature, and one which applies to all studies, is the need to consider the possibility that sample size is inadequate before accepting no difference between an interventive procedure as being the significant finding.

CRITIQUE OF A RANDOMIZED CONTROL TRIAL OF MANIPULATION IN LOW BACK PAIN

In the excellent review of ten trials by Evans (in this volume) perhaps the study most relevant to present considerations is the one by that author and his colleagues (Evans *et al.*, 1978) as being the one which employed a cross-over design. In the Cardiff Study, 32 patients with chronic low back pain were treated three times at weekly intervals with rotational manipulation. Background therapy of codeine phosphate was administered throughout. A cross-over design was employed as described in the undernoted trial timetable:

TRIAL TIMETABLE

				Trial Day				
GROUP	– 7	0	7	14	21	28	35	42
A	S F X	F M	 M	 M	F X A			F (X) A

Codeine Phosphate as Necessary

B	S F X	F			X A M	F M	(X) M	F A

Codeine Phosphate as Necessary

S = Screening	( ) = Only if Over 45 Years Old
F = Anterior Spinal Flexion Measured	M = Lumbar Spine Manipulation
X = Radiograph of Lumbar Spine	A = Assess

(after Evans et al., 1978)

Allocation to both groups was claimed to be equal for all major characteristics such as age, sex, etc. There were 4 (11%) defaulters.

The value of a cross-over design whereby all patients have all the treatments, has already been described. Not the least consideration is the ethical one of not depriving controls of treatment. The methods employed in the Evans's study are excellent in many respects. The criteria for selection and exclusion are defined. The objectivity of "before" and "after" assessments is described as being obtained by employing a single assessor unaware of the nature of the previous treatment. However, there are lessons to be drawn from this study for the design of future clinical trials of low back pain employing the cross-over approach.

Despite claims that the distributions of all parameters were similar in the two treatment groups for whom the only differences in treatment were to be that group A received 3 manipulations at a week's interval first, while both had codeine phosphate as necessary, there was great heterogeneity in the duration of pain, 0.2-31 years (with a median of 4 years), duration of current attack, 6-676 weeks (with a median of 39 weeks); and it is not clear whether the treated and control groups were matched for these factors. If on the other hand, as claimed, the characteristics of both groups did not differ significantly, one might wonder why advantage was not taken of the opportunity to pair like patients. However, age and sex as already stated, are major factors in determining disease and disability; and the extent to which such a small sample could standardize for these two variables alone, is to be questioned. Incidentally, the study provides no estimates of sample size.

A second area of concern is the truncated nature of the duration of the trial. Apart from the absence of an equivalent observation period of three weeks after manipulation of group B, (a period of observation which would have provided a better control and also post-manipulation observations), the overall duration of the trial seems inadequate to do anything more than explore the unstated hypothesis that manipulation benefits low back pain over a period of 49 days. More generally, low back pain is of high chronicity and characterized by spontaneous remission. Neither the Cardiff trial nor any of the others reviewed, had observation periods anything like adequate for studies of the natural history of remission.

The statement that patient pain scores were reduced to a significant degree within four weeks of starting treatment only in the group manipulated in the first treatment period, is to be questioned on the following grounds: firstly, that the controls would already have had one manipulation before the week of observation; and secondly, that the second group to be manipulated were not followed for more than one week beyond the end of their period of manipulation.

Finally, the conclusion that patients benefitting subjectively were likely to be older and to have had symptoms for a shorter time than those not deriving benefit, might be questioned on the grounds that the sample was too small for age specific analysis, and that this difficulty may have been increased by an eleven percent default rate.

It must be stressed that these observations in no way detract from the very high standards established by the investigators in this important study.

CONCLUSION

We may not have too much specific to learn today from James Lind but we can gather strength in our approach to low back pain from a few generalities. Although Lind is still cited as a celebrated scientist, it is as much for his method as for scurvy that he is remembered. Oranges and lemons were not luxuries to the world-wide navigators of his day. More than likely the antiscorbutic effect of fresh fruit was already part of the international nautical folklore of his day. The addition of a few tidbits from the captain's table might not have been much more than a commonplace and logical extension of what was readily available for use in a ship at sea to test out his "acidulate everything" hypothesis. Again, like so many "cures" in medical history, Lind knew nothing of Vitamin C nor the pathophysiological mechanism of its action in preventing scurvy. Despite a situation approaching eradiction of tuberculosis in some Western countries, the exact mechanism of the interaction between Mycobacterium tuberculosis and pulmonary tissues is still unknown. Lack of knowledge of the exact mechanism, however, should never be a deterrent to randomized controlled trials of low back pain or any other condition.

With regard to sample size, Lind's sample was most probably dictated by the number of sick seamen he could accommodate in the crowded fore-hold of the H.M.S. Salisbury. Despite these difficulties, however, he did try the experiment, and we should expect him to describe an equivocal or negative result if he had achieved one. Incidentally, a common thread between the scurvy experiment and low back pain is the same need to get incapacitated workers back to duty.

The answer to low back pain probably already lies somewhere in the international folklore of the condition that has accumulated over the past century. Perhaps all we have to do now is to select and study the right combination of hypothesis, method and intervention.

SUMMARY

Use of the randomized controlled trial would seem to be integral to the future development of our understanding, treatment and prevention of low back pain. Although there is always a place for unstructured studies of problems whose natural history is incompletely understood, ultimately such findings as emerge must be used to formulate a hypothesis and to design and conduct an experiment to decide whether or not the new theory can be accepted. At this stage, the principles of the randomized controlled trial must be rigorously applied.

Review of the scientific literature of low back pain suggests the need for more attention to methodology by investigators and insistence on more detail of methodology by editors. Hypotheses could be more clearly stated, and biologically plausible mechanisms to support them more frequently postulated. More detail is required of the type of population being studied, their demographic features, particularly socioeconomic class and the appropriateness and representativeness of samples—Are the subjects hospital outpatients or in primary medical care? Does their back pain represent the whole spectrum of symptomatology or just part of the distribution? Do patients all have the disability they are supposed to have and are the criteria reasonable? Are the techniques used for classifying subjects practical and reproducible?

There is need for more attention to the classification of low back pain in chronic rheumatoid arthritis and the 3 digit rubrics used to describe disorders of the spine by nosologists. The subjective nature of low back pain calls for review of recent technologic advances to identify new objective tests of disease and disability and validate their use by studies of sensitivity, specificity, reproducibility and predictive value.

The literature of low back pain often seems to lack information on how patients were recruited and informed of the nature of the experiments in which they are participating. It is rare to find in the literature particulars of the numbers eligible to enter a trial who consent to enter and then actually participate. Both factors can effect representativeness of, and introduce bias into, findings.

The method of randomization needs to be reported not just to satisfy skeptics but to provide estimates and sometimes possibilities of adjusting for bias later. From a practical viewpoint, the process of randomization must take account of major risk factors like obesity which can influence outcome of treatment. Standardized methods of "before" and "after" clinical assessment need to be used; and the method of "blinding" the assessor reported.

Sequential trials using paired and cross-over designs, seem particularly suitable for randomized controlled studies of treatment for low back pain where there is a strong clinical emphasis within a single center. Each patient acts as his own control and, with the cross-over design, each patient has his share of new and old treatments or placebo. The sequential cross-over design is particularly suitable for the chronic diseases, and for conditions which do not vary greatly in severity over time but which can undergo spontaneous remission without treatment, like arthritis and low back pain. On the other hand, closed as opposed to open designs are perhaps better for the multi-center trials which now may be indicated to complement the laboratory and clinically-oriented studies. These randomized controlled trials would require larger numbers drawn from many centers. The studies will need more simple assessment techniques and modalities of care, and much longer periods of observation to take into account the chronicity and remission patterns of low back pain. Experimental studies, with a more epidemiologic emphasis, can contribute to better understanding of the natural history and prevention of low back pain.

Finally, until the right combination of hypothesis, method and intervention come along, investigators must be on guard not to misinterpret a negative conclusion when all that may be wrong is too small a sample and too short a period of observation.

REFERENCES

Armitage, P. *Statistical Methods in Medical Research.* Blackwell Scientific Publications, Oxford, 1971.

Brockington, CF. The history of public health, in Hobson, W. (ed.) *The Theory and Practice of Public Health*, (3rd ed.), New York, Oxford University Press, 1969, p. 3.

Daniels, M. and Hill, AB. Chemotherapy of pulmonary tuberculosis in young adults: An analysis of the combined results of three Medical Research Council trials, *British Medical Journal, 1*:1162, 1952.

Evans, DP, Burke, MS, Lloyd, KN, Roberts, EE and Roberts, GM. Lumbar spinal manipulation on trial, Part I: Clinical assessment. *Rheumatology and Rehabilitation, 17*:40-53, 1978.

Evans, DP. The design and results of clinical trials of lumbar manipulation: A Review, in this volume.

Fisk, JW. The Passive Hamstring Stretch Test: Clinical Evaluation. *New Zealand Medical Journal*, 89 (Number 632):209-211, 1979a.

Fisk, JW. A controlled trial of manipulation in a selected group of patients with low back pain favoring one side. *New Zealand Medical Journal, 90* (Number 645):288-291, 1979b.

Gehlbach, SH. *Interpreting the Medical Literature.* Lexington, MA, The Collamore Press, D.C. Heath and Co., 1982.

Glover, JR, Morris, JG and Khosla, T. Back pain: A randomized clinical trial of rotational manipulation of the trunk. *British Journal of Industrial Medicine, 31*:59-64, 1974.

Hawthorne, VM. Preventing cardiovascular disease for the nineties: Practical policies for the present. *Scottish Medical Journal, 28*:7-16, 1983.

Medical Research Council. Report of medical research council working party on mild to moderate hypertension, randomized controlled trial of treatment for mild hypertension: Design and Pilot Trail, *British Medical Journal,, 1*:1437-1440, 1977.

Mosteller, F, Gilbert, JP and McPeek, B. Reporting standards and research strategies for controlled trials: agenda for the editor. *Controlled Clinical Trials: Design and Methods, 1*:37-58, 1980.

Robertson, JD and Armitage, P. Comparison of two hypotensive agents. *Anaesthesia, 14*:54-64, 1959.

Rose, GA and Blackburn, H. *Cardiovascular Survey Methods.* World Health Organization (WHO) Monograph Series, No. 56; Geneva, WHO, 1968.

World Health Organization. *Report of a Working Group: Studies on chronic rheumatoid arthritis and their relation to rheumatic complaints as a public health problem.* Regional Office for Europe of the World Health Organization, WHO, 1970, especially pp. 21-27.

CHAPTER ELEVEN

LOW BACK PAIN IN INDUSTRY:
A RANDOMIZED CLINICAL TRIAL

MARIANNE BERGQUIST-ULLMAN, Ph.D., M.D.

Introduction

VERY little is known about the value of different methods of treatment in patients with back pain. There is therefore a great need for controlled trials of different methods of treatment. It is known that mechanical, psychological and social factors influence the occurrence of low back pain (Nachemson, 1971; Westrin, 1970). The prognostic importance of these factors in the course of the condition has not previously been studied, however. A prospective three-year study of patients with acute low back pain was carried out at the Volvo factory in Gothenburg, Sweden, between 1974 and 1977 (Bergquist-Ullman and Larsson, 1977). One of the aims of the study was to compare the effect of the Back School (Lidstrom and Zachrisson, 1973) with physiotherapy and with low-voltage short-wave treatment as placebo therapy. A further aim was to elucidate the course of acute low back pain and to relate it to certain clinical, occupational and psychosocial factors. In this paper, only highlights of the original paper will be presented. Please refer to Bergquist-Ullman and Larsson (1977) for more complete information.

Patients and Procedure

Two hundred and seventeen patients were selected at Volvo's Medical Centre. They all had low back pain without radiation below the knee. The distribution is shown in Figure XI-1 (after Figure 2, page 45 in Bergquist-Ullman [1977]). The current period of pain had not lasted more than three months and the patients had not had back pain during the previous year.

All the patients had pain in the lumbar region. The pain was mainly located centrally in the lower lumbar area or in the paravertebral region as illustrated. Pain in the gluteal region or the thigh occurred in 26% of the patients. Pain was more common in the right gluteal region and thigh than on the left side.

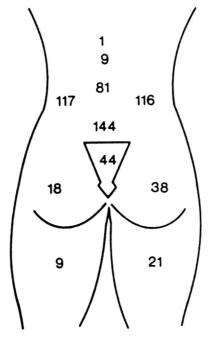

Figure XI-1. The distribution of pain in 217 back pain patients without pain below the knee.

Patients reporting discontent with their jobs were found to have a longer initial episode ($p < 0.05$) and a longer absence from work ($p < 0.05$) than the satisfied patients. Dissatisfaction with the working environment was also associated with a longer duration of absence both during the initial episode ($p < 0.01$) and during recurrences ($p < 0.05$). However, relations with colleagues and a desire to change jobs did not have any significant influence on the course of the disease.

The patients were examined by an orthopaedic surgeon, who used standardized questionnaires to register the clinical and psychosocial factors and forms for the registration of objective findings (Bergquist-Ullman and Larsson, 1977). Copies of these questionnaires and forms comprise Appendix A. After the examination, the patients were randomly allocated to one of the three methods of treatment, with about 70 patients in each group. All patients were re-examined by the same orthopaedic surgeon at five to seven predetermined points of time during one year. The course of the initial complaint and of relapses was registered. The *same* standardized forms were used for the registration of pain and objective findings as at the initial examination.

Also, according to the patients, their work tended to require bending, twisting, lifting and forceful movements. This data is shown in Table I (after Table 15, page 50 in Bergquist-Ullman [1977]). A high frequency of bending and twisting movements was reported by the manual workers while lifting and forceful movements were not considered to be necessary as frequently.

Table XI-1

Patient's answers regarding movements required during work.

Manual workers = m, office staff = o.

Type of movement	Often		Sometimes		Seldom	
	No.	% m, o	No.	% m, o	No.	% m, o
Bending forward	140	(81,19)	34	(14,21)	43	(5,60)
Twisting	140	(79,21)	37	(16,21)	40	(4,58)
Lifting (> 5kg)	66	(39,5)	62	(36,9)	89	(25,86)
Lifting (> 20kg)	25	(14,2)	37	(23,4)	155	(63,94)
Forceful movements	25	(15,2)	38	(24,0)	154	(61,98)

METHODS OF TREATMENT

The Back School

The Back School was initiated by Marianne Zachrisson-Forssell, RPT, in 1970 (Lidstrom and Zachrisson, 1973). The Back School is an educational sound-slide program based on research on the etiology of low back pain, intradiscal pressure measurements, EMG, and epidemiological studies. A group of six to eight patients take part in the Back School during four sessions of 45 minutes each under the supervision of a physiotherapist. (English versions of these four Back School Lessons may be available through the author.)

During the first lesson, the patients are taught the epidemiology of back pain, the anatomical structures of the spine and possible anatomical locations for the origin of pain. The lack of knowledge regarding the cause of low back pain is emphasized, consequently the patients recognize the lack of curative methods of treatment for low back pain. At this first lesson the patients are told that resting a painful back decreases the pain. This is applied practically by having the patients take part in the Back School in a supine position with hips and knees flexed to 90°, and supported by a chair or cushion.

The next two lessons continue with discussions regarding the biomechanics of the spine in various postures. The patients are informed that an increased strain on an already afflicted back increases the pain. The patients are taught why certain postures or movements increase the pain, and perhaps most importantly, how to avoid these stressful movements. Most of the third lesson is therefore spent encouraging the patient to apply practically the theoretical knowledge acquired in the Back School by using proper lifting techniques and working postures.

The fourth lesson consists of a repetition and summary of the previous lessons with emphasis on the importance of being in a good physical condition. The patients are guided to physical activities suitable to their back condition, and encouraged to use the knowledge gained in the Back School to change their working environment and to live well in spite of their back troubles.

In this trial an additional analysis of the working conditions was carried out by the physiotherapist on two occasions. Improper working postures were corrected the first time; two weeks later the second visit was spent to see whether the patient succeeded in following the instructions given.

If certain tasks of work could not be carried out in proper working postures, suggestions were made to the work managers to adjust these work sites to improve the conditions for the back. However, if immediate changes were not possible, attempts were made to transfer the patient to another job temporarily.

In this study seventy patients were allocated to the Back School at random.

Physiotherapy

The physiotherapy mainly comprised manual therapy supplemented with brief ergonomic counseling. The patients allocated to this group were treated by physiotherapists specially trained in manual therapy. A combination of methods was used by the physiotherapists to examine specifically the patient's musculoskeletal system and to individualize the treatment. For general diagnosis, the methods were largely based on those of Cyriax (1959); for examination and treatment, they were largely based on those of Kaltenborn (1975); for examination and diagnosis of the pelvis they were largely based on those of Lewit (1977); and for stretching exercises, they were largely based on those of Janda (1975). At the discretion of the physiotherapist giving treatment some form of manual therapy was used on most, but not all, patients randomly assigned to the physiotherapy group.

The patients were examined standing up, sitting with the pelvis fixed, lying prone, supine and in a lateral position. In every position the active and passive mobility of the spine and adjacent joints was examined as well as the length and strength of muscles (Bergquist-Ullman and Larsson, 1977). According to the physiotherapists, this examination was very important in order to locate the structure(s) causing the pain in the back. The treatment could thereafter be focused on the afflicted structure(s).

Patients who had hypomobile segments were treated with mobilization; only the hypomobile segment was moved passively (articulated), while the adjacent mobile segment was stabilized. The procedure was carried out with the patient lying in a lateral position.

Hypermobile segments were given stabilization exercises, starting with individual segments and gradually increasing the number of segments until all hypermobile segments were included.

Patients with a blocked sacroiliac joint were treated with "gapping." According to the physiotherapist "gapping" is performed to increase the mobility in the joint. The patient lies on the blocked side and the trunk is "rotated" forward.

Patients who were found to have a pelvis "rotated" forward or backward were treated with "articulation" resulting in a rotational movement of the sacroiliac joint.

Stretching exercises were given to patients who had "contracted postural muscles."

Placebo

Low-voltage heat treatment was administered by means of a shortwave apparatus without the presence of a physiotherapist.

Evaluation Variables

The following variables were used to compare the effect of the methods of treatment, and to correlate clinical, occupational and psychosocial factors with the course of the complaint:

(1) Duration of pain after the start of treatment.
(2) Duration of the first registered period of pain.
(3) Length of sick-leave during the first period of pain.
(4) Duration of relapses during one year.
(5) Length of sick-leave for relapses during one year.

SOME RESULTS

The course of the patients' complaint was in accordance with previous retrospective studies (Horal, 1969). Thirty-five percent of the patients had recovered within one month, 70 percent were free from symptoms within two months, and 86 percent had no low back pain after three months. Only four percent of the patients had a longer duration of low back symptoms than one year. Eighty-five percent of all patients were on sick-leave at some time during the initial episode of pain.

Sixty-two percent relapsed. The median number of relapses was 1.3 during the year of observation. The duration of the recurrences of pain was shorter than the initial episode of pain. The median duration of all recurrences in one year was 27 days. The corresponding sick-leave due to recurrences was 16 days. Among the 134 patients who relapsed during the year, 50 percent were at some time absent from work.

Comparison of the three methods of treatment showed that the patients who had attended the Back School or received physiotherapy had a considerably shorter duration of pain than those given low-voltage short-wave treatment (Table XI-2).

There were also considerable differences in the length of sick leave during the first registered period of pain. The patients attending the Back School had, on average, one week shorter sick-leave than the other patients (Table XI-3). The patients were equally distributed between the three groups as regards the time of sick-leave in relation to the date of onset of symptoms.

Table XI-2

Duration of pain after the first treatment. The length of sick-leave is calculated from the day of onset of pain, whereas the duration of pain below is calculated from the first treatment.

	Means
Back School	14.8 days
Physiotherapy	15.8 days
Placebo	28.7 days

Table XI-3
Length of sick-leave during the first period of pain.

	Means
Back School	20.5 days
Physiotherapy	26.5 days
Placebo	26.5 days

When comparing the three groups regarding relapses, no significant difference was detected in favour of any treatment.

Of the other factors studied during the one-year follow-up period, occupational factors had the greatest influence on the course of the complaint. Patients whose jobs entailed bending and twisting movements during a large part of the working day had both longer periods of pain and longer sick-leave during the observation period. Lifting movement, on the other hand, did not influence the course.

DISCUSSION

This investigation clearly shows that early initiation of treatment of patients with acute low back pain in the form of the Back School or physiotherapy accelerates recovery. The length of sick-leave can also be markedly reduced by the Back School. Unfortunately, this study does not permit conclusions concerning causal associations between the treatment given and the cause of back pain, as the etiology is still unknown. An investigation of a multifactorial disorder like low back pain may be characterized by an abundance of soft variables, the influence of which is not always easy to determine. Examples of the confounding factors influencing these results are shown in Table XI-4 (after Table 27, pages 70 and 71 in Bergquist-Ullman [1977].

The positive results of the Back School and physiotherapy are probably related to increased individual contact with the therapist. This is probably not, however, the only explanation for the earlier recovery, as each patient who received individual treatment by the physiotherapist had considerably more contact with the therapist than patients who attended the Back School in groups. Individual treatment should then give a shorter period of pain than the Back School, which was not found in our study.

In addition, the individual treatment within the physiotherapy group did not appear to reduce the rate or duration of relapses, in spite of the fact that patients who received physiotherapy during the first period of pain received the same treatment when they relapsed. The patients who received low-voltage short-wave treatment during the first attack also received the same treatment during relapses. The patients who attended the Back School, on the other hand, only received this treatment during the first period of pain, because it was not practical to have patients attend the Back School more than once.

Whatever the explanation for the effect of the different methods of treatment, the Back School is advantageous from an economic point of view; the same effect on the duration of pain as was achieved with a patient given physiotherapy could be achieved with six to eight patients at the same time with the Back School. Furthermore, the patients who attended the Back School were able to return to work one week earlier, on the average, than the patients who received physiotherapy or low-voltage short-wave treatment.

This study has also shown that patients whose jobs necessitated frequent bending and twisting movements had both a longer duration of pain and longer periods of sick-leave during the one-year observation period. It is therefore very important that such work places are subjected to ergonomic analysis and improvements are made wherever possible. It may otherwise be impossible to apply the ergonomic principles taught at the Back School.

Table XI-4

The confounding factors found to be related to the course of disease. Definitions: * = p < 0.05, ** = p < 0.01, *** = p < 0.001

Confounding factors	Duration of initial episode	Duration of sick-listing during initial episode	Duration of relapses	Duration of sick-listing during relapses
History of back pain				
Onset of symptoms	*			
Pain index				
Initially		*		
After ten days	***	***		
Objective findings				
Pain on percussion		**		
Straight Leg Raising Test		**		
Vocational factors				
Category of employment	**	***		**
Sitting	*	***		
Fixed posture	*		**	
Bending forward	**	***		*
Twisting movements	*	**		**
Lifting (> 5kg)		**		
Forceful movements				*
Fatigue back	**			
Fatigue after work	*			
Repetitive	***	*		
Monotonous work	**			
No need to concentrate		*		
Satisfaction with work tasks	**	*		
Satisfaction with working environment		***		*
Nervousness after work			**	

Table XI-4 (continued)

Vocational factors manual workers separately

Fatigue back	*				
Repetitive work	**				
Monotonous work	*				
Sitting (< 2 hours)			*		

Psychological factors

MMPI-test: Hy-scale	*		*		
Eysenck-test: Extroversion-scale				*	

Social factors

Tendency to report sick			***		
Contacts with social welfare authorities	**				

Demographic factors

Age	*				*

REFERENCES

Bergquist-Ullman, M.: *Acute Low Back Pain in Industry: A controlled prospective study with special reference to therapy and vocational factors.* (A privately published summary of Bergquist-Ullman & Larsson [1977]), Goteborg, 1977.

Bergquist-Ullman, M. and Larsson, U.: Acute Low Back Pain in Industry: A controlled prospective study with special reference to therapy and confounding factors. *Acta Orthopaedica Scandinavica, Supplementum 170*, 1977.

Cyriax, J.: *Textbook of Orthopaedic Medicine,* (2nd ed.), London, Cassell, 1959.

Horal, J.: The Clinical Appearance of Low Back Pain Disorders in the City of Gothenburg, Sweden. Comparisons of incapacitated probands with matched controls. *Acta Orthopaedica Scandinavica, Supplementum 118*, 1969.

Janda, V.: Muskelfunktionsdiagnostik. *Studentlitteratur (Lund)*, 12-23:266-275 and 278, 1975.

Kaltenborn, F.M.: *Test segmenti mobilis. Columna vertebralis. Course 1*:44-57, Bygdy Alle 14, Oslo 2, Norway, 1975.

Lewit, K.: *Manuelle Medizin im Rahmen der Medizinischen Rehabilitation, 2*, Leipzig, Johann Ambrosius Barth, 1977.

Lidstrom, A. and Zachrisson, J.: Ryggskolan: Ett forsok till mer rationell fysikalisk terapi. *Socialmed tidskrift, 7*:419-422, 1973.

Nachemson, A.: Low back pain: Its etiology and treatment. *Clinical Medicine, 78*:18-24, 1971.

Westrin, C-G.: Low back sick listing: A nosological and medical insurance investigation. *Scandinavian Journal of Social Medicine, Supplement 7*, 1970.

CHAPTER TWELVE

A RANDOMIZED CLINICAL TRIAL
OF MANIPULATION: DIAGNOSTIC CRITERIA
AND TREATMENT TECHNIQUES

G. RASMUSSEN, M.D.

IN spite of the fact that manipulation of the spine has been described clinically since the days of Hippocrates, there is still relevant discussion possible about the scientific foundations of the indications for and the effects of manual therapy.

The randomized double blind clinical trial is usually the only acceptable documentation for diagnostic and treatment techniques in modern medicine (Buerger, 1980).

Very few clinical trials had been published about manipulation for low back pain at the time this study was carried out (e g. Doran and Newell, 1975; Evans et al., 1978; Glover et al., 1974), although the empiric literature is rather huge. Furthermore some of these trials failed to demonstrate the effects of manipulation.

This study (Rasmussen, 1979) attempted to test the following hypothesis: Manipulation has a certain effect in treatment of low back pain superior to other modalities of treatment. As a control group short wave diathermy was chosen.

The trial was designed and carried out in 1975-76 at the Department of Physical Medicine and Rheumatology in Aalborg in Northern Jutland, Denmark.

METHODS

Former clinical trials were not conclusive mainly because non-homogenous patient populations were used; hence a very strictly defined patient population was chosen.

Male outpatients who:

(1) were between 20-50 years,
(2) had low back pain without any signs of root compression with a duration of less than 3 weeks, and;
(3) of course, demonstrated no contraindication to manipulation or traction. The patients were referred acutely from general practitioners to the rheumatological department and had received no treatment other than analgesics.

The first day the patients were examined by the rheumatologist and had x-rays taken of the lumbo-sacral spine. Then, if no contraindication to the protocol or manipulation was found and formal consent was given, the patients were allocated at random to either group A: manipulation 3 times a week for 14 days or group B: short wave diathermy 3 times a week for 14 days.

The manipulation was performed by a skilled physiotherapist. The patients were examined formally by the rheumatologist on day 1, day 8 and day 15.

In the clinical investigation the following parameters were noted:

(1) the patients' evaluation of feeling (a) pain or (b) no pain at all,
(2) fitness for work or still unable to do it.

The subjective parameters should in this way be very reliable.

In the clinical examination a modification of Schober's test was made measuring the difference in distances between spinous processes of C7 through S1 during standing and during forward bending. An ordinary examination of the back and a neurological examination were also performed.

There was no blind observer. (This is a critical point.) Very clear criteria were registered as markers, that is the patients were declared fully restored if they fulfilled all the following criteria:

(1) no pain at all,
(2) normal function of the spine,
(3) no objective signs of disease,
(4) fit for work.

The trial was stopped if:

(1) the criteria above (1-4) were fulfilled,
(2) complications occurred, or
(3) after 14 days according to the protocol.

Manipulation was performed as a part of manual therapy which always included rotational manipulation in each session of treatment, that is soft tissue treatment was given first, then articulation leading directly into rotational manipulation. After the trial all patients were instructed in ergonomic principles in an individual back school.

The manual techniques were as follows:

(1) Soft tissue treatment was performed both with the patient lying forward and in a side-lying position.

(2) In the forward lying position the manipulator used push and draw with the four ulnar fingers of one hand and the thenar of the other hand on the cranial and caudal part of the muscles, kneading the muscle transversely.

(3) In the side-lying position the manipulator used the four ulnar fingers near the spinous processes and then drew the erector spinae muscle away from the midline. Simultaneously the spine was stretched and deflected by the pressure of the manipulator's forearms on the thorax and pelvis.

Articulation was performed in several ways:

(1) Ventral flexion and articulation in side-lying position with flexion of the knee joints and hips. The manipulator then fixed the thighs and directed flexion with one hand on the pelvis and the other on the lumbar spine.

(2) Side-flexion and articulation in side-lying position was performed by accentuating the concavity of the spine with one of the manipulator's hands and the other hand palpating cranial to the segment to be articulated.

(3) Side-flexion and articulation was done with the patient sitting; the manipulator had his (her) front against the side of the patient with one arm around the thorax under the patient's arm and with the manipulator's axilla over the patient's nearest shoulder which was pressed down. The concavity of the spine was overaccentuated by the free hand of the manipulator.

(4) Rotational articulation in the sitting position was done with the manipulator in the same position; the free hand of the manipulator accentuated the articulation by pressure on transverse process of the other side of the patient.

(5) Rotational articulation in the side-lying position was done in the pain-free direction by rotating the upper part of the patient's body away from the manipulator, who pressed one hand on the pectoral region and the other against the spinous process caudal to the segment to be articulated.

Rotational manipulation was done as was an advanced and more specific procedure with the patient and manipulator in the same relative positions as above. The manipulator fixated the patient's pelvis with his forearm while the patient's torso was rotated and fixed by the other forearm. The manipulation was performed specifically by the second finger of one hand and the first finger of the other against each side of the spinous process adjacent to the segment being manipulated.

In the control group, short wave was given for 15 minutes 3 times a week to the control group.

Twenty-six patients were admitted to the trial. Two dropped out, one because of neurological signs of root compression. The other patient strayed after a few short wave treatments.

Twenty-four patients remained who fulfilled the criteria of acute low back pain described above. Their mean age was 34.9 years with a standard deviation of 7.3. They were randomized in two groups of 12 patients each.

RESULTS

The Table XII-1 shows the time required for cessation of all symptoms. All restored patients fulfilled the four criteria listed above.

The Table XII-2 shows the improvement in mobility of the spine measured by a modified Schober's test.

Table XII-1.

Time to cessation of all symptoms:

	short wave	manipulation
1 - 7 days	2	7
8 - 14 days	1	4
Total within 14 days	3	11

P < 0.01, Mann Whitney rank-sum test.

Table XII-2.

Time of restorment of all symptoms.

	short wave	manipulation
Improvement	6	12
No Improvement	6	0

Chi square = 7.5, p < 0.01, Yates' corrected chi-square test

Ninety-two percent of the manipulated patients were totally restored within 14 days whereas only 25% were restored in the short wave group. Improvement in the mobility of the spine was seen in all manipulated patients but in only 6 of the 12 patients in the short wave group.

A written inquiry was performed after a year, and all restored patients were free of symptoms for at least this year.

Discussion:

The main purpose of this work has been to investigate if manipulation has any effect on low back pain, as this had not previously been demonstrated in a randomized clinical trial. The spontaneous prognosis in acute low back pain is rather good, whereas results of treatment in chronic back pain are well-known to be dubious (e.g. Sloop et al., 1982).

For ethical and practical reasons, acute low back pain with a very clear cut definition and observation time was chosen. One might discuss the choice of the control group, as detuned short-wave diathermy might be considered a better control than short-wave diathermy. Short-wave diathermy was considered a treatment with no effect, in order to give patients in both groups the same amount of placebo effect. The patients were informed that we were comparing two different modalities of treatment of low back pain.

In this study two main points are emphasized:

(1) Manipulation does have some effect.
(2) Manipulation abbreviates the duration of acute low back pain.

The latter is a crucial point because McGill (1968) has shown that one-half of patients with sick leave for more than 6 months did not return to work.

Further studies are called for to demonstrate further indications and to explore the pathophysiological background. It is the author's opinion that manipulation is a main modality of treatment for acute low back pain but is only a supportive modality in chronic low back pain and in some cases of disc herniation. In the latter circumstance, it should only be used under strict surveillance. Under such cases manipulation might be useful as a diagnostic tool—if no effect of manipulation is found the suspicion of a prolapsed disc may be enhanced.

REFERENCES

1. Buerger, A.A.: A controlled trial of rotational manipulation in low back pain. *Manuelle Medizin, 2*:17-26, 1980.
2. Doran, D.M.L. and Newell, D.J.: Manipulation in Treatment of Low Back Pain: A Multicenter Study. *British Medical Journal, 2*:161-164, 1975.
3. Evans, D.P., Burke, M.S., Lloyd, K.N., Roberts, E.E. and Roberts, G.M.: Lumbar spinal manipulation on trial part K — Clinical assessment. *Rheumatology and Rehabilitation, 17*:46-53, 1978.
4. Glover, J.R., Morris, J.G. and Khosla, T.: Back pain: a randomized clinical trial of rotational manipulation of the trunk. *British Journal of Industrial Medicine, 31*:59-64, 1974.
5. McGill, C.M.: Industrial back problems: A control program. *Journal of Occupational Medicine, 10*:174-178, 1968.
6. Rasmussen, G.G.: Manipulation in treatment of low back pain — A randomized clinical trial. *Manuelle Medizine, 1*:8-10, 1979.
7. Sloop, P.R., Smith, D.S., Goldenberg, E. and Dore, C.: Manipulation for chronic neck pain, a double-blind controlled study. *Spine, 7*:532-535, 1982.

CHAPTER THIRTEEN

THE SELECTION AND TREATMENT OF PATIENTS
TO BE INCLUDED IN CLINICAL TRIALS
OF LUMBAR MANIPULATION

M.S. BURKE, M.B., B.Ch.

REPORTS of clinical trials on the effectiveness of manipulation in the treatment of low back pain are limited, although such reports as have been published certainly suggest that, at least in the short term, manipulation is superior to most, if not all, other forms of treatment with which it has been compared. However, it is difficult to find adequate criteria for entry into or exclusion from such a trial except in the report of the trials themselves. These, of course, vary according to the likes and dislikes of the organizers of the trial. This paper is an attempt to provide such data.

Statistics in back pain can be very misleading as so often assessment of the numbers concerned can take into account only special groups, as for example, that of Glover et al (1974), but it has been estimated by some observers that 80% of the population, at some time or other, suffer an attack of back pain. In 1977, a Working Group was set up by the Department of Health and Social Security (Report of the Working Group on Back Pain, Her Majesty's Stationary Office, 1978) in Great Britain. In their report, they stated that while back pain imposes a substantial economic and financial cost to the community, unrecorded sickness and reduced work effectiveness can only be quantified to the vaguest degree, but based on official statistics, they estimate that back pain costs the British community 220 million pounds per annum in lost output alone. Add to this the cost of lost taxes, social security payments, drugs, etc. and the figure obviously becomes very much higher. To put this in perspective, one should multiply these figures by a factor of 4 to give us roughly the equivalent of the cost in the United States. Furthermore, the Working Group claim that the major impact of back pain appears to be experienced by those in the

179

most active years of life, a claim with which I think we would all agree. There are of course many gaps in our knowledge and understanding of the frequency and occurrence of back pain. What is certain, however, is that it is widespread, unpleasant and occasionally serious and that it imposes a considerable burden on society.

Low back pain, of course, is not a disease but a symptom, and may be defined as pain occurring between the level of the inferior angle of the scapula down to and including the sacrum. Many attempts have been made to define the cause of back pain but none that I have seen account for the great variety of symptoms (especially neurological symptoms) which so often occur in association with low back pain. The commonest theories given include facet joint malfunction, disc degeneration, nipping of synovial membrane and ligamentous strain — if I have left out any of your own favorite pet theories, I crave forgiveness. I repeat, not one of these theories, in my opinion, accounts for the variety of symptoms that occur and particularly those of nerve root irritation, which are so often relieved by manipulation. All can explain one or more of the symptoms but none explain them all. Furthermore, I have never been satisifed with the theory that nerve root irritation can be caused by pressure on the nerve as it leaves the spinal column. Surely any movement at the joint, sufficient to produce such an effect would be so great that it would have to show up on x-ray. If, however, we re-examine the problem while looking at the area as a whole, instead of in sections, then perhaps a clearer picture of the basic cause of back pain may emerge. Movement of any facet joint must cause movements of any of the other three facet joints, forming part of the same vertebra, in turn setting up pressure on the intervertebral disc. Furthermore, there will be tension of the ligaments on one side with relaxation of the opposing side. Any malfunction or displacement of ligaments, facet joints in intervertebral disc must inevitably affect all the other parts described and I suggest that we should forget the concept of backache being due to individual areas such as the facet joint and consider backache as being due to a malfunction of the intervertebral joint, that being the sum of all its parts. This concept of the intervertebral joint being the cause of backache would I believe explain the whole range of symptoms, which occur in relation to back pain.

We can now look at the patients who would or would not be suitable for inclusion in a proposed trial. They would consist of ambulant outpatients (male or female) over the age of 18 years, complaining primarily of lower back pain of moderate to severe intensity. The presence of sciatic or femoral root pain in addition to lumbar pain would not exclude entry into the trial. The nature and objects of the trial must of course be explained to the patient and their consent in writing must be obtained. However, there are certain criteria which may be used in the assessment of the suitability (or unsuitability) of patients for entry into such a trial and these criteria may be divided into three groups:

(1) Manipulation is completely contra-indicated,

(2) Manipulation is unlikely to be of value,

(3) Manipulation is likely to be of value.

The first group would include the rheumatoid group of diseases together with any concomitant disease, e.g., severe cardiac or respiratory disease, severe gastro-intestinal disease, liver or renal disease, osteomyelitis, tuberculosis or carcinoma, and to put these groups into perspective, they would comprise probably far less than 10% of all patients presenting with back pain, and whilst some of these *might* benefit from manipulative treatment, I would consider them completely contra-indicated from taking part in a clinical trial. I would add to this group also the pregnant patient with backache. While I do not consider pregnancy a bar to manipulation, it would be unwise to admit them to a clinical trial, not least being the reason that one can never be sure that the patient could complete the trial.

The second group consists of a number of conditions which often present with back pain but again I would exclude them for any trial of manipulation. These include osteoporosis, Scheuermann's disease or osteochondritis, psychiatric conditions, myelographic evidence of disc herniation, central nervous disorders, spinal distortion and a straight leg raising of less than 40°. One further group I would exclude would be anyone who had previously been treated by manipulation, primarily because he would know the type of treatment he is receiving which may affect the opinion of the assessor. Apart from patients who have received previous manipulation, the main reason for the exclusion of these patients from the proposed trial is that they would all respond badly, if at all, to manipulation unless there was the added complication of sudden onset of back pain associated with loss of mobility. These criteria for both exclusion and inclusion into a clinical trial of manipulation in low back pain are comparable with the criteria exhibited in many of the trials that have been performed, for example, Buerger (1980) in a report of a controlled trial of manipulation, gives an almost identical list of criteria as do Coxhead (1981), and Doran and Newell (1975) in their trials. Edwards (1969) however gives a less restricted list while in the trial undertaken by Glover (1974) and associates, he was looking for unilateral pain, apart from the fact that his group of patients were all in acute pain whose symptoms developed while at work and were seen more or less the same day.

Others who have written on controlled clinical trials in manipulation include Jayson (1981) and others, Hoehler (1981)* and others, Maitland (1957) and Stoddard (1960), all of whom give similar reasons for inclusion or exclusion of patients from controlled clinical trials.

These then are the patients presenting with back pain who would be considered unsuitable for entry into a clinical trial. All other patients presenting with back pain of short or long duration could be expected to be admitted. They

---

*Editors Footnote: See footnote to the first page of the paper by D.P. Evans.

would present with symptoms which have been described as acute, chronic or acute on chronic back pain. The pain may be confined to one segment or could spread up the back or radiate into the thighs and could be associated with symptoms of nerve root irritation, for example sciatic or femoral radiation of pain and also associated with paraesthesia and/or numbness. In most, if not all, of these cases, there would be in addition limitation of movement in one or more directions. Naturally a careful assessment of each patient must be undertaken. In this trial, incidentally, and working in close conjunction with Dr. Geraint Roberts (Roberts et al., 1978) of the Radiology Department of the University Medical School in Cardiff, we were able to show that response to treatment cannot be assessed radiologically either before or after treatment, so that while radiological assessment may be necessary prior to manipulation, especially for medico-legal reasons, there would appear to be no point in continual radiological assessment of such patients.

I have already said that in the selection of patients, they would show some degree of limitation of movement in one or more directions. Such restricted mobility at one point will call for increased mobility elsewhere and will also produce compensatory problems—a point to which I will return shortly. There is, of course, nothing new about manipulative treatment for back pain. If it is true that all medicine started with Hippocrates, then manipulation is no exception as Schiotz and Cyriax (1975) show in their book on the history of manipulation.

Manipulation can be divided into three main commonly used methods of treatment, namely, osteopathic, chiropractic and vertebral manipulation, the latter first described by Maitland (1977). Although often thought of by their advocates as separate and distinct methods of treatment, and indeed the first two have at times been thought of as different types of medicine, they are all in my opinion methods of manipulation and are or should be complementary to each other. In our own clinical trial, we described our technique as being a rotational-thrust with distraction. This, of course, tends towards the long-lever type of movement of the osteopath as opposed to the direct thrust of the chiropractioner. Vertebral manipulation consists of repetitive gentle oscillatory movements within the normal range of movement. However, in any clinical trial, I would suggest that any or all of these types of treatment may be used, that is, one should use the treatment most suited to a patient, remembering that it is manipulation that is on trial, not a particular category. Alternatively, any clinical trial set up could include osteopathy or chiropractice as separate entities, enabling them to be compared with each other as well as comparing them with any alternative method of treatment selected.

I have some doubts, however, of the value of oscillatory manipulation *a la* Maitland in the complete relief of pain. I believe it to be of some value in the patient with acute symptoms, but, at least in my hands, I have never been able to achieve the relief that a rotational thrust so often gives.

I have already referred to the fact that any patient with back pain is likely to set up compensatory changes elsewhere in the spine and such areas are, of course, a potential source of pain. For this reason, I always examine and, if necessary, treat the whole spine, not just the part of which the patient complains. It is surprising how often this helps to give complete and lasting relief.

These, then, are the criteria for inclusion into a trial of manipulation and the treatments available, but one further aspect should be considered and that is the length of the trial and the number of treatments to be given. Obviously, these will vary with the design of the trial and the individual patient but we found that in general, two treatments at one week's interval were sufficient. Our own trial (Evans et al., 1978, Roberts et al., 1978) was based on three weeks each of manipulation and placebo, but we found this to be unnecessarily long and we now believe that two visits at one week's interval would be sufficient to give results which would be adequate to assess the value of the manipulative techniques we used. There would of course be the need for follow-up assessments, although most trials that have been conducted tend to show that there is little difference between the different forms of treatment for back pain by the end of approximately three months.

Before finally concluding, may I digress somewhat from the main theme of the validation of manipulation in the treatment of low back pain. In fact, although the emphasis has been on low back pain, there is nothing in the title of this volume to suggest why this should be. If, in fact, we want to prove the value of manipulation, then I would suggest that a clinical trial of manipulation in the treatment of pain of cervical origin would be much easier to establish. Furthermore, it would provide two additional values:

(1) The problem of setting up a valid trial of manipulation is that of finding a suitable alternative treatment with which to compare it. In the treatment of pain of cervical origin, however, there is a ready-made alternative and well established treatment, that of using a cervical collar, and the provision of a protocol comparing manipulation with the wearing of such a collar; for example, two weeks should not present any real difficulty.

(2) There is also the added advantage of using either still or cine x-rays. I have been told by experts in the field that apart from the fact that no vital parts are subjected to radiation, the actual amount of radiation exposure of the cervical spine is far less than at the lumbar spine. It is therefore considered safe to use either cine x-rays or still x-rays before and after manipulation to show the difference in range of movement achieved by this method of treatment.

In conclusion, then, I consider that this would be a viable alternative method of validating the use of manipulation in back pain.

REFERENCES

Buerger, A.A.: A controlled trial of rotational manipulation in low back pain. *Manuelle Medizin, 2*:17-26, 1980.

Coxhead, C.E., Inskip, H., Mead, T.W., North, W.R.S., and Troup, J.D.G.: Multicentre trial of physiotherapy in the management of sciatic symptoms. *Lancet, 1*:1065-1068, 1981.

Doran, E.M.L. and Newell, D.J.: Manipulation in the treatment of low back pain: A multicentre study. *British Medical Journal, 2*:161-164, April 26, 1975.

Edwards, B.C.: Low back pain and pain resulting from lumbar spine conditions: A comparison of treatment results. *Australian Journal of Physiotherapy, 14*:104-110, 1969.

Evans, E.P., Burke, M.S., Lloyd, K.N., Roberts, E.E., and Roberts, C.M.: Lumbar spinal manipulation on trial: Part I — Clinical Assessment. *Rheumatology and Rehabilitation, 17*:46-53, 1978.

Glover, J.R., Morris, J.G., and Khosla, T.: Back Pain: A randomized clinical trial of rotational manipulation of the trunk. *British Journal of Industrial Medicine, 31*:59-64, 1974.

Greenland, S., Reisbord, L.S., Haldeman, S., and Buerger, A.A.: Controlled trials of manipulation: A review and a proposal. *Journal of Occupational Medicine, 22*:670-676, 1980.

Hoehler, F.K., Tobis, J.S., and Buerger, A.A.: Spinal manipulation for low back pain. *Journal of the American Medical Association, 245*:1835-39, 1981.

Jayson, M.I.V., Sims-Williams, H., Young, S., Baddeley, H., and Collins, E.: Mobilization and manipulation for low back pain. *Spine, 6*:409-416, 1981.

Maitland, G.D.: Low back pain and allied symptoms and treatment results. *The Medical Journal of Australia, 44*:851-854, 1957.

Maitland, G.D.: *Vertebral Manipulation (4th ed.).* London and Boston, Butterworths, 1977.

Report of the Working Group on Back Pain. Issued by Her Majesty's Stationery Office, 1978.

Roberts, G.M., Roberts, E.E., Lloyd, K.N., Burke, M.S., and Evans, D.P.: Lumbar spinal manipulation on trial, Part II — Radiological Assessment. *Rheumatology and Rehabilitation, 17*:54-59, 1978.

Schiotz, E.H. and Cyriax, J.: *Manipulation: Past & Present.* London, William Heinemann, 1975.

Stoddard, A.: Manipulation for low backache. *Rheumatism, 16*:20-24, January 1960.

CHAPTER FOURTEEN

CONTROLLED TRIALS OF MOBILIZATION AND MANIPULATION FOR GENERAL PRACTITIONER AND HOSPITAL PATIENTS

S.M.S. YOUNG, M.C.S.P.

THE work presented was carried out in Bristol in collaboration with two rheumatologists—Malcolm Jayson and Heather Sims-Williams; a radiologist—Hiram Baddeley; and a statistician—Elizabeth Collins. Much of this research has been published previously (Sims-Williams et al., 1978, 1979; Jayson et al., 1981).

Two classes of patients were assessed. In the first class there were 94 patients referred from their general practitioners; and in the second class there were 94 patients referred from hospital orthopaedic and rheumatology clinics. The patients were aged 20-65 years. They were patients with non-specific lumbar pain (although many of these had referred symptoms, including some with true sciatic radiation and therefore were not comparable with those who only had back pain). The patients were required to attend for treatment daily for one week, then 3 times a week until they were symptom free or had completed 12 treatments.

Exclusions from the trial were:

(1) gross psychological disturbances,
(2) pregnancy,
(3) previous spinal surgery,
(4) inflammatory or other specific disorders of the spine such as ankylosing spondylitis, Paget's disease, vertebral collapse, bladder or bowel disturbance, muscle wasting,
(5) any other medical disorder that might contra-indicate the forms of treatment used, and
(6) if it was thought that mobilization should not be the first choice of treat-

ment, i.e., those who required re-education for postural problems.

Both classes participated in a double-blind controlled trial comparing mobilization with placebo physiotherapy. Treatment in detail is described later.

Initial assessment was carried out by a rheumatologist who also assessed the patients blind after one month of treatment, again two months later and finally by postal questionnaire after one year. Patients who failed to answer the questionnaire were visited at home.

Subjective assessments were made of:

(1) pain,
(2) return to normal activity,
(3) opinions of the value of treatment, and
(4) the need for further treatment.

Objective measurements were made of spinal mobility and straight leg raising.

Table XIV-1

PATIENTS ASSESSMENT OF PAIN AT 1 MONTH

	IMPROVED	NOT IMPROVED
Group I (Treatment)	39 (29)	4 (18)
Group II (Control)	32 (25)	12 (18)

PATIENTS ASSESSMENT OF ACTIVITY AT 1 MONTH

	NORMAL WORK	LIGHT WORK	UNABLE TO WORK
Group I (Treatment)	22 (19)	16 (14)	5 (13)
Group II (Control)	19 (20)	11 (8)	14 (15)

PATIENTS ASSESSMENT OF TREATMENT AT 1 MONTH

	HELPED	NOT HELPED
Group I (Treatment)	38 (36)	5 (12)
Group II (Control)	31 (28)	13 (16)

Assessments one month after exposure to either mobilization sometimes with manipulation (Group 1) or microwave at its lowest setting (Group 2). The first number is that for general practice patients, the second number in parentheses is that for hospital patients. See text for details.

Eighty-seven patients attended the one month follow-up from the general practitioner group, and 92 from the hospital group (Table XIV-1). In the general practitioner series, the treated patients showed a slightly better improvement than the controls. In the hospital series they both showed some improvement, though in each group there was a higher number who found the control useless.

Two months later, 83 of the General Practitioner and 82 of the hospital patients were reassessed and the results were fairly similar except that in the general practitioner series those in the treatment group thought that they had gained more benefit than those in the control group (Table XIV-2).

Table XIV-2

PATIENTS ASSESSMENT OF PAIN AT 3 MONTHS

	IMPROVED	NOT IMPROVED
Group I (Treatment)	26 (28)	14 (14)
Group II (Control)	22 (27)	21 (13)

PATIENTS ASSESSMENT OF ACTIVITY AT 3 MONTHS

	NORMAL WORK	LIGHT WORK	UNABLE TO WORK
Group I (Treatment)	25 (26)	9 (8)	5 (8)
Group II (Control)	19 (23)	13 (10)	11 (7)

PATIENTS ASSESSMENT OF TREATMENT AT 3 MONTHS

	HELPED	NOT HELPED
Group I (Treatment)	38 (36)	5 (12)
Group II (Control)	31 (28)	13 (16)

Assessments as in Table XIV-1 except at 3 months.

At one year information was obtained from 90 of the general practitioner patients and 80 of the hospital patients. The majority of patients in both groups showed some improvement (Table XIV-3).

PHYSIOTHERAPY

A. Mobilization and Manipulation

The area of pain was recorded on a body chart indicating areas of greatest intensity and whether the symptoms were constant or intermittent, the type of pain and whether there was any paraesthesia or anaesthesia.

The subjective examination included careful questioning on the behavior of symptoms: how they were aggravated or eased, how they were during the night or with particular activities such as sitting, coughing, etc.

Special questions were asked to eliminate any dangers associated with treatment such as cauda equina involvement, malignancy, etc. These questions are mandatory to this approach despite the fact that the patient has already been seen by a doctor because there could be a change in symptoms even in a few days. A detailed history is then taken of the onset of the present attack: how the pain has altered since the initial onset and whether at the time of examination the symptoms are getting better, worse, or remaining unchanged. This is followed by questions on the past history to establish the first attack in detail and then a brief account of subsequent attacks, noticing particularly how frequently they occur, how readily they settle, how they are brought on and whether the patient has had any previous physiotherapy, and whether it was helpful and finally whether the pain was the same or different in any previous attack. These are all factors which will help guide the choice of treatment technique and the likely effect of treatment and whether one should be prepared to change treatment techniques quickly or not.

This is followed by an objective examination of the patient, noticing their posture, and testing the standard active movements of flexion, extension, lateral flexion and rotation, noticing not only the range of movement but also the behavior of pain during movement. This will be retested after treatment and it

Table XIV-3

1 YEAR FOLLOW UP

	BETTER		SAME		WORSE	
Group I (Treatment)	30	(15)	11	(15)	4	(9)
Group II (Control)	28	(29)	12	(9)	5	(3)

PHYSICAL ACTIVITY LIMITED BY BACK AT 1 YEAR						
	NOT AT ALL		SLIGHTLY		SERIOUSLY	
Group I (Treatment)	13	(6)	23	(23)	9	(10)
Group II (Control)	10	(5)	29	(27)	5	(9)

PATIENTS OPINION OF TREATMENT AT 1 YEAR						
	LASTING VALUE		HELPED AT THE TIME		NO VALUE	
Group I (Treatment)	13	(5)	21	(26)	11	(8)
Group II (Control)	11	(14)	30	(17)	4	(8)

Assessments at 1 year; see Table XIV-1 and text for details.

may be found that the range remains unchanged but the pain may not radiate so far, thus indicating some improvement. The quality of movement is important, i.e. does the movement occur uniformly throughout the lumbar spine or is there an area which remains stiff? Routine tests of passive neck flexion, straight leg raising and sacroiliac compression and distraction are carried out as well as neurological testing and a brief examination of hip joints when relevant.

Palpation is a very important aspect of the examination. With the patient lying prone, the vertebrae are palpated for position and any para-vertebral thickening or spasm. The accessory movements at each level are then tested by means of oscillatory pressures over each spinous process noticing the relationship of pain and range with postero-anterio central vertebral pressures, i.e. whether one can palpate to the end of range and, if not, how far in one direction one can go and at the same time where this causes pain and whether it is the same as the presenting pain. Where there are no limiting factors such as pain or spasm, one can determine the "end-feel" of the movement. Unilateral and transverse pressures are also used to test each level. In some cases a particular level may appear stiffer rather than painful but one always needs to see whether the palpation findings are comparable and compatible with the patient's area of pain so that treatment is directed to the correct level(s). Tenderness on its own can be misleading.

Each time the patient attends, a subjective assessment is made not only of how the patient feels but whether the pain still radiates so far, whether it is still constant, etc. Then the most significant of the movements is checked and the pain range relationship is recorded. They are then assessed following each mobilization technique as only in this way can one determine whether to continue, stop or change. As patients do not always notice small percentages of improvement, it is very important for the physiotherapist to notice these. Patients should be treated daily for the first week and then three times a week until they have completed twelve treatments, or discontinue sooner if symptoms disappear. By treating patients daily initially, it is easier to notice slight improvement. If the patient comes back feeling worse, it is important to question them carefully to find out why they are worse. It may be that the treatment was too vigorous but it may also be that the patient was better for several hours until doing some strenuous activity such as gardening. If the treatment had helped initially it would be worth continuing with the same technique.

The main techniques used were derived from Maitland (1977) and were in the form of rotation, postero-anterior central vertebral pressures (accessory movements) or traction which was used as sustained or intermittent treatment depending on the symptoms using a friction free traction bed (Figure XIV-1).

Sometimes manipulation was used. Although this term can be synonymous with mobilization, it is used here to indicate a small amplitude high velocity thrust.

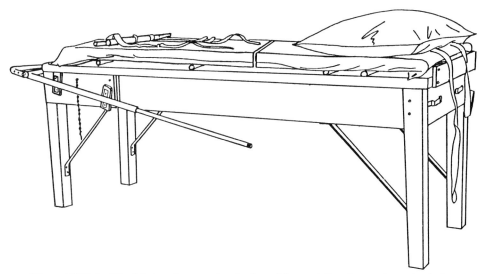

Figure XIV-1. The friction free traction bed used for mobilization and manipulation.

Active exercises were occasionally used to maintain the range gained but were never used in the first instance until the effect of mobilization had been evaluated. Abdominal exercises were considered important and were given where necessary. Posture correction and lifting advice were also given as necessary.

B. Minimal Microwave

For the control group the same method of examination was used including the same assessment before each treatment. These patients were given microwave on its lowest setting. The patients were told that they were receiving a special heat treatment. They were treated lying prone unless their pain was made worse in that position. The machine was switched on and the output control was kept at minimal. They were treated for 15 minutes. When they asked what the treatment was doing (because they could not feel anything) they were told that heat is a form of pain relief and that the machine was a method of giving heat.

SUMMARY

There is a definite need for more research in this area. I can see many limitations in this trial which I would like to put forward in the hope that this will be of some help in future research. The trial was started in 1975 and therefore with a further eight years experience there are many things that I would now do differently.

Examination procedure could have been more precise leading to a greater accuracy in treatment. I was too cautious initially and sometimes overlooked the importance of stiffness. It is sometimes necessary to go into the painful range when using thumb pressure techniques and with careful questioning the pain gradually recedes and one can go in more deeply and therefore obtain a quicker result.

At that stage there was very little research done by physiotherapists and I was lacking in guidance in how to go about it.

Although the title was Back Pain, many of the patients had referred symptoms as well as true sciatic radiation which means that they were not a totally comparable group.

There was too wide an age range for true comparison.

Are we defeating our own ends in assessing the value of treatment in non-specific pain? Should we now try and find a category which does respond so that treatment can be given where applicable and not waste time where it is not, because we already know that there are many patients who are less likely to respond?

How does one compare return to normal activity in such widely differing groups as manual workers and sedentary workers? What is improvement? If some patients are sufficiently better to return to work after one month rather than lose their job, does this not mean that something has been achieved?

Those with a history of pain of less than one month duration usually did better than those with a history of longer than one month. Does this indicate that we should treat patients earlier — though not too early before spontaneous recovery has taken place.

CONCLUSION

In conclusion, this trial shows that mobilization is of some benefit in patients with non-specific back pain. I feel that there are changes that could be made in the approach that could make future trials more penetrating and therefore more worthwhile. It is very important that any trial must be a controlled trial.

Although spontaneous resolution is common there is a need for further longer trials and tighter definition of diagnostic sub-groups. However, from this trial it appears that many patients will recover without treatment but that there are still a great many who will be helped by the right treatment given at a fairly early stage in their problem. No two patients are identical which makes direct comparisons very difficult.

REFERENCES

Jayson, M.I.V., Sims-Williams, H., Young, S., Baddeley, H., Collins, E.: Mobilization and manipulation for low-back pain. *Spine,* 6:409-416, 1981.

Maitland, G.D.: *Vertebral Manipulation*, 4th ed., London, Butterworths. 1977.

Sims-Williams, H.L., Jayson, M.I.V., Young, S.M.S., Baddeley, H., Collins, E.: Controlled trial of mobilization and manipulation for patients with low back pain in general practice. *British Medical Journal, 2*:1338-1340, 1978.

Sims-Williams, H.L., Jayson, M.I.V., Young, S.M.S., Baddeley, H., Collins, E.: Controlled trial of mobilization and manipulation for low back pain: Hospital patients. *British Medical Journal, 2*:1318-1320, 1979.

CHAPTER FIFTEEN

A "DOUBLE-BLIND" RANDOMIZED CLINICAL TRIAL OF ROTATIONAL MANIPULATION FOR LOW BACK PAIN

A.A. BUERGER, Ph.D.

INTRODUCTION

PAIN is the most common presenting complaint for all clinicians. However, it is an unreliable diagnostic tool. Hence the reasons why a patient hurts can be a subject of endless clinical debate. The discussions can be especially confusing when the clinicians involved do not share common terminologies and/or training. This difficulty is especially clear in the study of back pain when its diagnosis by palpation and its treatment by manual means are being discussed.

Consider the following clinical problem:

A patient expressed pain on palpation but the pain appeared to move from place to place. However, the pain could occasionally be relieved by careful manual treatment(s).

You may have been thinking that I was describing back pain, but in fact, I was describing appendicitis or "ileitis" as it was then usually called from the point of view of a physician somewhere between 1650 and 1900. The exact date would depend on the physician.

From a more modern perspective, as demonstrated by the excellent book on the diagnosis of the acute abdomen by Sir Zachary Cope (1968), pain due to the appendix tends to start in the region immediately above the umbilicus and to migrate to the lower right quadrant, where palpable rebound tenderness is common. As we all know, with the advent of general anesthesia, appendicitis has become a clearly recognizable and treatable entity. However the kinds of debates that we are currently experiencing concerning back pain are very similar to those that took place concerning appendicitis between approximately 1600 and 1850. For example, appendicitis was ascribed to an inflamed caecum by many physicians for at least 150 years and the exact location of the various placements of the appendix caused almost endless debate (Deaver, 1914; De-Moulin, 1975; Meade, 1963). The book by Deaver (1914) and the paper by DeMoulin (1975) are especially useful in following the debate concerning "ileitis".

Given the fact that there are severe differences of clinical opinion concerning back pain, the randomized clinical trial is probably the most efficient mechanism for distinguishing differences between two or more treatments. However, it is interesting to note that the problem of "ileitis" was settled without any clinical trial being conducted, at least according to a computer search by the National Library of Medicine, including its historical archives.

At the present time, the weight of the evidence from randomized clinical trials suggests that patients with relatively "acute" problems are helped. The weight of the evidence for patients with more "chronic" problems is still unproven; furthermore this problem appears not to have been examined in a randomized clinical trial. In the light of these comments, I will now discuss a randomized clinical trial which was carried out at the California College of Medicine, associated with the University of California, Irvine. Some results of this trial have been published elsewhere, e.g., Buerger, (1980, 1981), Hoehler et al. (1981), and Hoehler and Tobis (1982).

STUDY DESIGN

Figure XV-1 is a flow chart of the organization of this trial. Patients were drawn from the out-patient clinic pool at the University of California, Irvine, Medical Center. They were given x-ray examinations for obvious radiographic diagnoses. They were assessed by a screening manipulator and then split into one of three groups; that is patients were:

  (1) accepted into the study (this group will be described in more detail subsequently);
  (2) treated by manipulation *but were not accepted* into the study, or;
  (3) referred elsewhere.

Patients who were accepted into the study were randomly divided into two groups. One group received rotational manipulation of the lumbosacral spine and whatever additional manual treatment(s) the manipulator treating these patients felt was required. These treating manipulators were always different physicians than the screening manipulator who selected the patients for treatment and who re-evaluated them at the end of the study.

The other randomly selected portion of this group received soft-tissue massage from one of the same treating manipulators mentioned above. Some

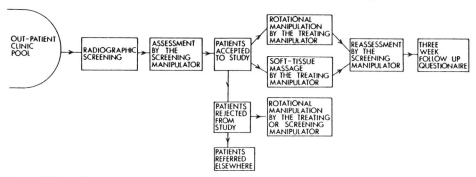

Figure XV-1. Flow chart of the progress of patients through the Back Clinic and through the double-blind clinical trial. Note that comparisons can be made not only between rotationally manipulated and soft-tissue massaged patients but also between these patients and the less ideal patients rejected from this study but given both rotational manipulation and soft-tissue massage (from Buerger, 1980).

details of these treatments and their effects can be obtained from previous publications (Buerger, 1980; Buerger, 1981; Hoehler et al., 1981; Hoehler and Tobis, 1982). After the treating manipulators felt that treatment had been successful, these patients were re-assessed by the screening manipulator. Also, in an attempt to equalize the typical duration of treatment in the two groups, the members of the control group with whom this member of the experimental group was originally "matched" was also referred to the screening manipulator. However, as will be shown later, this attempt was not particularly successful. After this reassessment there was a follow-up by questionnaire in three weeks. However, patient compliance with answering this questionnaire was not particularly successful.

It is important to note that the number of patients who were actually included in the study was a very small percentage of the total clinic census.

Figure XV-2 shows the data for a typical year. The total census determined from billing activity is represented by T. The total census determined from the number of forms filled out within the back clinic is represented by F. The total number of patients reported manipulated within the clinic is represented by M and the total number of patients involved in the study is represented by S. It is obvious that the percentage of study patients is quite small. The percentage of patients involved in the study at the University of California, Irvine, is approximately 5%. It is my feeling that most of these patients would be termed "acute" by most osteopathic manipulators, but this is not provable.

RESULTS

There have been several concerns expressed about the kinds of patients who are susceptible to manipulation. One of those is that they have some psychological deviation from the norm.

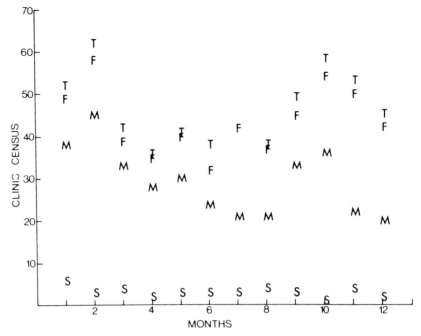

Figure XV-2. The clinic census by month in a typical year. T indicates the total census; M, the number of manipulated patients and S, the patients included in the study (from Buerger, 1981).

Figure XV-3 shows the results of a Mini-Mult examination which was ad-ministered to almost all manipulated and un-manipulated study patients and many other manipulated patients. It is compared to other medical patients. The means are very close together and the standard deviations overlap on every portion of the Mini-Mult scale. The results clearly suggest that there were no sizable psychological differences between the manipulated patients, the study patients and other medical patients.

One difference that did appear in the study at the University of California, Irvine, was that the study patients tended to be significantly *younger* than the non-study patients. Figure XV-4 shows a histogram by decade of the non-study patients and the study patients. As you can see, the difference between the distributions is significant, at well over the 0.5 level.

For this reason and others, we decided to adopt an unusual procedure for comparing the study and non-study groups. We constructed a computer pro-gram which selected from the original randomized patients matched pairs of patients who were comparable for age, number of treatments, and duration of treatment. I am still not sure if this was a valid approach, but a significant dif-ference between the *originally randomized patients* and the subsequently *matched pairs* suggests very strongly that rotational manipulation has a different effect than soft tissue massage.

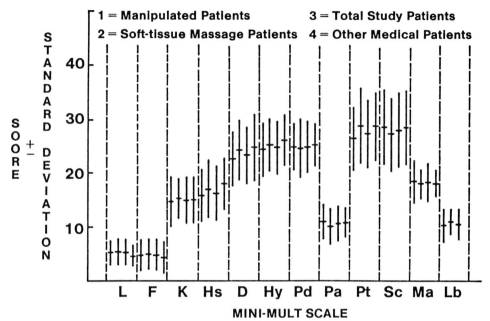

Figure XV-3. The mean and standard deviation of the various scales of the Mini-Mult and the Low Back Scale (Lb) for the rotationally manipulated and the soft-tissue massaged study patients, as well as for a previously published sample of other medical patients (from Buerger, 1980).

Figure XV-5 shows the comparison for patient age. As will be true of the following few figures, the original random pairs are shown on the right hand side. The difference between the matched pairs is the greatest for age among the three variables for which they were matched. As you can see, even in this case, ages for the matched pairs were remarkably close.

As Figure XV-6 shows, for the original random pairs, there was a very large difference in the distribution of the duration of treatment. However, for the matched pairs this difference was markedly diminished. In fact, the means and standard deviations were essentially identical.

And as Figure XV-7 shows, there was a somewhat worrisome difference in the number of treatments for the original random pairs, but for the matched pairs there was essentially no difference.

Unfortunately, the only results of the study were *subjective*; that is, they were based on questions such as those shown in the following figures.

The patients were asked:

"Can you do any of the following more easily or better after today's back clinic treatment?

- walking,
- bending or twisting,
- reaching,

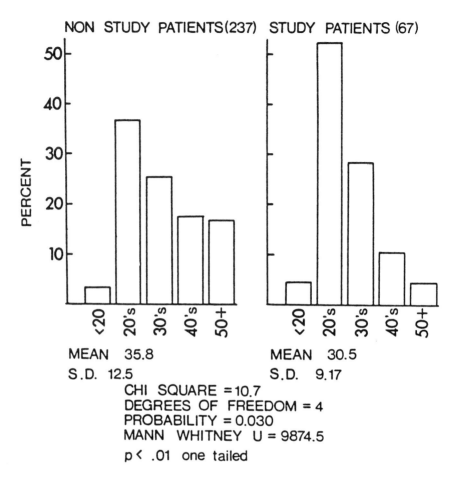

Figure XV-4. The age distributions by decade of the study and non-study patients (from Buerger, 1981).

- sitting down or getting up from a chair,
- sitting up from a lying position as in bed,
- dressing or
- other"

and the possible answers were

"1) yes

2) no change;

3) no worse."

The lower part of Figure XV-8 shows the responses for bending or twisting. As you can see for both the original random pairs and the matched pairs, these differences are significant at least at the .05 level.

This data suggests the rotational manipulation and the other forms of

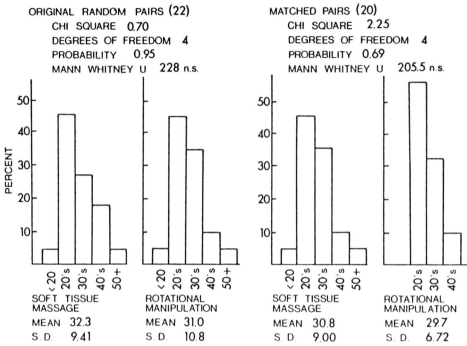

Figure XV-5. The age distributions by decade of the "original random pairs" and the "matched pairs." See text for details (from Buerger, 1981).

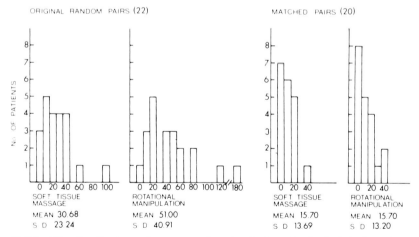

Figure XV-6. The distributions of treatment duration in days for the "original random pairs" and the "matched pairs" (from Buerger, 1981).

manipulative treatment which were delivered to these patients did improve the patients' impressions of their ability to bend or twist.

In addition, Figure XV-9 suggests that these patient's ability to sit down or get up from a chair was improved because both of these differences were

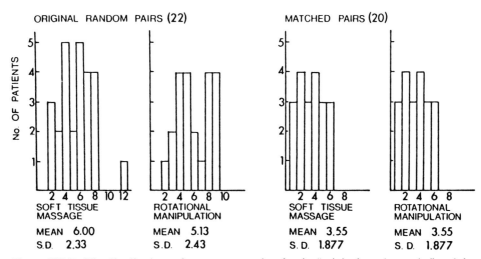

Figure XV-7. The distributions of treatment number for the "original random pairs" and the "matched pairs" (from Buerger, 1981).

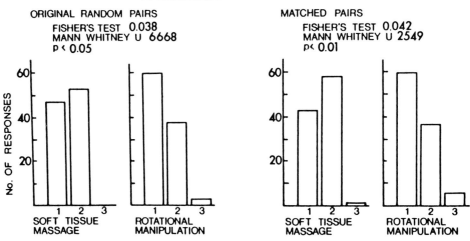

Figure XV-8. The effects of manipulation upon patients' reports of their ability to bend or twist. See text for details (from Buerger, 1981).

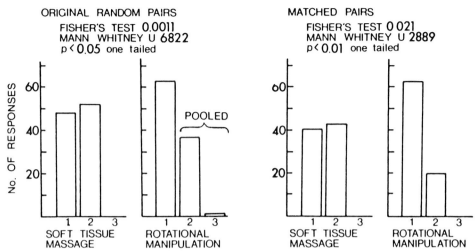

Figure XV-9. The effects of manipulation upon patients' reports of their ability to sit down or get up from a chair (from Buerger, 1981).

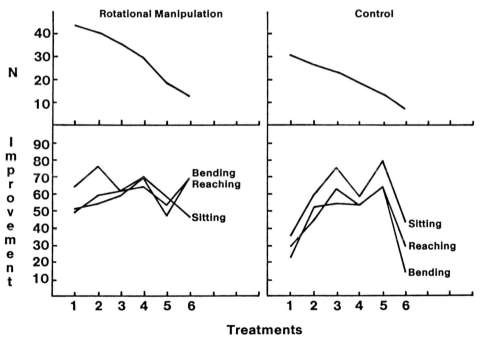

Figure XV-10. The effect of treatment number upon patient number (N) and upon patients' reports of the effects of manipulation upon their ability to bend, reach and sit. See text for details (from Buerger, 1981).

significant at the point of .05 level.

However, the situation is much more complicated than has been suggested in the previous figures. For example, if you plot the number of treatments versus the patients' impression of improvements, not only does the number of patients fall for both groups but it is also clear that the effective difference between the rotational manipulation group and the sham-message group appears to occur within the first two or three treatments (Figure XV-10). The reasons for these differences are unclear, especially because the number of patients falls markedly with increasing treatment number.

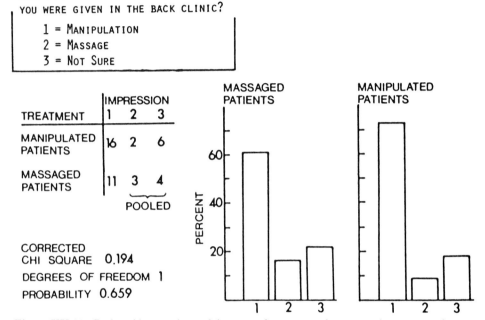

Figure XV-11. Patients' impressions of the type of treatment they were given versus the type they actually received for the massaged control group and the manipulated experimental group (from Buerger, 1981).

Figure XV-11 raises an important but confusing point. When one is dealing with a treatment which is delivered by a pill, it is possible to achieve four levels of blinding in a randomized clinical trial; that is, one can arrange things such that:

(1) the patients may not know what treatment they received,
(2) the evaluating clinicians may not know what treatment the patients received,
(3) the treating clinicians (that is, the deliverer of the pill) may not know what treatments the patients received, and finally
(4) the re-evaluating clinicians (that is, the clinician appraising the effects of treatment) may not know what treatment the patients received.

However, when you are dealing with a treatment such as surgery or any other manual procedure such as manipulation of the back, it is obviously impossible to arrange the design such that the treating clinician does not know what treatment the patient has received. Hence the maximum number of blindings that one can achieve in such a situation is 3, i.e.:

(1) the patients may not know what treatment they received,
(2) the evaluating or screening clinicians may not know what treatment the patients received and
(3) the re-evaluating clinicians may not know what treatment the patients have received.

There has been some discussion as to whether it is possible to arrange a clinical trial design of manipulation in which the patient did not know what treatment they received. As shown in Figure XV-11, after patients had completed the experiment at the University of California, Irvine, they were asked, as shown in the upper left hand corner:

"Which form of treatment you feel you were given in the back clinic:

(1) manipulation,
(2) massage,
(3) not sure."

There was no statistically significant difference between the massaged patients and the manipulated patients. It is possible that if the number of patients who have been asked these questions had been large, a difference might have emerged. But at least at this point it is theoretically possible to construct an experimental design which is blind to three out of these four possibilities.

One other point, which may be even more important, is the question: Can an experienced manipulator predict whether an individual patient will respond to manipulation?

Figure XV-12 shows a comparison between two questions; the first question was asked of the screening manipulator. It was:

"How good a candidate is this patient for manipulation?

A) very good;
B) good;
C) fair;
D) poor."

The second question was asked of patients after each of their treatments. It was:

"How does your present back pain or discomfort compare with the way you felt before you saw the doctor today?

1) much better;
2) somewhat better;
3) no change;
4) somewhat worse;
5) much worse."

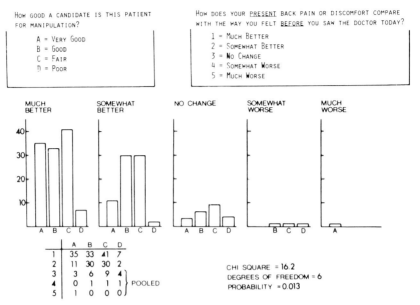

Figure XV-12. Histograms and table showing the relation between (1) the screening manipulator's prediction of a patient's susceptibility to successful manipulative treatment and (2) the patient's impression of the effects of manipulative treatment (from Buerger, 1981).

Those patients who were rated very good or good or reported much better effects of treatment than the patients rated as fair or poor candidates for manipulation, and an appropriate Chi square test on this data is significant above the 0.05 level.

This effect is even more strongly shown when the predicted effect of treatment is plotted against patients' responses on the sitting and bending and reaching questions defined earlier (Figure XV-13). It appears that not only were the responses to the sitting, bending and reaching questions better for patients rated very good or good, but also the responses of patients fair and poor were somewhat more erratic. Furthermore, the effect is strongest during the early treatments. The effect is even more strongly shown when treatments are plotted against patients' responses to the sitting and bending and reaching questions which were described above. It again appears that not only are the responses to the sitting, bending and reaching questions better for patients rated good and very good, but also the responses of patients graded fair and poor are somewhat more erratic.

DISCUSSION AND CONCLUSION

As this and the related papers published in this volume show, the randomized clinical trial is a useful tool for investigating the effects of manipula-

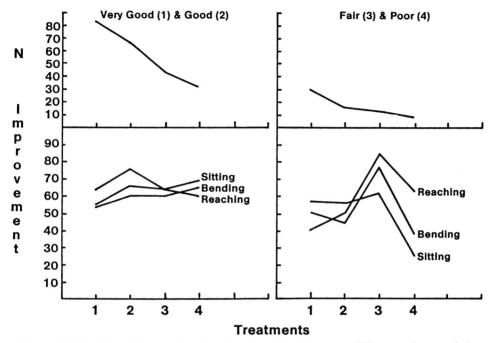

Figure XV-13. Plots of the number of patients receiving treatment (N) versus the cumulative number of treatments and the patients' perception of improvements in bending, sitting, and reaching for the rotationally manipulated patients rated as very good or good candidates for manipulation on the left side and patients rated as fair or poor candidates for manipulation on the right side (from Buerger, 1981).

tion upon back pain. Unfortunately, the bulk of the data concerning the effects of manipulation on back pain is *subjective*. A concerted effort to develop consistent objective measures of the effects of manipulation on back pain is necessary; unfortunately this effort is likely to be complex and frustrating, but it must be made.

A problem with most 'objective' tests relevant to low back pain is that they retain a considerable element of subjectivity. This is partially due to the fact that (a) thepatient must determine the criteria for 'maximal' effort or motion (e.g., active tests of strength or mobility), (b) the patient must determine the criteria for 'pain' (e.g., passive tests of mobility) or (c) the physician must assess subtle palpatory cues (e.g., the straight leg raising test of hamstring tightness).

An example of the frustration which can accompany an effort to find objective signs diagnostic of a manipulable lesion and/or changeable by manual means is shown in Table XV-1. Several "quasi-objective" measures which have been widely regarded to be related to the diagnosis and treatment of low back pain are listed (Hoehler and Tobis, 1982). This data was collected from the same clinic and from essentially the same patient population as the study presented above.

As stated by my former colleagues, their "study investigated several possible quasi-objective measures of low back pain, and attempted to answer the following questions: (1) Do the measures distinguish subjects with low back pain from subjects without low back pain? (2) Can the measures be obtained reliably by separate examiners? (3) Are the measures systematically affected by time or testing? (4) Can the measure be used to predict the results of spinal manipulation? (5) Can the measures be used to assess the effects of spinal manipulation?"

Table XV - 1

"Quasi-Objective" Measures of Low Back Pain
and the
Effects of Manipulation

	Patients with and without Low Back Pain (Means ± Standard Deviations)			Reliability			Before and After Treatment (Means ± Standard Deviations)		
	With low back pain	Without low back pain	t	Mean absolute error (degrees or cm)	Standard score of absolute error	r	Pretreatment	Post-treatment	t
Number of subjects	19	8					11	11	
Percentage of males	42	63							
Age (years)	32 ± 10	27 ± 4	1.41						
Tests of flexibility:									
Anterior flexion (cm)	5.5 ± 1.8	7.8 ± 2.5	2.70*	1.7	0.66	0.50**	6.8 ± 1.4	7.1 ± 1.5	0.55
Lateral flexion	23 ± 8	30 ± 11	1.83	5.6	0.55	0.71**	25 ± 9	26 ± 9	0.38
Hamstring tightness	56 ± 10	61 ± 6	1.18	9.0	0.97	0.36*	52 ± 8	57 ± 10	3.95**
Passive SLR	65 ± 15	77 ± 7	2.29*	8.0	0.52	0.78**	69 ± 10	74 ± 10	3.69**
Voluntary SLR	63 ± 21	79 ± 7	2.20*	4.7	0.24	0.95**	69 ± 13	73 ± 12	3.59**
Foot eversion	45 ± 11	44 ± 18	0.17	9.9	0.77	0.63**	50 ± 9	50 ± 11	0.08
Tests of asymmetry:									
Lateral flexion	3.7 ± 2.7	3.4 ± 2.4	0.31	4.4	0.78	0.23	5.0 ± 3.7	6.5 ± 7.5	0.52
Hamstring tightness	3.0 ± 3.0	2.1 ± 1.3	0.76	3.4	0.67	-0.04	5.0 ± 3.1	3.1 ± 2.8	1.56
Passive SLR to pain	4.8 ± 2.8	3.5 ± 2.5	1.19	6.0	0.99	0.32	8.4 ± 5.0	5.9 ± 6.0	1.85
Active SLR to pain	4.5 ± 6.0	4.0 ± 6.2	0.19	3.5	0.41	0.44*	6.3 ± 4.2	2.3 ± 2.1	3.35**
Foot eversion	6.9 ± 4.4	3.3 ± 2.9	2.15*	5.0	0.63	0.38*	10.4 ± 4.5	10.6 ± 6.9	0.13
Malleolar levels (cm)	0.33 ± 0.31	0.24 ± 0.19	0.71	0.35	0.79	0.33	0.25 ± 0.38	0.06 ± 0.18	1.43
Iliac levels (cm)	1.6 ± 1.3	1.3 ± 1.2	0.74	1.9	0.89	0.37*	2.0 ± 1.9	2.0 ± 1.8	0.00
Scapular levels (cm)	1.8 ± 1.6	2.3 ± 2.6	0.58	2.5	0.91	0.43*	2.6 ± 2.3	2.0 ± 2.1	1.67

Measures are in degrees unless otherwise noted.
*P < 0.05; **P < 0.01.
t is Student's t
r is the Pearson r coefficient of correlation   modified from Hoehler and Tobis, 1982
SLR is straight leg raising.

Table XV-1. The predictive ability, the reliability on the effect of manipulative treatment on pain (after Hoehler and Tobis, 1982).

Of the measures listed in Table XV-1, only the active and passive straight leg raising tests as a measure of flexibility approached these four ideals, although even these tests have a marked tendency to vary with time and repetition. These displayed high agreement between examiners, significant restriction in low back pain patients and significant improvement following manipulation. However these tests vary with time and repetition. In contrast, although the anterior flexion test and asymmetry of foot eversion distinguished low back pain patients from other patients, they were not greatly effected by manipulation. In conclusion, of the tests listed in Table XV-1, the most useful are the measures of the angle of passive or voluntary straight leg raising required to produce pain. The hamstring tightness test can be used only when conformity between examiner(s) can be demonstrated, while the measures of anterior flexion and foot eversion may be used with the understanding that they are not greatly affected by a successful spinal manipulation, but do aid the selection of patients with low back pain. The relations among straight leg raising tests, hamstring tightness and manipulation have been studied in detail by Fisk (e.g., 1978, 1979). It is important to note that a straight leg raising test was also found to have significant prognostic value in an independent study of low back pain by Roland and Morris (1983). Hence, the careful investigation of the usefulness of straight leg raising tests in clinical research, originally pursued by Fisk, requires careful continued investigation.

Another problem which has to be dealt with in the near future is the nature of the patient population which is affected by manipulative treatments. One position is that only patients with relatively acute problems are helped by manipulative treatments; the other position is that patients with much longer term problems are also helped. Objective data on the latter question are not available. However at the current time, the weight of the evidence from randomized clinical trials *suggests* that patients with relatively acute problems are helped by rotational lumbo-sacral manipulation, but the effect of manipulation upon patients with more "chronic" problems is still unproven.

REFERENCES

Buerger, A.A.: A controlled trial of rotational manipulation in low back pain. *Manuelle Medizin, 2*:17-26, 1980.

Buerger, A.A. and others: Klinische Untersuchungen zur Wirksamkeit der Manuellen Therapie in *Theoretische Fortschritte und praktische Erfahrungen der Manuellen Medizin.* Herausger (Publisher) H-D Neumann, Buhl, West Germany. pp. 194-214, 1981.

Cope, Z.: *The Early Diagnosis of the Acute Abdomen.* London, Oxford University Press, 1968.

Deaver, J.B.: *Appendicitis. Its History, Anatomy, Clinical Aetiology, Pathology, Symptomatology, Diagnosis, Prognosis, Treatment, Technic of Operation, Complications and Sequels.* Philadelphia, P. Blakiston, 1914.

DeMoulin, D.: Historical notes on appendicitis, *Archivum Chirurgicum Neerlandicum, 27*:97-102, 1974.

Fisk, J.W.: *The Significance of Disordered Muscle Activity in the Perpetuation and Treatment of Low Back Pain, with Particular Reference to the Effect of Manipulation.* M.D. Thesis, University of Edinburgh, 1978.

Fisk, J.W.: A controlled trial of manipulation in a selected group of patients with low back pain favouring one side. *New Zealand Medical Journal, 90*:288-91, 1979.

Hoehler, F.K.; Tobis, J.S. and Buerger, A.A.: Spinal manipulation for low back pain. *Journal of the American Medical Association, 245*:1835-1839, 1981.

Hoehler, F.K. and Tobis, J.S.: Low back pain and its treatment by spinal manipulation: Measures of flexibility and asymmetry. *Rheumatology and Rehabilitation, 21*:21-26, 1982.

Meade, R.H.: The evolution of surgery for appendicitis. *Surgery, 55*:741-752, 1963.

Roland, M., Morris, R.: A study of the natural history of back pain. *Spine, 8*:141-150, 1983.

CHAPTER SIXTEEN

A MULTICENTER TRIAL OF THE PHYSIOTHERAPEUTIC MANAGEMENT OF SCIATIC SYMPTOMS*

CHRISTENE E. O'DONAGHUE NÉE COXHEAD
M. PHIL., M.C.S.P.

THE history of treatment for back and sciatic pain dates back to the ancient Pharaohs; the first known mention of a treatment for back pain describes a diet of fresh meat and honey and is found in the Edwin-Smith Papyrus (16th Century B.C.). Treatment throughout the ages has been almost entirely empirical. It was therefore decided to evaluate various techniques being used in physiotherapy departments in a randomized controlled study to compare the therapeutic value of four kinds of treatment in terms of both symptom relief and capacity for work (Coxhead et al., 1981). They were:

    a. lumbar traction,
    b. manipulation,
    c. exercises, and
    d. corsets.

These were compared with a control group given a common treatment which was also given to all the groups in the study.

The results of each type of treatment were compared when given alone and in all the possible combinations. The study was funded by the Department of Health and Social Security and took place at eight hospitals in the greater London area. Three were teaching hospitals, and five were district general hospitals.

A total of 334 patients were admitted to the study. There were no differences between the patient population from any of the hospitals on matching

*Thanks are due to Dr. J.G.D. Troup for advice in preparing this paper.

for age, sex, and occupation.

METHODS

Patient Selection

Before patients were admitted to the study, they had to meet certain criteria which included:

1. *Age*. Male or female patients between the ages of 20 years and 65 years.
2. *Presentation*. Out-patients, complaining of back pain and/or pain and paraesthiae compatible with a sciatic distribution in the lower limb, radiating at least as far as the buttock crease.
3. *Treatment*. Patients should not have had any previous form of physiotherapy in the present episode before admission to the trial. There should be no obvious preference or dislike on the patients' part for one type of treatment.
4. *Exclusions*. Metastases and malignant disease, gynecological disorders, pregnancy or being post-partum less than 3 months, post-operative cases up to 3 months after post-surgery, surgery to the spine (e.g., panniunectomy), sacroiliac disease (e.g., ankylosing spondylitis, osteitis condensans ilii), vertebral collapse, gross structural abnormalities (e.g., spondylolisthesis, osteoarthritis of the hips), infective diseases of the spine or sacroiliac joints, and finally, all women of child bearing age whose expected menstrual period was overdue by more than nine days.

All patients, therefore, had lumbar spinal derangements with pain compatible with a sciatic distribution, and all were deemed suitable for physical therapy irrespective of their diagnostic subgroup.

Therapeutic Groups and Methods of Allocation

Types of therapy in common use in physiotherapy departments were compared with a "control" treatment. They were as follows:

1. *Manipulation*. Physiotherapists practicing within the National Health Service most commonly use a regime of manipulation based on the work of Maitland (1977). It has the advantage that the techniques are carefully graded according to the force applied and, therefore, allow quantification of the treatment given and standardization of treatment from center to center. The manipulative procedures and grades used were recorded at each treatment, and the effects in terms of pain and range of movement, were also recorded.
2. *Traction*. Intermittent rhythmic motorized lumbar traction was used; all the centers were supplied with identical 'Tru-Trac' machines (Manufac-

turer — Tru-Eze Manufacturing Co., Burbank, California, USA). The treatment varied according to the severity of symptoms and was at the discretion of the physiotherapist. Both force and duration of treatment were recorded at each session.

3. *Exercises*. A catalogue of exercises was produced for the purposes of this study. All the exercises were graded according to the tension developed in the muscles and the range of movement. The exercises were classified into four grades ranging from easy to difficult.

Grade I: Exercises with minimal resistance
Grade II: Exercises with resistance due to the effect of gravity on a limited part of the body.
Grade III: Exercises with the resistance due to the effect of gravity on any part of the body.
Grade IV: Exercises involving external work with resistance due to the effects of gravity on the body and the loads handled.

The exercises were catalogued under the following headings:
a. flexor
b. extensor
c. lateral flexor, and
d. rotator.

The physiotherapists taking part in the study were free to select exercises suitable for the patient from the catalogue, progressing through the grades according to the ability of the patient. Each session included some exercises from each range of motion, but at no time was the patient made to work through pain. At each session, all the exercises performed were recorded, together with the total amount of time spent exercising.

4. *Corsets*. Half the patients in the study wore corsets of the 'ready made' instant variety. Allocation was random throughout the treatment groups.

5. *Common "Control" Treatment*. A treatment having a minimal mechanical effect on the patient was selected for the control group which was given to every patient in the trial. Short-wave diathermy using an induction coil was used for 20 minutes. This treatment also included a "back care" lecture containing advice on posture and lifting related to the patients' work and daily living activities. So as to standardize any beneficial effect *this treatment* may have had, it *was given to every patient in the trial*. This was done for two reasons; firstly, it was felt that patients given no active treatment would be lost to the trial; also because physiotherapists were reluctant to take part in a study where all treatment was withheld from patients. Hence a treatment of minimal mechanical input to the patient was chosen. By comparing all those patients who had any one treatment with those who did not have it, a 'control' was achieved.

Control of the Flow and Treatment of Patients

Four treatments were given, either alone or in combination, giving eight treatment groups; in addition, half the patients were allocated an 'instant' lumbar corset giving a total of 16 treatment groups in a 2 to the power of 4 design which unfortunately is difficult to represent in a two dimensional figure. The 16 groups were:

1. Control
2. Control and corset
3. Control and exercises
4. Control, exercises and corset
5. Control and manipulation
6. Control, manipulation and corset
7. Control, manipulation and exercises
8. Control, manipulation, exercises and corset
9. Control and traction
10. Control, traction and corset
11. Control, traction and exercises
12. Control, traction, exercises and corset
13. Control, traction and manipulation
14. Control, traction, manipulation and corset
15. Control, traction, manipulation and exercises
16. Control, traction, manipulation, exercises and corset

The duration of all treatments used in the study was given at the discretion of the physiotherapists. Details were recorded at each attendance on structured forms so as to minimize omissions. The statistician provided each center with a series of envelopes to be opened consecutively, so as to ensure the random allocation to treatment groups. The patients, who as mentioned above were suitable for any or all of the treatments used in the study, were admitted to the trial by clinicians in orthopaedic and rheumatology outpatient clinics. Initially, patients were given a daily appointment; attendances were reduced at the physiotherapists' discretion as the symptoms settled.

In all the centers patients underwent the following procedures:

1. Initial examination by physician.
2. Initial examination by physiotherapist.
3. Allocation to treatment group.
4. Standardized x-ray examination.
5. Therapy program.
6. Assessment one month from beginning of study by physician and physiotherapist.
7. Assessment four months from entry to study.
8. Postal follow-up sixteen months from entry.

If patients became worse, the physiotherapist referred the patient back to the doctor, when necessary before the completion of the four-month therapy program. When patients improved quickly, therapy was also stopped before the end of the four week period. In either case for which therapy was stopped before the four week assessment, the interview and examination normally carried out at one month was completed.

Monitoring the Progress of Patients

The patients' progress was assessed by the following measures:

a) Pain severity using an analogue scale,
b) Return to physical activity and work,
c) Mobility tests,
d) Dynamic strength tests, and
e) Radiographic measurements. These measures are described in more detail below:
a) *Pain Analogue*. Patients were asked by the physiotherapist to assess their improvement on a three point scale, "better," "no change" or "worse." This assessment was repeated at the end of each weeks treatment. A further assessment was made by the physician at the one month assessment — patients were asked to rate their improvement or deterioration on a percentage scale from minus 100% to plus 100%.
b) *Return to Physical Activity and Work*. The postural stress and occupational activity of every patient in the study was coded on a four-point scale based on the job descriptions taken at the initial interview. The number of days lost from work in the current episode was recorded throughout the study. In addition, at the year follow-up patients were asked if they were in the same job; if not, if the change was due to their back problem. The patient's ability to perform certain activities was recorded, including:

- Lifting,
- Bending,
- Sitting still,
- Standing,
- Stairs,
- Walking,
- Leaning over working surfaces, and
- Pushing and pulling activities.

Patients were asked if these activities were painful: if so, whether these activities could be performed despite pain; or if they had to stop doing them; or if they were no problem at all. This enabled an assessment of the change in the capacity for these activities to be made and used as a measure of improvement or deterioration.
c) *Mobility Tests*. An assessment of mobility was made by measuring the

extremes of movement with a spirit goniometer (Figure XVI-1). Measurements of spinal mobility were made using skin marks placed over bony landmarks, i.e., a vertical line between the spinous processes of T12 and L1 and in inverted 'T' at the lower margin of the posterior superior iliac spines (Figure XVI-2). Hip flexion was measured using a horizontal line marked on the lateral aspect of the thigh.

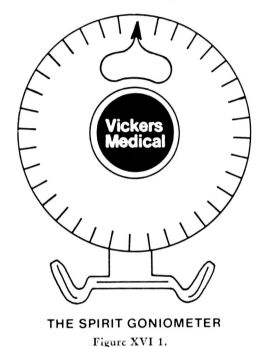

THE SPIRIT GONIOMETER
Figure XVI 1.

The following measurements were made:

    a) lumbar sagittal mobility (Figure XVI-3)
    b) lumbar lateral mobility (Figure XVI-4)
    c) hip flexion (Figure XVI-5)
    d) hip rotation (Figure XVI-6)
    e) straight leg raising (Figure XVI-7)

All measurements were made before treatment commenced and again after one and four months.

    d) *Dynamic Strength Tests*. Two dynamic strength tests were carried out, before and after the therapy program had been carried out.

    1. The Arch-up (Figure XVI-8), and
    2. The Sit-up (Figure XVI-9).

    e) *Radiographic Measurements*. Before each patient was treated, a standard set of radiographs were taken including:

    1. An erect postero-anterior view with the patient weight bearing. The

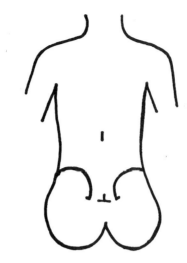

SKIN MARKS
FOR MEASURES OF LUMBAR POSTURE
Figure XVI-2.

view from T-12 to include both femoral heads. (Posterior-anterior films were taken rather than anterior-posterior films in order to observe obliquity of the rays through the disc spaces).

2. A lateral view of the flexed lumbar spine from L-3 to the tip of the sacrum. For this view the patient was seated on a high stool (standardized in each center) and was asked to flex as much as possible in order to obtain maximal flexion without undue pain.

3. A lateral view of the extended lumbar spine from L-1 to the tip of the sacrum with the patient seated and maximally extended.

4. An antero-posterior view of the lower three lumbar vertebrae and sacro-iliac joints taken with the patient supine and the x-ray tube at an angle of 30° to the vertical.

All the x-rays taken were coned to the limits of the views required in order to minimize radiation. The films to tube distance was one meter.

The following measurements were made of the lower three vertebrae levels:

a) Interpedicular distance (A in Figure XVI-10)

b) Interarticular distance (B in Figure XVI-10)

c) Midsagittal diameter (A in Figure XVI-11)

d) Foraminal anterior-posterior distance (B in Figure XVI-11), and

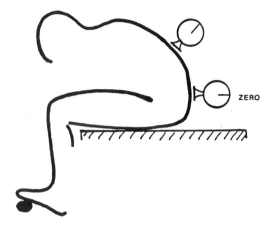

FLEXED POSTURE

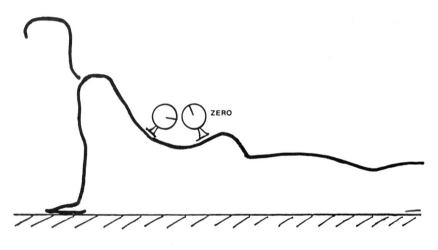

EXTENDED POSTURE
Figure XVI-3.

e) Pedicular length (C in Figure XVI-11).

Anterior and posterior disc heights were measured from the lower three disc spaces. Flexed and extended films were traced, then superimposed to allow a measurement of intervertebral mobility to be made (Figure XVI-12).

A number of other assessments were made such as the presence of abnormalities of both vertebral bodies and synovial joints, the presence of sacralization and spina bifida and the presence of lateral curvature and pelvic tilt.

Reproducibility of Measurements

Approximately every six months the reliability of measurements made by the therapists was assessed. A major testing session was also held in each center

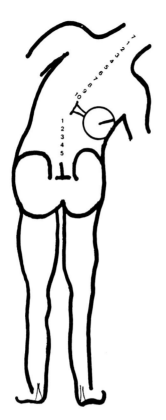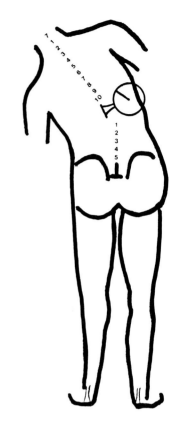

LUMBAR LATERAL FLEXION

Figure XVI-4.

from which intern-observer errors were assessed.

Statistical Analysis

A factorial design was adopted so as to study each of the four treatments at two levels — given and not given — resulting in a 2^4 design. This type of analysis required an equal number of patients in each of the treatment groups. As this was not achieved due to the poor recruitment of patients at several centers, a multiple regression analysis was used to compensate for this inequality.

Patients lost to the Study

From a total of 334 patients admitted to the study, a number had to be

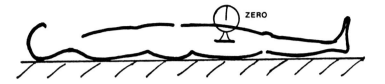

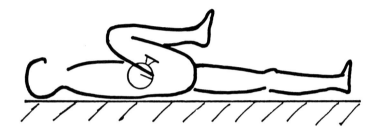

HIP FLEXION
Figure XVI-5.

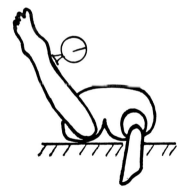 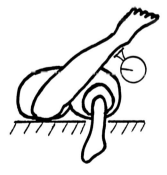

HIP ROTATION
Figure XVI-6.

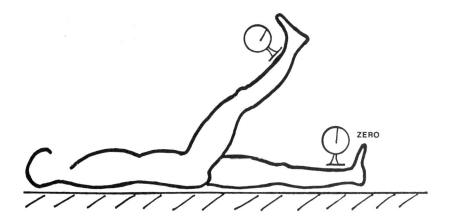

STRAIGHT LEG RAISING

Figure XVI-7.

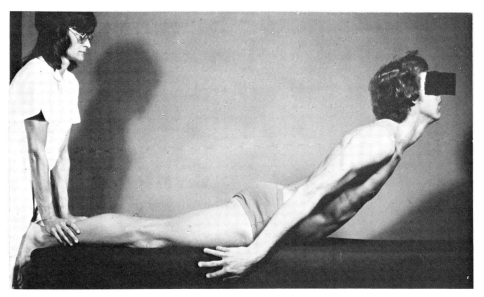

Figure XVI-8.

taken out after admission because they did not fulfill the criteria for entrance, also a number failed to complete the course of treatment and finally a number were withdrawn because they were either better or worse. Details can be seen in Table XVI-1.

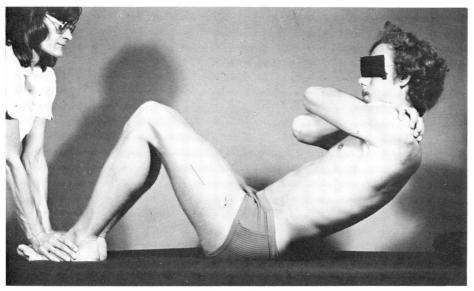

Figure XVI-9.

RESULTS

Preliminary Data

There was no significant difference in duration of symptoms between the hospitals taking part in the study. The overall duration of symptoms prior to admission to the study was 14.3 weeks. There was a significant difference in the mean duration of symptoms between those who were withdrawn from the trial because they were "worse" and those who were "better."

	Withdrawn "Worse"	Withdrawn "Better"
Mean no. of weeks since attack began	11.9 weeks	5.1 weeks
Standard deviation	± 10.9	± 4.9
Total	19	10
	$d = 6.8$, $t = 2.31$, $p < 0.05$	

There was a significant relationship between the number of activities causing pain and the patient's ability to work:

No. of activities causing pain	Able to work normally	Able to work with difficulty	Unable to work
0-4	72	63	73
5-9	15	19	40
	$X^2[2°] = 8.936$, $p < 0.02$		

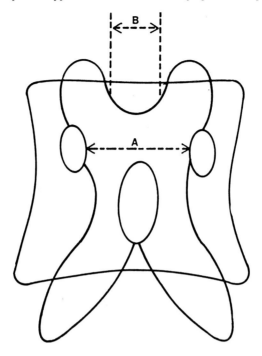

MEASUREMENTS FROM
ANTERIOR - POSTERIOR
RADIOGRAPHS
Figure XVI-10.

130 patients had right sided sciatica and 132 left-sided symptoms, 24 patients had bilateral symptoms. On admission, 22 patients had pain as far as the buttock or groin; 81 as far as the knee; 70 as far as the calf and 135 as far as the foot.

Changes in knee and ankle jerks on admission to the study are shown below.

	Exaggerated	Normal	Diminished	Absent	Total
Right knee jerk	24	250	23	10	307
Left knee jerk	17	250	31	10	308
Right ankle jerk	5	230	38	32	306
Left ankle jerk	3	221	40	42	306

Response to Treatment

Overall Results (Pain)

The overall results after one and four months on the better, same, worse

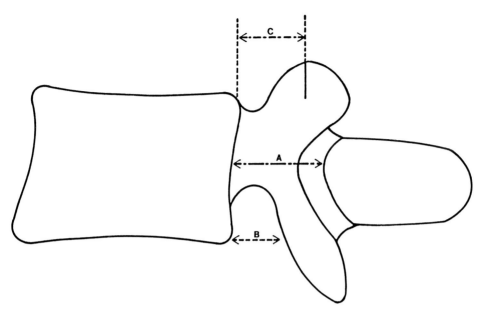

MEASUREMENTS FROM LATERAL RADIOGRAPHS

Figure XVI-11.

analogue were as follows:

	Better	Same	Worse
1 month	78.0%	16.3%	5.7%
4 months	72.1%	20.4%	7.5%

On the percentage scale, the average improvement at one month was 49.4% (S.D. ± 23.64). At sixteen months 72 (27.9%) patients had remained pain free between four and sixteen months, 186 (72.1%) reported some residual pain, 43.5% of patients had further treatment between one and four months; 56.6% had no further treatment; 23.8% of patients had treatment between four and sixteen months and 76.2% did not.

Two-fifths of all the patients in the study remained at work during the first month; by the end of four months, four-fifths were back at work.

Overall Results (Mobility)

Mobility showed no significant changes at either the one or four month assessments. Most patients were able to perform the arch-up and sit-up test. The average percentage improvement reported by patients in relation to the sit-up test was:

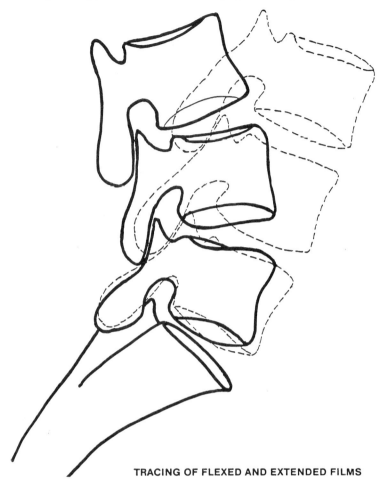

TRACING OF FLEXED AND EXTENDED FILMS

Figure XVI-12.

TABLE XVI-1

	WRONGLY ENTERED	WITHDRAWN WORSE	WITHDRAWN BETTER	DROPPED OUT WORSE	DROPPED OUT UNKNOWN	DROPPED OUT BETTER	COMPLETED 3/12 & 15/12	COMPLETED 15/12 Only	
MT. VERNON	1	1	4	2	6	1	99	0	114
BARTS	1	1	1	0	3	0	19	1	26
KINGS	0	0	0	1	0	0	3	0	4
ASHFORD	1	1	0	2	1	0	8	0	13
Q. MARYS	0	0	1	1	1	0	13	2	18
LEWISHAM	0	3	1	2	0	0	19	2	27
DARTFORD	1	2	0	0	1	0	19	0	23
RFH	4	4	2	9	12	2	72	1	106
TOTALS	8	12	9	17	24	3	252	6	331

(Number in nil data category equals three)

Initial Assessment	Able	Unable	Able	Unable
	changed to	changed to	changed to	changed to
One Month Assessment	Unable	Unable	Able	Able
Percent improvement	45%	28%	59.3%	71.7%

Results of Individual Treatment Groups

The difference between any of the treatments was not significant (NS) on the outcome relating to changes on the better/worse/same scale both at one and four months. The mean improvement at one month on the percentage scale showed a significant trend for manipulation; the effects of the other treatments were not significant (NS).

	Traction		Manipulation		Exercises		Corset	
	Yes	No	Yes	No	Yes	No	Yes	No
Percent improvement at one month	51.1	45.4	52.6	42.2	49.0	46.3	49.8	46.1
Standard Deviation (S.D.)	± 37.9	± 40.3	± 36.9	± 40.9	± 40.0	± 38.2	± 37.9	± 40.0
	NS				NS		NS	

$$t = 2.30, p < 0.05$$

When considering only those patients who were off work at the commencement of treatment, there were no significant differences between the numbers returning to work for any of the treatments used in the study. Nor was there any significant difference between the treatments for those patients who had further treatment nor those who did not.

At sixteen months, the assessment on the basis of the patients' ability to continue in the same job showed a significant trend in favor of those receiving manipulation during the therapy period.

	Traction		Manipulation*		Exercise		Corset	
	Yes	No	Yes	No	Yes	No	Yes	No
same job	86	86	103	69	90	82	73	99
changed	28	28	19	37	29	27	23	33

$$*X^2 = 11.44, p < 0.001$$

Number of Treatments by Outcome Measures

Further analysis was carried out on the basis of the number of treatments each patient received irrespective of the type of treatment. When comparing those who were better with those who were the same or worse, there was a significant trend in favor of an increasing number of types of treatment. Using the method of Armitage (1955), the chi squared for trend when comparing those patients who were better with those who were the same or worse equaled 7.31 and was significant at the 0.05 level. See Table XVI-2.

A similar trend was seen for assessment on the basis of return to work, although it did not reach significant levels.

The fewer the number of types of treatments received during the initial therapy program, the higher was the proportion of patients who received further treatment between the one and four month assessment periods. Using method similar to that in Table XVI-2 this result was statistically significant (Table XVI-3).

TABLE XVI-2

PATIENT'S ASSESSMENT AT 4 WEEKS BY NUMBER OF TYPES OF TREATMENT

	NONE	ONLY 1	ANY 2	ANY 3	ALL 4
Better	14 (70%)	54 (69%)	81 (78%)	64 (86%)	14 (88%)
Same	5 (25%)	19 (24%)	17 (16%)	5 (7%)	1 (6%)
Worse	1 (5%)	5 (6%)	6 (6%)	5 (7%)	1 (6%)
Total	20	78	104	74	16

$\chi^2(1) = 7.31$, p<0.05. See text for details.

TABLE XVI-3

PATIENT'S RECEIVING FURTHER TREATMENT BETWEEN 1 AND 4 MONTHS BY NUMBER OF TYPES OF TREATMENT RECEIVED INITIALLY

	NONE	ONLY 1	ANY 2	ANY 3	ALL 4
Further Treatment	12	38	33	24	4
	67%	34%	38%	35%	29%
No Further Treatment	6	34	53	44	10
	33%	47%	62%	65%	71%

$\chi^2(1) = 9.41$, p<0.01. See text for details.

A significant number of patients who were unable to sit-up at the initial assessment had to have further treatment between four and sixteen months.

Treatment between 4 & 16 months	Initially able to sit-up	Initially unable to sit-up
No treatment	169 (80.1%)	54 (68.4%)
Further treatment	42 (19.9%)	25 (31.6%)
	$X^2 = 4.46$, $p < 0.05$	

Patients with neurological deficit responded neither better nor worse than those with no such deficit. Nor was there any difference in terms of resolution of signs or gains in mobility.

Radiological Results

A total of 158 radiographs were measured. None of the measurements showed any significant relationship to duration of symptoms, sickness absence, diminution or absence of tendon jerks, incidence of back pain at 16 months, incidence of leg pain at 16 months or reports of further treatment between 4 and 16 months.

The most significant results related to the sit-up test. Interarticular measurements were significantly reduced in those patients who were unable to sit-up at all levels. See Table XVI-4. Those patients with diminished sensation on the right side together with right sided sciatica had a significantly reduced mid-sagittal diameter.

	Diminished Sensation on the Right	Normal Sensation
Mean	21.35 mm	23.25 mm
SD	± 3.061	± 2.726
Total	17	51
	difference (d) = 1.9mm, t = 2.27, p < 0.05	

DISCUSSION AND CONCLUSIONS

There was no attempt in this study to establish a requirement for "blindness" on the part of either the physiotherapist, doctor or patient. In a study by Doran and Newell (1975) in which a double-blind trial was attempted, the assessing physician inadvertently discovered the treatment used in 10% of the patients. It was impossible for the physiotherapist and patient to remain

Table XVI-4

L-3 Interarticular Distance
Ability to sit-up at one month assessment.

	Able	Unable
Mean	20.59mm	19.04mm
S.D.	2.99	3.37
Total	125	25
d = 1.55mm	5 = 2.87,	p<0.005

L-4 Interarticular Distance
Ability to sit-up at one month assessment

	Able	Unable
Mean	20.82mm	19.44mm
S.D.	3.33	2.82
Total	125	25
d = 1.38mm	t = 2.16	p<0.05

L-5 Inarticular Distance
Ability to sit-up at initial assessment

	Able	Unable
Mean	23.22mm	20.12mm
S.D.	4.21	4.61
Total	125	25
d = 3.10mm	5 = 3.13	p<0.005

S-1 Inarticular Distance
Ability to sit-up at one month assessment

	Able	Unable
Mean	28.99mm	26.72mm
S.D.	5.0	4.8
Total	125	25
d = 2.27mm	t = 2.14	p<0.05

ignorant of the treatment used. However, patients with a particular preference for treatment were eliminated from the study and this was as much as could be done in the circumstances of this clinical trial.

After the study had commenced, Bergquist-Ullman and Larsson (1977) published work that showed "Back School" therapy to be at least equivalent to "combined physical therapy." The back lecture used in this study covered essentially the same material and may account for the absence of a significant difference between any of the treatments and the control treatment.

There was a significant benefit from manipulation in the first month in only one method of assessing progress. Cyriax (1977) and many others suggest that manipulation is more effective in certain types of patients although their characteristics were not objectively defined. None of the clinical characteristics of the patients in this study was associated with a tendency to do well or badly with any of the treatments used.

There is little evidence that therapy had a long-term effect. Despite 72.1% reporting persistent symptoms at 16 months, only 23.8% had actually sought further treatment.

The radiological results show the mid-sagittal diameters of patients in this study to be less than a group of normal spines measured by Roberts (1978). These results are consistent with the report of Parker et al. (1980) of fringing of narrow canals in subjects with sciatic symptoms.

In conclusion, this study showed a significant advantage in relation to manipulation but only for one outcome measure. In addition, there was a significant improvement shown with increasing numbers of therapies. None of the results reported here give any indication that experienced physiotherapists should not be allowed to exercise their discretion in the management of patients with sciatic symptoms. The results indicate that active physiotherapy with several treatments including manipulation are of benefit in the out-patient management of patients with sciatica, at least in the short term.

REFERENCES

Armitage, P. Test for linear trends in proportions and frequencies. *Biometrics, 11*:375-386, 1955.

Bergquist-Ullman, J. and Larsson, U. Acute Low Back Pain in Industry. *Acta Orthopaedica Scandinavica, Supplementum, 170*, 1977.

Coxhead, C.E., Inskip, H., Mead, T.W., North, W.R.S., Troup, J.D.G. Multicentre trial of physiotherapy in the management of sciatic symptoms. *The Lancet*, 1, 1065-1068, 1981.

Doran, D.M.L. and Newall, D.J. Manipulation in treatment of low back pain: A multicentre study. *British Medical Journal, 2*:161-164, 1975.

Maitland, G. *Vertebral Manipulation*, 4th Ed., Butterworth, London, 1977.

Parker, R.W., Hibbert, C. and Wellman, P. Backache and the Lumbar Spinal Canal. *Spine, 5*:99-105, 1980.

Roberts, G.M. *Lumbar Stenosis*. M.D. Thesis, London University, 1978.

CHAPTER SEVENTEEN

THE DESIGN AND RESULTS
OF CLINICAL TRIALS
OF LUMBAR MANIPULATION:
A REVIEW

DAVID P. EVANS, M.Sc., M.D.

WHEN a treatment is tested to evaluate its effectiveness, it must be compared against an alternative therapy except in those rare cases where the natural history of the disease is well-defined. This can be done retrospectively by surveying the results of treatments, or prospectively by means of a clinical trial. The inclusion of the alternative therapy, whether this be placebo or some supposedly active regimen, bedecks the prefix 'controlled' to the clinical trial. Kane et al. (1974) have described a retrospective survey comparing the effectiveness of physician and chiropractic care, but the clinical trials I am reviewing here have been controlled, prospective studies.

If an untested treatment were to be compared with "no treatment," any response obtained could not be differentiated from a "placebo" response. This is especially relevant to trials of spinal manipulation as the "laying-on-of-hands" may well provide a substantial placebo effect. Ebbets (1975) has said that a placebo manipulation is impracticable, but some investigators (Buerger, 1980; Hoehler et al., 1981)* have approached the ideal situation by using a 'sham manipulation' of soft tissue massage. In many cases, the patient was unaware whether manipulation was performed or not, and so remained 'blind' to the treatment given. If the assessor is also unaware which treatment the patient received, the trial is said to "double-blind." Most controlled trials have not been blind as far as the patient was concerned, but have been 'single-blind' in the

---

*Editor's Footnote: These two reports are different analyses of essentially the same data base; the paper of Buerger in this volume is another analysis of this data base.

sense that the observer was kept ignorant of the patient's treatment.

If the treatments being compared are given during the same trial period, the trial is said to be 'parallel-group.' Allocation to treatment group should be made according to some pre-determined key drawn-up randomly.

I have reviewed eleven trials of lumbar spinal manipulation. A more extensive analysis of some of the early trials may be found in Evans (1982).

The trial of Chrisman et al. (1964) was not controlled but is included because myelography was undertaken before and after manipulation. This provided some interesting results which may have a bearing on the syndrome most likely to benefit from manipulative therapy. This trial also differs from the other ten because manipulation was carried out under general anesthesia. The remaining ten trials are all prospective, controlled trials; nine being parallel-group and the other a 'cross-over' in which each patient received both the comparative treatments, one after the other.

Bergquist-Ullman and Larsson (1977) wrote that since the etiology is not known in most cases of low back pain, the classification of the disease must be based upon symptoms and clinical findings. The eleven trials reviewed here have been undertaken in patients with low back pain and/or sciatic pain. The trial of manipulation under general anesthesia (Chrisman et al., 1964) specified inclusion of patients with severe symptoms of a herniated intervertebral disc, and a myelogram was performed to show whether a herniated disc was present or not.

In some of the trials the manipulation was rotational and in others it was mobilization. Sometimes both forms of manipulation have been used together. I have not tried to separate the effects of the two types of therapy, but if the results are subsequently analyzed by this factor one should not forget the almost equally great effect caused by differences between individual practitioners when performing the same type of manipulation.

Having established the design of the trial, the symptoms of the patients and the type of manipulation employed, one must examine the control treatments. In the trial of Coxhead et al. (1981) the treatments were not only given singly but also in combination. Soft tissue massage, detuned short-wave diathermy and lowest level microwave radiation have all been employed as placebo treatments. Analgesics, physiotherapy, corsets and Back School training have been used as active controls. Table XVII-1 lists the trials analyzed below and assigns identification numbers to them. Table XVII-2 lists those features of the clinical trials already mentioned together with the number of patients in each trial.

Table XVII-3 lists the times of post-treatment assessments. Patients suffering from low back pain often have a high rate of spontaneous recovery, so it is important to know the periods on which the results, also shown in Table XVII-3, are based. The results are those conclusions drawn by the authors of the trials. Significant refers to statistical significance at a level of $p < 0.05$.

Tables XVII-2 and XVII-3 contain an abundance of information from

TABLE XVII-1

1.	BERGQUIST-ULLMAN AND LARSSON	(1977)
2.	BUERGER	(1980)
3.	CHRISMAN ET AL	(1964)
4.	COXHEAD ET AL	(1981)
5.	DORAN AND NEWELL	(1975)
6.	EDWARDS	(1969)
7.	EVANS ET AL	(1978)
8.	GLOVER ET AL	(1974)
9.	HOEHLER ET AL	(1981)
10.	JAYSON ET AL	(1981)
11.	RASMUSSEN	(1979)

well-designed and well-executed clinical trials. What conclusions can we draw from this information?

I have listed the effects, drawn from the results in Table XVII-3, in the first hours, first days, first weeks, first months and first years after manipulation.

Table XVII-4 shows the results in the first hours. Without exception when assessments were made in the first hours post-treatment manipulation was more effective than the control. Interestingly, the control in these comparisons was always placebo-sham-manipulation or detuned short-wave diathermy.

Table XVII-5 shows the results in the first days post-treatment. Here the effect of manipulation was variable and did not depend upon whether the control was placebo or active. In the trial of Evans et al. (1978) daily pain scores were recorded and the first week after manipulation was associated with more pain than the first week in the control group. They found benefit from manipulation within weeks rather than days after starting treatment and this effectiveness in the early weeks was also reported in most of the other trials (Table XVII-6).

TABLE XVII - 2 CLINICAL TRIALS REVIEWED (Part 1)

Trial	Criteria of Patients	No. of Patients	Manipulation	Control	Design	Blinding
1. Bergquist-Ullman and Larsson (1977)	Lumbosacral back pain of less than 3 months duration ± sciatic radiation.	217	Combined physical therapy. (postural instruction ± mobilization ± exercises ± rotational.	1. Back School. 2. Placebo (lowest intensity short-wave). 3. Physiotherapy.	Prospective. Parallel-group. Randomized. One-centre.	Non-blind. (Suggestion only assessor unaware of treatment).
2. Buerger (1980)	Low back pain ± sciatic radiation. Areas of vertebral immodility.	83	Rotational manipulation.	1. Sham manipulation (soft-tissue massage).	Prospective. Parallel-group. Randomized. One-centre.	Single-blind. (Assessor unaware of treatment. Almost double-blind).
3. Chrisman et al (1964)	Severe symptoms of herniated intervertebral disc. (Low back pain with sciatic radiation, pain on one of the sciatic-nerve stretch tests and at least one unequivocal objective neurological sign).	39	Rotational manipulation under general anaesthesia.	22 patients with similar symptoms. No general anaesthesia.	Prospective. Uncontrolled. One-centre. Myelography before & after manipulation.	Non-blind.
4. Coxhead et al (1981)	Sciatic pain with or without back pain.	322	Mobilization. (Alone and with control treatment).	1. Traction. 2. Exercises. 3. Corset Treatments singly and combined.	Prospective. Parallel-group. Randomized. Multi-centre.	Non-blind.
5. Doran and Newell (1975)	Low back pain without sciatic pain. Age 20-50 years. Painful limitation of movement.	456	Any type of manipulation or mobilization.	1. Physiotherapy. 2. Corset. 3. Analgesics.	Prospective. Parallel-group. Randomized. Multi-centre.	Single-blind.

+ plus analgesics (paracetamol) if needed +

TABLE XVII - 2 CLINICAL TRIALS REVIEWED (Part 2)

Trial	Criteria of Patients	No. of Patients	Manipulation	Control	Design	Blinding
6. Edwards (1969)	Low back pain + sciatic radiation.	184	Mobilization.	1. Heat, massage and exercise.	Prospective. Parallel-group. Not known if randomized. Four centres.	Non-blind.
7. Evans et al (1978)	Low back pain of more than 3 weeks ± sciatic radiation.	32	Rotational manipulation plus codeine phosphate.	1. Codeine phosphate alone.	Prospective. Cross-over. Randomized. One-centre.	Single-blind. (assessor unaware of treatment).
8. Glover et al (1974)	Unilateral low back pain + hyperaesthesia + limitation of movement.	84	Unilateral rotational manipulation plus detuned short-wave diathermy.	1. Detuned short-wave diathermy.	Prospective. Parallel-group. Randomized. One centre.	Single-blind. (Assessor unaware of treatment)
9. Hoehler et al (1981)	Low back pain. Hyperalgesia or restricted or painful range of vertebral motion.	95	Rotational manipulation.	1. Soft tissue massage.	Prospective. Parallel-group. Randomized.	Single-blind. (Assessor unaware of treatment).
10. Jayson et al (1981)	Patients with low back pain thought suitable for mobilization. (a) General Practitioner patients. (b) Hospital patients.	(a) 94 (b) 94	Mobilization.	1. Lowest level microwave radiation.	Prospective. Parallel-group. Randomized. One-centre.	Single-blind. (Assessor unaware of treatment).
11. Rasmussen (1979)	Low back pain without signs of root pressure of less than 3 weeks. Males aged 20-50 years.	26	Rotational manipulation in pain-free direction.	1. Short-wave diathermy.	Prospective. Parallel-group. Randomized. One-centre.	Non-blind.

TABLE XVII - 3 RESULTS OF MANIPULATION (Part 1)

Trial	Post-treatment assessments	Results

1. Bergquist-Ullman and Larsson (1977)	10 days
	3 weeks
	6 weeks
	3 months
	6 months
	1 year
		(1) Duration of symptoms after first treatment - Back School mean 14.8 days
		  - Physiotherapy mean 15.8 days
		  - Placebo mean 28.7 days
		
		(2) Patients attending Back School had shorter duration of sick leave than patients in other two groups.
		
		(3) Enough evidence to conclude that Back School and combined physiotherapy are superior to placebo.

2. Buerger (1980)	Immediate 1 hour 4 hours 1 day 4-5 days	(1) Immediately after treatment and during first hour manipulated patients felt better than control patients. (2) 30% of manipulated patients felt worse after 4-5 days. (3) Significantly (P < 0.025) longer pain relief in manipulated patients (mean 8.0 days) than in control patients (mean 2.9 days). (4) Significant (P < 0.05) improvement in manipulated group in sitting, reaching and bending. (5) The percent of patients reporting improved ability in manipulated group remained constant over the first six treatments; in the control group the percent increased over the first three treatments until it approximated percent in manipulated group. (6) Patients who responded to manipulation tended to be older when their pain started. (7) Conclusion that in the short-term manipulation superior to control.
3. Chrisman et al (1964)	2-4 days 6-8 weeks 5-12 months 3 years	(1) Significant benefits of manipulation were its rapid effect on leg pain, list, and straight leg raising. (2) Patients showing the most benefit from manipulation were those who had no myelographic evidence of disc protrusion. (3) Manipulation did not change the appearance of the myelogram.
4. Coxhead et al (1981)	4 weeks 4 months 16 months	(1) At 4 weeks each treatment slightly better than spontaneous improvement. (2) For manipulation significant benefit on pain analogue scale. (3) Significant increase in symptomatic improvement with increasing numbers of treatments in combination. (4) No beneficial effects at 4 months or 16 months.

TABLE XVII - 3 RESULTS OF MANIPULATION (Part 2)

(continued)

Trial	Post-treatment assessments	Results
5. Doran and Newell (1975)	3 weeks 6 weeks 3 months 1 year	(1) A few patients responded well and quickly to manipulation, but no way of identifying those patients in advance. (2) More patients in manipulation group were markedly improved and completely relieved, but the number was not significantly higher than in other groups.
6. Edwards	During and at the end of course of treatment. Probably 1-2 weeks after starting course.	(1) The results achieved in the two groups were not significantly different but the number of treatments required to obtain an acceptable result by manipulation and mobilization was approximately half the number when treated by heat, massage and exercise.
7. Evans et al (1978)	3 weeks 6 weeks	(1) Spinal flexion significantly increases during manipulative treatment, but decreases quickly afterwards. (2) Pain scores significantly decrease within four weeks of starting course of manipulation. (3) First week after manipulation associated with more pain than first week in control group. (4) Responders significantly older than non-responders. (5) Responders had significantly later age of onset of low back pain.
8. Grover et al (1974)	Immediate 3 days 7 days 1 month	(1) In patients suffering first episode of low back pain, significantly more pain relief in manipulated group than in control group immediately after treatment. (2) No significant differences between groups in pain relief thereafter. (3) Patients with less than a week's history improved more rapidly than those with more than a week's history.
9. Hoehler et al (1981)	Immediate On discharge 3 weeks later	(1) Immediately after first manipulation more improvement than in control group in 4 of 6 parameters measured. (2) Immediately after first manipulation significantly (P < 0.05) more relief from pain than in control group. (3) No difference between groups thereafter.

Nevertheless the beneficial effect seems to wear off after a month or so, and both trials with assessments months and years after treatment showed manipulation to be without long-term effectiveness (Tables XVII-7 and XVII-8).

The effect of manipulation on symptoms and signs is shown in Table XVII-9. Hints at the diagnoses which may be responsive to manipulation are shown

TABLE XVII - 3 RESULTS OF MANIPULATION (Part 3)

(continued)

Trial	Post-treatment assessments		Results
10. Jayson et al (1981)		At 4 weeks: ·	
		(1) General Practitioner patients	- some advantage in favor of patients in mobilization group.
		(2) Hospital patients	- no difference between groups.
		(3) General Practitioner patients	- decrease in spinal flexion in controls; no in treated group.
	4 weeks 3 months 1 year		- both groups had significant improvement in spoinal extension. - straight leg raising improved significantly in treated group.
		(4) Hospital patients	- no changes in spinal flexion. - both groups had significant improvement in spinal extension. - straight leg raising improved significantly in treated group.
		At 3 months: ·	
		(5) No differences between treatment groups.	
		At 1 year: ·	
		(6) No differences between treatment groups.	
11. Rasmussen (1979)	1 week 2 weeks	(1) Significantly (P · 0.01) more patients pain-free, normal function and fit to work in manipulated group (92% restored to full function) than in control group (25% restored). (2) Significantly (P · 0.01) more patients had increased mobility in the manipulated group than in the control group.	

TABLE XVII-4

EFFECT WITHIN FIRST HOURS AFTER MANIPULATION

	TRIAL
IMMEDIATELY AFTER TREATMENT AND DURING FIRST HOUR MANIPULATED PATIENTS FELT BETTER THAN CONTROL PATIENTS.	(2)
IN PATIENTS SUFFERING FIRST EPISODE OF LOW BACK PAIN, SIGNIFICANTLY MORE PAIN RELIEF IN MANIPULATED GROUP THAN IN CONTROL GROUP IMMEDIATELY AFTER TREATMENT.	(8)
IMMEDIATELY AFTER FIRST MANIPULATION MORE IMPROVEMENT THAN IN THE CONTROL GROUP IN 4 OF 6 PARAMETERS MEASURED.	(9)
IMMEDIATELY AFTER MANIPULATION SIGNIFICANTLY MORE PAIN RELIEF THAN IN CONTROL GROUP.	(9)

in Table XVII-10.

These statements can be combined in the conclusion:

Manipulation is effective in a condition that exists in older patients suffering from low back pain, but one giving symptoms of recent onset. This con-

TABLE XVII-5

EFFECT WITHIN FIRST DAYS AFTER MANIPULATION

	TRIAL
SIGNIFICANTLY LONGER PAIN RELIEF IN MANIPULATED PATIENTS (MEAN 8.0 DAYS) THAN IN CONTROL PATIENTS (MEAN 2.9 DAYS).	(2)
THE PERCENT OF PATIENTS REPORTING IMPROVED ABILITY IN MANIPULATED GROUP REMAINED CONSTANT OVER THE FIRST SIX TREATMENTS: IN THE CONTROL GROUP THE PERCENT INCREASED OVER THE FIRST THREE TREATMENTS UNTIL IT APPROXIMATED THE PERCENT IN THE MANIPULATED GROUP.	(2)
THE RESULTS ACHIEVED IN THE TWO GROUPS WERE NOT SIGNIFICANTLY DIFFERENT BUT THE NUMBER OF TREATMENTS REQUIRED TO OBTAIN AN ACCEPTABLE RESULT BY MANIPULATION AND MOBILIZATION WAS APPROXIMATELY HALF THE NUMBER WHEN TREATED BY HEAT, MASSAGE AND EXERCISE.	(6)
NO SIGNIFICANT DIFFERENCE BETWEEN GROUPS IN PAIN RELIEF AT 3 DAYS AND 7 DAYS.	(8)
30% OF MANIPULATED PATIENTS FELT WORSE AFTER 4-5 DAYS.	(2)
FIRST WEEK AFTER MANIPULATION ASSOCIATED WITH MORE PAIN THAN FIRST WEEK IN CONTROL GROUP.	(7)

dition is almost certainly NOT a prolapsed intervertebral disc. After treatment patients exhibit more spinal mobility and straight leg raising may be increased. The beneficial effect of manipulation is time-dependent. Manipulation is effective in the first hours, days and weeks after a treatment, but ineffective from one month post-treatment onwards. It is not possible to distinguish between the effectiveness of mobilization and manipulation in the controlled trials reported in the literature.

TABLE XVII-6

EFFECT WITHIN FIRST WEEKS AFTER MANIPULATION

	TRIAL
DURATION OF SYMPTOMS AFTER FIRST MANIPULATION (MEAN 16 DAYS) SHORTER THAN AFTER PLACEBO (29 DAYS).	(1)
AT 4 WEEKS EACH TREATMENT SLIGHTLY BETTER THAN SPONTANEOUS IMPROVEMENT.	(4)
FOR MANIPULATION THERE WAS A SIGNIFICANT BENEFIT ON PAIN ANALOGUE SCALE.	(4)
A FEW PATIENTS RESPONDED WELL AND QUICKLY TO MANIPULATION, BUT NO WAY OF IDENTIFYING THOSE PATIENTS IN ADVANCE.	(5)
MORE PATIENTS IN THE MANIPULATION GROUP WERE MARKEDLY IMPROVED AND COMPLETELY RELIEVED, BUT THE NUMBER WAS NOT SIGNIFICANTLY HIGHER THAN IN THE OTHER GROUPS.	(5)
PAIN SCORES SIGNIFICANTLY DECREASED WITHIN FOUR WEEKS OF STARTING COURSE OF MANIPULATION	(7)
NO SIGNIFICANT DIFFERENCE BETWEEN GROUPS IN PAIN RELIEF AT 1 MONTH.	(8)
NO DIFFERENCE BETWEEN GROUPS ON DISCHARGE AND 3 WEEKS LATER.	(9)
AT FOUR WEEKS IN GENERAL PRACTITIONER PATIENTS, SOME ADVANTAGE IN FAVOUR OF PATIENTS IN MOBILIZATION GROUP.	(10)
AT FOUR WEEKS IN HOSPITAL PATIENTS, NO DIFFERENCE BETWEEN GROUPS.	(10)
SIGNIFICANTLY MORE PATIENTS PAIN-FREE, NORMAL FUNCTION AND FIT TO WORK IN MANIPULATED GROUP THAN IN CONTROL GROUP.	(11)

TABLE XVII-7

EFFECT WITHIN FIRST MONTHS AFTER MANIPULATION

	TRIAL
NO BENEFICIAL EFFECTS AT 4 MONTHS.	(4)
AT 3 MONTHS NO DIFFERENCES BETWEEN TREATMENT GROUPS.	(10)

TABLE XVII-8

EFFECT WITHIN FIRST YEARS AFTER MANIPULATION

TRIAL

NO BENEFICIAL EFFECTS AT 16 MONTHS.   (4)

AT 1 YEAR NO DIFFERENCES BETWEEN TREATMENT GROUPS.   (10)

TABLE XVII-9

EFFECT ON SYMPTOMS AND SIGNS

TRIAL

SIGNIFICANT IMPROVEMENT IN MANIPULATED GROUP IN
SITTING, REACHING AND BENDING.   (2)

SPINAL FLEXION SIGNIFICANTLY INCREASES DURING
MANIPULATIVE TREATMENT, BUT DECREASES QUICKLY
THEREAFTER.   (7)

GENERAL PRACTITIONER PATIENTS –
    –   DECREASE IN SPINAL FLEXION IN CONTROLS:
        NOT IN TREATED GROUP.
    –   BOTH GROUPS HAD SIGNIFICANT IMPROVEMENT IN
        SPINAL EXTENSION.
    –   STRAIGHT LEG RAISING IMPROVED SIGNIFICANTLY
        IN TREATED GROUP.   (10)

HOSPITAL PATIENTS –
    –   NO CHANGES IN SPINAL FLEXION.
    –   BOTH GROUPS HAD SIGNIFICANT IMPROVEMENT IN
        SPINAL EXTENSION
    –   STRAIGHT LEG RAISING IMPROVED SIGNIFICANTLY
        IN TREATED GROUP.   (10)

SIGNIFICANT EFFECTS OF MANIPULATION WERE ITS RAPID
EFFECT ON LEG PAIN, LIST AND STRAIGHT LEG RAISING.   (3)

SIGNIFICANTLY MORE PATIENTS HAD INCREASED MOBILITY
IN THE MANIPULATED GROUP THAN IN THE CONTROL GROUP.   (11)

TABLE XVII-10

SUGGESTIONS HINTING AT DIAGNOSES RESPONSIVE TO MANIPULATION

	TRIAL
PATIENTS SHOWING THE MOST BENEFIT FROM MANIPULATION WERE THOSE WHO HAD NO MYELOGRAPHIC EVIDENCE OF DISC PROTRUSION.	(3)
MANIPULATION DID NOT CHANGE APPEARANCE OF MYELOGRAM.	(3)
PATIENTS WITH LESS THAN ONE WEEK'S HISTORY IMPROVED MORE RAPIDLY THAN THOSE WITH MORE THAN ONE WEEK'S HISTORY.	(8)
PATIENTS WHO RESPONDED TO MANIPULATION TENDED TO BE OLDER WHEN THEIR PAIN STARTED.	(2)
RESPONDERS HAD SIGNIFICANTLY LATER AGE OF ONSET OF LOW BACK PAIN.	(7)
RESPONDERS SIGNIFICANTLY OLDER THAN NON-RESPONDERS.	(7)

REFERENCES

Bergquist-Ullman, M. and Larsson, U.: Acute low back pain in industry: A controlled prospective study with special reference to therapy and confounding factors. *Acta Orthopaedica Scandinavica, Supplementum 170*:1-117, 1977.

Buerger, A.A.: A controlled trial of rotational manipulation in low back pain. *Manuelle Medizin, 2*:17-26, 1980.

Chrisman, O.D.; Mittnacht, A. and Snook, G.A.: A study of the results following rotatory manipulation in the lumbar intervertebral-disc syndrome. *Journal of Bone and Joint Surgery, 46-A*:517-524, 1964.

Coxhead, C.E.; Inskip, H.; Meade, T.W.; North, W.R.S. and Troup, J.D.G.: Multicentre trial of physiotherapy in the management of sciatic symptoms. *Lancet, 1*:1065-8, May 16, 1981.

Doran, D.M.L. and Newell, D.J.: Manipulation in the treatment of low back pain: A multicentre study. *British Medical Journal, 2*:161-164, April 26, 1975.

Ebbets, J.: Manipulation in the treatment of low back pain. *British Medical Journal, 2*:393, May 17, 1975.

Edwards, B.C.: Low back pain and pain resulting from lumbar spine conditions: A comparison of treatment results. *Australian Journal of Physiotherapy, 15*:104-110, 1969.

Evans, D.P.; Burke, M.S.; Lloyd, K.N.; Roberts, E.E. and Roberts, G.M.: Lumbar spinal manipulation on trial: Part I — Clinical assessment. *Rheumatology and Rehabilitation, 17*:46-53, 1978.

Evans, D.P.: *Backache: Its Evolution and Conservative Treatment.* MTP Press, Lancaster, England, 1982, especially pp. 221-228.

Glover, J.R.; Morris, J.G. and Khosla, T.: Back pain: A randomized clinical trial of rotational manipulation of the trunk. *British Journal of Industrial Medicine, 31*:59-64, 1974.

Hoehler, F.K.; Tobis, J.S. and Buerger, A.A.: Spinal manipulation for low back pain. *Journal of the American Medical Association, 245*:1835-38, 1981.

Jayson, M.I.V.; Sims-Williams, H.; Young, S.; Baddeley, H. and Collins, E.: Mobilization and manipulation for low-back pain. *Spine, 6*:409-416, 1981.

Kane, R.L.; Leymaster, C.; Olsen, D.; Woolley, F.R. and Fisher, F.D.: Manipulating the patient: A comparison of the effectiveness of physician and chiropractor care. *Lancet, 1*:1333-1336, June 29, 1974.

Rasmussen, G.G.: Manipulation in treatment of low back pain (A randomized clinical trial). *Manuelle Medizin, 1*:8-10, 1979.

Section 5
OVERVIEWS — INTRODUCTION

I T is an unfortunate fact that randomized clinical trials are ultimately unable to "prove" anything, although they are the most potent available approach to vindicating clinical techniques. To assure scientific acceptance one must have a theoretical explanation for any particular clinical treatment which encompasses the bulk of the evidence available from clinical trials and the evidence from other experiments in the basic and clinical sciences, and is therefore accepted by a significant proportion of the scientific community, both basic and clinical.

The fundamentals of this difficult problem can be easily understood when one remembers that if one runs 1000 statistical tests *merely by chance* 50 of them will be significant at the 0.05 level and 10 of them, at the 0.01 level. Hence, when one conducts a clinical trial it is essential that most of the reportable results which approach or surpass statistical significance fall into a pattern explainable by a theory well founded in the basic and clinical sciences.

It is for this reason that we feel the papers of Drs. Dvorak and Neumann are especially important because they begin to put the current evidence in theoretical perspectives which integrate much of the available knowledge.

CHAPTER EIGHTEEN

NEUROLOGICAL AND BIOMECHANICAL
ASPECTS OF BACK PAIN

J. DVORAK, M.D.

1. INTRODUCTION

IN 1955 Gutzeit identified two important historical starting points essential in documenting the importance of the spinal disorders and in understanding their clinical appearance:

(1) the operation for the herniated intervertebral disc by Mixter and Barr (1934) by which the "rheumatic" ischialgia could be cured,

(2) the perception by osteopathic physicians and chiropractors that pain caused by the joints of vertebrae can be influenced through manual treatment of the spine.

Both points are still significant. Diagnosis of the objective radicular failure or breakdown, clarification through radiology including myelography, CT-scan with its three dimensional reconstructive recordings (Glen et al., 1979), as well as precise palpatory examination of the spine and the neighboring soft tissue are all prerequisites for the establishment of a clear decision as to what procedure or procedures are to be applied. These procedures are (1) the surgical removal in a radicular compression syndrome (be it the result of a herniated intervertebral disk or bony new growth), (2) the manual treatment of the spine when a spondylogenic or pseudoradicular pain syndrome is present, and/or (3) pharmaceutical therapy.

As a result of their palpatory experience, manual therapists (Lewit, 1977; Maigne, 1970), osteopathic physicians (Mitchell et al., 1979; Jones, 1981), and chiropractors (Walther, 1981) have contributed to the field of functional diagnosis of the musculoskeletal system, especially of the spine and its sur-

In patients suffering from an acute radicular syndrome, there is little diagnostic difficulty. Again, the neurophysiological explanation of radicular pain is well known. This is not true of patients suffering from chronic back pain. Especially in these individuals, the differentiation for further therapy is very important but not always simple.

Different authors with extensive clinical experience have tried to systematize the painful soft tissue changes (often described as non-inflammatory soft tissue rheumatism) found in chronic back pain and have tried to correlate these with functional disturbances of the vertebral column or peripheral joints (e.g. Bruegger, 1962; Dvorak and Dvorak, 1983; Feinstein, 1977; Jones, 1981; Simons, 1981; Sutter, 1974; Tilscher, 1981; Travell, 1981). Even though the same or similar phenomena were described, the language used by these authors was different and depended on each individual's training and understanding. Due to this diverse terminology and also due to divergent neurophysiological theories, these valuable clinical observations were accepted by organized medicine only under certain conditions and in a limited fashion.

However, new neurophysiological work substantiates these previous empirical observations of the non-radicular pain syndrome of the vertebral column (e.g. Eldred et al., 1976; Howard, 1982; Jowett and Fidler, 1975; Korr, 1975; Richmond and Abrahams, 1979; Schmidt et al. 1981; Simons, 1976; Wyke, 1979; Zimmermann, 1981). Articular neurology, as presented by Wyke, contributes valuable findings and is especially useful in understanding of the non-radicular pain syndrome of vertebral and para-vertebral structures as well as in understanding manipulative medicine.

1.1 SPONDYLOGENIC REFLEX SYNDROME

The clinical literature has presented many concepts of the referred pain in connection with the vertebral structures (Bruegger, 1962; Feinstein, 1977; Jones, 1981; Kellgren, 1977; Simons, 1976; Travell and Rinzler, 1952). From this point on, only the concept of the Swiss School for Manipulative Medicine is explained further.

Sutter (1974) observed relationships between the vertebral column with its soft tissues and the peripheral soft tissue which could not always be attributed to radicular, vascular and humoral causes. These empirically found relationships are defined as spondylogenic reflex syndrome. Being mediated through the reflexogenic paths of the central nervous system, it is defined as the reproducible, causative relationship between the reciprocal functionally abnormal position or segmental dysfunction of skeletal parts of the axial skeleton and the local, and anatomically determined noninflammatory-rheumatic soft tissue changes. The term "functionally abnormal position" or segmental dysfunction is understood to be disturbance of the so-called "inner function" of the vertebral unit as described by Junghans (1976).

The segmental dysfunction in a vertebral unit results in a reflexogenic pathological change of the soft tissue, the most important being the myotendinosis. Myotendinosis is characterized by permanently increased tone, elevated consistency, resistance and decreased plasticity.

A clinically demonstrable manifestation of the segmental dysfunction is the zone of irritation according to Caviezel (1973) and Sutter (1974), or the paravertebral joint as described by Maigne (1970). These are swellings painful upon pressure which can be palpated and are found at topographically well defined sites in the musculo-fascial tissue (i.e. Figure XVIII-1: zone of irritation at the cervical spine). Their size ranges between 0.5 to 1.0 cm. The zone of irritation is directly related to the duration and quality of the segmental dysfunction in the vertebral unit. As long as a disturbance exists, zones of irritation can be shown which, however, disappear after successful treatment. To date no anatomic or histological substrate of the zone of irritation could be found.

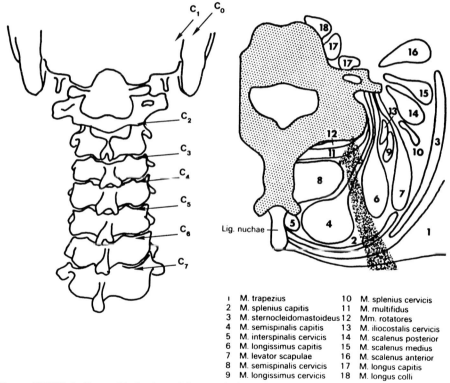

1	M. trapezius	10	M. splenius cervicis
2	M. splenius capitis	11	M. multifidus
3	M. sternocleidomastoideus	12	Mm. rotatores
4	M. semispinalis capitis	13	M. iliocostalis cervicis
5	M. interspinalis cervicis	14	M. scalenus posterior
6	M. longissimus capitis	15	M. scalenus medius
7	M. levator scapulae	16	M. scalenus anterior
8	M. semispinalis cervicis	17	M. longus capitis
9	M. longissimus cervicis	18	M. longus colli

Figure XVIII-1. Zone of irritation of the cervical spine (left). Cross section of the central cervical spine (right). Access to the zone of irritation is indicated by arrow (from Dvorak and Dvorak, 1983).

The segmental dysfunction in the vertebral unit causes reflexogenic and pathological changes in the soft tissue of which the most important are the myotendinoses. These can be discriminated by palpation.

1.2 MYOTENDINOSES ("HARTSPANN")

Myotendinosis is characterized by increased permanent tone, elevated consistency, resistance and decreased plasticity. They are termed "Hartspann" in German. A whole muscle or only a few segments in the longitudinal direction can be affected. When palpating perpedicularly with average pressure, myotendinosis is painful and can easily be differentiated from the unaffected surrounding area of the same muscle. "Nervous misinformation" of certain muscle bundles arriving in the reflexogenic pathway may be responsible for the origin of the involuntary isometric increase of tonus in the muscle bundle (Fassbender, 1980).

After a latency period myotendinosis leads to the formation of myoses in the muscles, and tendinoses of the tendons at the origins and insertions (Table XVIII-1). A segmental dysfunction in one vertebral unit causes simultaneous myotendinosis in the related myotendons. Since the spondylogenic-reflexogenic myotendinoses can be located with regularity, they are correctly termed "systematic myotendinoses" (Sutter, Sutter and Frohlich, 1981; Dvorak and Dvorak, 1983).

Figures XVIII-2, XVIII-3, XVIII-4 illustrate the complete spondylogenic reflex syndromes correlated with segmental dysfunctions in the vertebral unit C_2, C_5 and L_3 respectively. Again, it should be noted that these are empirical, clinical findings; neurophysiological findings and speculations are currently insufficient and only partially successful.

2. NEUROPHYSIOLOGICAL ASPECTS OF BACK PAIN

The following presentation deals with two aspects of the non-radicular back pain caused by somatic dysfunction:

(1) pathology due to articular neurology, and
(2) functional pathology of paraspinal and peripheral muscles.

It is conceivable that a disturbance in both the region of the fibrous joints capsule of the upper apophyseal joints and the back musculature can lead to a pathological (dysharmonic) motion in the individual vertebral segments (Figure XVIII-5).

2.1 ARTICULAR NEUROLOGY

2.1.1. Innervation of the Apophyseal Joints

The joint capsule of the apophyseal joints is supplied by the dorsal rami of the spinal nerves. The articular rami of a nerve root not only contribute to one

Myotendinoses

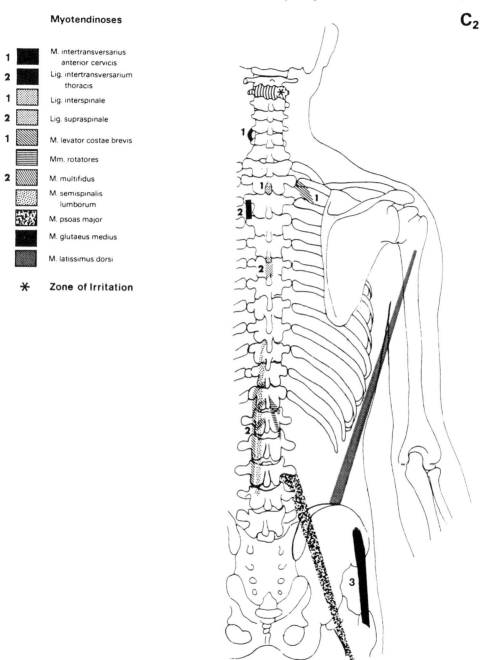

C_2

1		M. intertransversarius anterior cervicis
2		Lig. intertransversarium thoracis
1		Lig. interspinale
2		Lig. supraspinale
1		M. levator costae brevis
		Mm. rotatores
2		M. multifidus
		M. semispinalis lumborum
		M. psoas major
		M. glutaeus medius
		M. latissimus dorsi
∗		**Zone of Irritation**

Figure XVIII-2. Spondylogenic reflex syndrome with segmental dysfunction of the second cervical vertebra (from Dvorak and Dvorak, 1983).

segmental joint capsule, but collateral rami lead to one to two joints above and below (Wyke, 1967). This pluri-segmental innervation is of clinical importance. Recent anatomical and physiological studies are in agreement for the

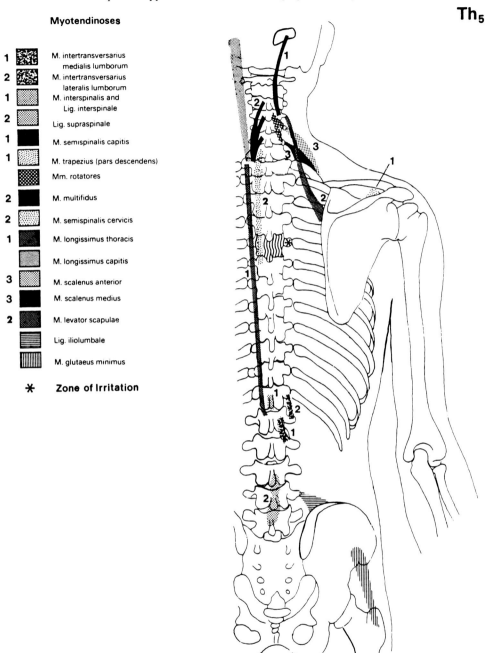

Myotendinoses

1		M. intertransversarius medialis lumborum
2		M. intertransversarius lateralis lumborum
1		M. interspinalis and Lig. interspinale
2		Lig. supraspinale
1		M. semispinalis capitis
1		M. trapezius (pars descendens)
		Mm. rotatores
2		M. multifidus
2		M. semispinalis cervicis
1		M. longissimus thoracis
		M. longissimus capitis
3		M. scalenus anterior
3		M. scalenus medius
2		M. levator scapulae
		Lig. iliolumbale
		M. glutaeus minimus

✳   Zone of Irritation

Th₅

Figure XVIII-3. The spondylogenic reflex syndrome caused by segmental dysfunction of the fifth thoracic vertebra (from Dvorak and Dvorak, 1983).

main part (Clark, 1975; Clark and Burgess, 1965; Freeman and Wyke, 1967; Grigg, 1977; Pollacek, 1966; Wyke, 1979, 1981). These joint capsule receptors share a certain similarity with the Ruffinian and Pacinian corpuscles, but as

Myotendinoses

L₃

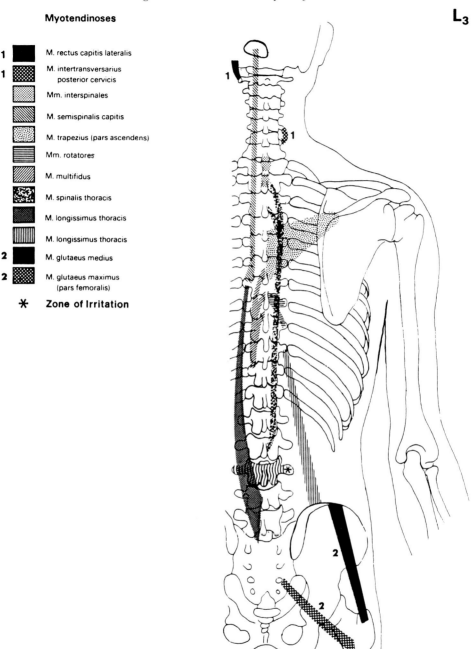

1	■	M. rectus capitis lateralis
1	▨	M. intertransversarius posterior cervicis
	▨	Mm. interspinales
	▨	M. semispinalis capitis
	▨	M. trapezius (pars ascendens)
	▤	Mm. rotatores
	▨	M. multifidus
	▨	M. spinalis thoracis
	▨	M. longissimus thoracis
	▥	M. longissimus thoracis
2	■	M. glutaeus medius
2	▨	M. glutaeus maximus (pars femoralis)
	✱	**Zone of Irritation**

Figure XVIII-4. The spondylogenic reflex-syndrome caused by segmental dysfunction of the third lumbar vertebra (from Dvorak and Dvorak, 1983).

suggested by Brodal (1981), the description of receptors should be used which was coined by Freeman and Wyke (1967). Freeman and Wyke divide the receptors of the fibrous joint capsules into four groups (Types I through IV) ac-

TABLE XVIII-1

DEVELOPMENT OF MYOTENDINOSIS.

(A) PATHOGENESIS OF THE NON-INFLAMMATORY SOFT TISSUE RHEUMATISM

(AFTER FASSBENDER, 1980).

(B) DEVELOPMENT IN MUSCLE

(C) DEVELOPMENT IN TENDINOUS PORTIONS

(AFTER DVORAK AND DVORAK, 1983 AND FASSBENDER, 1980).

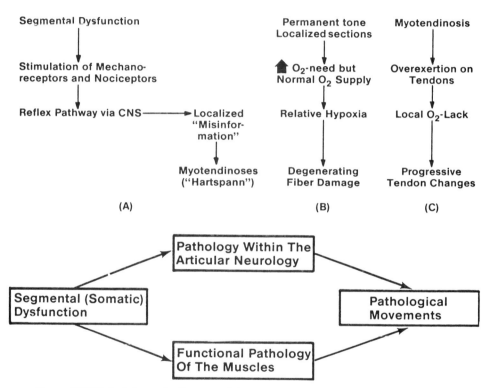

Figure **XVIII-5.** Schematic diagram of the consequences of segmental dysfunction.

cording to their neurohistological properties (Table XVIII-2, Figure XVIII-6). Every group seems to serve a specific function, whereby all react upon changes in pressure and tension.

TYPE I RECEPTOR (MECHANORECEPTORS)

This type of mechanoreceptor consists of multiple (3-8), thinly encapsulated, globular corpuscles (about 100 micrometers by 40 micrometers) which are found in the outer layer of the fibrous joint capsule. The afferent nerve fibers are thinly myelinated, that is, they are 6-9 micrometers in diameter.

These Type I Mechanoreceptors have three functions:

TABLE XVIII-2

MORPHOLOGICAL AND FUNCTIONAL CHARACTERISTICS OF THE RECEPTORS OF JOINT CAPSULES

Type	Morphology	Location	Parent Nerve Fibers	Behavioral Characteristics	Function
I	Thinly-encapsulated globular corpuscles (100 × 40 μm) in clusters of 3-8	Fibrous capsulae of joint (super-layers)	Small myelinated (6-9 μm)	Static and dynamic mechanoreceptors: low threshold, slowly adapting	Tonic reflexogenic effects on neck, limb, jaw and eye muscles. Postural and kinesthetic sensation. Pain suppression.
II	Thickly encapsulated conical corpuscles (280 × 100 μm) singly or in clusters of 2-4	Fibrous capsulae of joint (deeper layers) Articular fat pads	Medium myelinated (9-12 μm)	Dynamic mechanoreceptors: low threshold, rapidly adapting	a) Phasic reflexo-genic effects on neck, limb, jaw and eye muscles. b) Pain suppression
III	Fusiform corpuscles (600 × 100 μm) usually singly, also in clusters of 2-3.	Ligaments, also in related tendons	Large myelinated (13-17 μm)	Mechanoreceptor, high threshold, very slowly adapting	Unknown
IV	Three-dimensional plexus of unmyelinated nerve fibers	Entire thickness of fibrous capsulae of joint. Walls of articular blood vessels. Articular fat pads	Very small myelinated (2-5 μm), and unmyelinated	Nociceptive (pain-provoking). High threshold, non-adapting	a) Tonic reflexogenic effects on neck, limb, jaw and eye muscles b) Evocation of pain c) Respiratory and cardiovascular reflexogenic effects

(after WYKE) The Neurology of Joints. Annals of the Royal College of Surgeons, Edinburgh, 41 : 25-60, 1966.

a) These slowly adapting receptors control tension of the outer layers of the joint capsule.

b) They inhibit, via a synapse, the centripetal flow of the activity from the nociceptive afferent receptors (Type IV nociceptors), or in other words, they inhibit the impulses arising from pain receptors (Figure XVIII-7).

c) They have tonic reflex effects on the motoneurons of the neck, limbs, jaw, and eye muscles.

TYPE II RECEPTORS (MECHANORECEPTORS)

Type II receptors consist of oblong, conicle, thickly encapsulated corpuscles (about 280 micrometers by 100 micrometers), which appear most often singly in the deep layers of the fibrous joint capsule. These receptors are connected with articular rami through thickly myelinated fibers.

These Type II mechanoreceptors also have three functions:

a) They are rapidly adapting (less than 0.5 seconds) mechanoreceptors with a low threshold reaction to changes in tension of the fibrous joint capsule.

b) They have phasic reflex effects on neck, limb, jaw and eye muscles.

c) They reduce, via presynaptic inhibition, the nociceptive activity of the joint capsule.

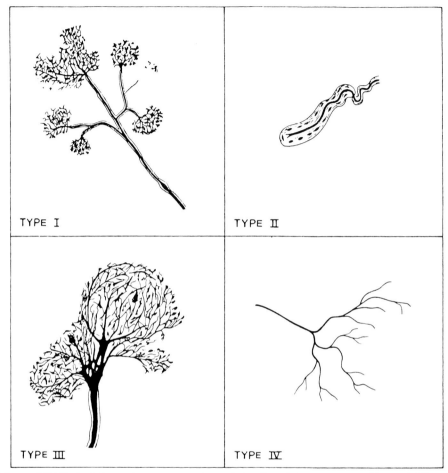

Figure XVIII-6. Schematic representation of the four joint receptors (Types I-IV, after Polacek, 1966; Wyke, 1979).

TYPE III RECEPTORS (MECHANORECEPTORS)

Type III mechanoreceptors are the typical receptors of the ligaments and tendons; they are found close to the joint capsule but are not found in the joint capsule itself. They do, however, have an important role in relation to the function of the joint. Histologically, they consist of broad fusiform corpuscles (about 700 micrometers by 100 micrometers) and usually appear singly. Type III receptors are innervated by large myelinated (13-17 micrometers in diameter) fibers and are connected with the articular branches. They resemble the ligamentous receptors of the Golgi's corpuscles; thus one can assume that they have the same function, that is that these slowly adapting receptors have an inhibitory effect on motoneurons.

TYPE IV RECEPTORS (NOCICEPTORS)

Type IV, the nociceptors, are very thinly myelinated or non-myelinated plexiform nerve endings. They are ubiquitous in the fibrous portion of the joint capsule, the ligaments and the subsynovial capsule. Depolarization occurs (1) with constant pressure on the joint capsule (due to non-physiological position, abrupt motions, etc.), (2) with narrowing of the intervertebral disc, (3) with fracture of the vertebral body, (4) with dislocation of the apophyseal joints, or (5) with chemical irritation (e.g. increased potassium, lactic acid, 5-hydroxy-tryptamine, histamine), as well as with interstitial edema of the joint capsule in acute or chronic inflammatory processes.

These Type IV nociceptors have three functions:

a) They have tonic reflex effects on neck, limb, jaw and eye muscles.
b) They evoke pain.
c) They have reflex respiratory and cardiovascular effects.

In addition to these four receptor types, sympathetic nerve fibers are found in the joint capsule.

It is obvious that the central nervous system continuously receives information about position and changes of position through the receptors of the joints. However, in the entire sequence of motion muscle spindles and Golgi-organs play a role as important as the joint receptors, but a definitive order of importance has not yet been established.

2.2.2 Clinical Correlations of the Reflexes Associated with Mechanoreceptors and Nociceptors

According to Wyke (1975, 1979a, 1979b), the results of experiments in

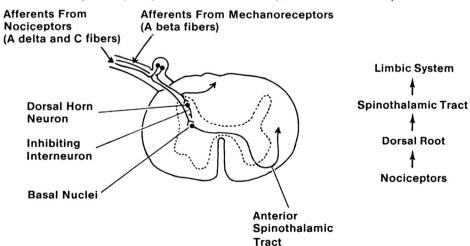

Figure XVIII-7. Simplified representation of the afferent fibers in the region of the dorsal root (after Wyke, 1979).

articular neurology yield new views which may contribute significantly to the diagnostic and therapeutic understanding of manipulative medicine.

According to a clinical study among adolescents, the absence of pain is not identical with absence of soft tissue changes. Systematic myotendinoses can often be detected by palpation in individuals subjectively free of complaints. It is our understanding that this situation is to be considered pathological and could be correlated with a latent state of the intervertebral insufficiency as described by Schmorl and Junghanns (1968).

To correlate this clinical observation with the experimental work of Wyke, one would equate myotendinoses with the tonic reflexogenic influence of Type I mechanoreceptors upon motoneurons of the axial musculature and the musculature of the extremities. The fact that pain inducing nociceptors demonstrate a significantly higher threshold than mechanoreceptors explains the time delay of the subjective perception of pain by the patient. In this situation as well, however, the nociceptors input can be presynaptically inhibited by adequate stimuli of the mechanoreceptors, especially Type II.

It is very probable that this neurophysiological mechanism plays as important a role in the manual-therapeutic treatment as in the mechanical correction of the segmental dysfunction. Tables XVIII-3 and XVIII-4 attempt to present this model schematically.

2.2 FUNCTIONAL PATHOLOGY OF THE MUSCLES

2.2.1 Morphology and Physiology of Slow and Fast Twitch Fibers

Human skeletal muscles are composed of thousands of individual muscle fibers. One single muscle fiber is approximately the thickness of one hair and can reach a length of 10-15 centimeters depending on the size of the muscle.

Two types of muscle fibers are differentiated. The so-called slow twitch fibers (Type I-fibers) and fast twitch fibers (Type II-fibers). In addition to these two important fiber types, so-called intermediary types (IIA, IIB) are found. A histochemical examination primarily with ATP-ase stains makes it possible to discriminate the slow and fast twitch portions of an individual muscle.

Postural muscles are mainly composed of slow twitch fibers in contrast to phasic muscles which are primarily composed of fast twitch fibers. As seen by their name, these slow twitch fibers contract more slowly (in approximately 100 milliseconds), in contrast to the fast twitch fibers which contract in about 7-milliseconds. The slow twitch fibers obtain their energy mainly from glycogen and fat with high oxygen consumption and minimal lactic acid production, is in contrast to the fast twitch fibers which receive their main energy from glucose from the anaerobic cycle with rapid production of lactic acid. The capil-

TABLE XVIII-3

MODEL OF FUNCTIONAL RELATIONSHIPS BETWEEN RECEPTORS OF JOINT CAPSULES
AND CORRECT POSITION OF VERTEBRAE. (AFTER DVORAK AND DVORAK, 1983)

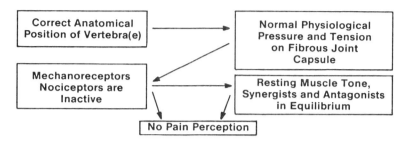

TABLE XVIII-4

FUNCTION AND ACTIVITIES OF RECEPTORS OF JOINT CAPSULES
DUE TO SEGMENTAL DYSFUNCTION IN A VERTEBRAL UNIT.
A MODEL OF A POSSIBLE ROLE OF MANIPULATION (AFTER DVORAK AND DVORAK, 1983).

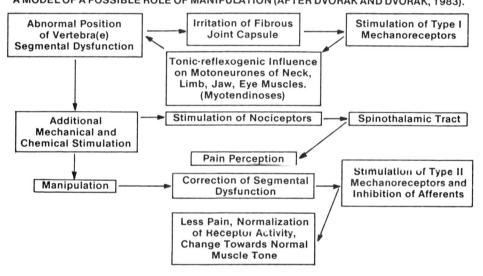

lary supply of slow twitch fibers is significantly higher (approximately 4.8 capillaries per fiber) than that of fast twitch fibers (approximately 2.9 capillaries per fiber). The slow twitch fibers fatigue after several hundred contractions in comparison to fast twitch fibers which fatigue after a few contractions. These slow twitch fibers are primarily innervated by alpha-two motoneurons and have a great supply of muscle spindles. The fast twitch fibers are innervated by alpha-one motoneurons and have only a few muscle spindles (Richmond and Abrahams, 1979). The fact that muscle spindles are not randomly distributed seems to have a significance in the development of the functional pathology of muscles. Table XVIII-5 shows the important differences between the slow twitch and fast twitch fibers.

TABLE XVIII-5

MAIN CHARACTERISTICS OF SLOW TWITCH AND FAST-TWITCH FIBERS

	Slow Twitch (I)	Fast Twitch (II)
Function	Phasic Fatigue Slowly	Tonic Fatigue Fast
Reaction	Slow	Fast
Color	Red	White
Spindle	Many	Few
Innervation	Alpha-2-Motoneuron	Alpha-1-Motoneuron
Tendency	Shortening	Weaking

Examinations of top athletes show (Billeter and Howald, 1981; Hintermann and Hintermann, 1983) that the ratio between slow twitch and fast twitch fibers is not fixed in one muscle and thus can be changed by different exercises. The quadriceps muscle of a marathon runner consists of up to 93 percent of slow twitch fibers while the musculature of an untrained person consists only of 48 percent of slow twitch fibers (Billeter and Howald, 1981).

The histochemical study by Jowett and Fidler (1975) indicates that hypomobility of the lumbar spine and compressions of the nerve roots can lead to changes of the slow twitch to fast twitch ratio inthe multifidous muscle, by decreasing the fast fibers. The same study shows that patients with idiopathic scoliosis have more slow twitch fibers on the side of the convexity than on the concave side.

No histochemical study has yet shown that morphological transformation of the individual muscle fibers takes place in patients with so-called functional muscular imbalance, even though it is assumed that a clinically shortened muscle (mainly postural muscle) shows a significantly higher number of slow twitch fibers than the normal muscle.

Figure XVIII-8 shows the possibilities of transformation of individual muscle fibers when stimulated with different electrical currents or with different types of training.

2.2.2 Muscle Receptors

Five different types of receptors are found in voluntary muscles:

(1) muscle spindles
(2) Golgi tendon organs
(3) Vater-Pacinian corpuscles
(4) free nerve endings (Type IV nociceptors, according to Wyke)

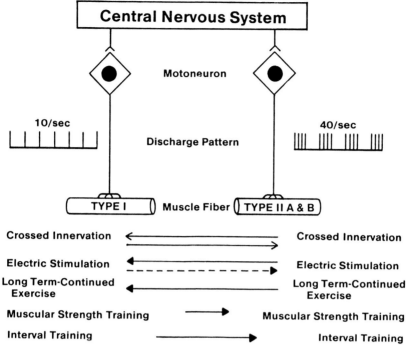

Figure XVIII-8. Transformation by the motor unit of slow-twitch and fast-twitch fibers (after Billeter and Howald, 1981).

(5) synovial joint capsule receptors (Type III mechanoreceptors, according to Wyke)

The three dimensional free nerve endings have been described above. The Type III mechanoreceptors are primarily found at the junction of tendon and the periosteum and have also been described in Section 2.1 on articular neurology. In the following the two most important receptors, the muscle spindles and tendon organs of Golgi, are emphasized.

a) Muscle Spindles

Morphological studies (Richmond and Abrahams, 1981) clearly demonstrate that the distribution of muscle spindles in the voluntary musculature is quite variable. Muscles which are responsible for very delicate and precise movements show significantly higher numbers of muscle spindles than those which deal with gross movements.

Fifty muscle spindles are found in one gram of the rectus femoris muscle; in contrast the small suboccipital muscles have 150-200 muscle spindles per gram of muscle tissue. The paraspinal musculature, such as the intertransverse muscles in the cervical regions, has as many as 200-500 muscle spindles per gram of tissue. Muscle spindles are usually found in proximity of the slow twitch fibers (Richmond and Abrahams, 1981). These findings significantly aid in understanding the behavior of postural muscles when overly used. As was mentioned above, the individual muscles show a higher proportion of slow twitch fibers in postural muscles. Clinical observation indicates that these muscles tend to be able to continue to shorten, while phasic muscles which primarily consist of fast twitch fibers tend to fatigue.

The muscle spindles contain 3-8 narrow muscle fibers which are also known as intrafusal muscle fibers. These intrafusal muscle fibers are parallel to the normal skeletal musculature or the so-called extrafusal muscle fibers (refer to Figures XVIII-9A through C). When the extrafusal muscle fibers contract, tension in the portion of that muscle spindle which does not contract decreases. When the muscle is stretched, tension in both intrafusal and extrafusal fibers increases.

The center of the muscle spindle is "sensory", not contractile and harbors

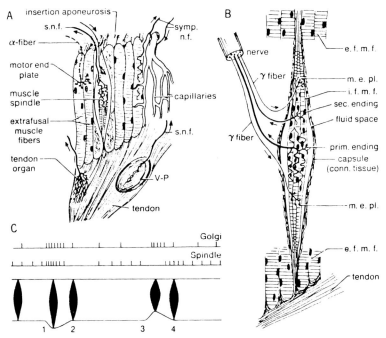

Figure XVIII-9. A. Diagrams of the three main receptors in skeletal muscles: a muscle spindle, a tendon organ, and a Vater-Pacinian corpuscle (V-P). Note that the spindle is arranged in parallel with the extrafusal muscle fibers, while the tendon organ is arranged in series with them. This has important consequences for their function.

B. Very simplified diagram of a muscle spindle to show its principle components (see text). Abbreviations: e.f.m.f., extrafusal muscle fibers; i.f.m.f., intrafusal muscle fibers; m.e.pl., motor endings; s.n.f., sensory nerve fiber.

C. A diagram illustrating the response of a Golgi tendon organ and a muscle spindle ending during stretch and contraction of the muscle. The muscle is drawn below in black, between lines indicating its insertion. Action potentials are shown in two top lines. Further explanation in text. (Fig. C from Granit, 1955) (from Brodal, 1981).

many nuclei. They are surrounded by spirally coursing nerve fibers, the primary sensory or annulospiral endings. A secondary sensory ending (flowerspray ending) may be present amongst the 3-8 narrow muscle fibers mentioned in the preceding paragraph at one or both sides of the annulospiral ending. In addition, the muscle spindles receive a motor innervation by fine nerve fibers (gamma fibers or fusimotor fibers), whose cell bodies are within the ventral horn of the spinal cord. They terminate in the distal cross-striated parts of the contractile intrafusal fibers. Hence a contraction of the distal parts of the intrafusal fibers in response to impulses in the gamma fibers will result in a stretching of the central "sensory" part of the intrafusal fibers, with a consequent stimulation of sensory endings, just as will the stretching of the entire muscle (after Brodal, 1981). (See Figure XVIII-10.)

b) Golgi Tendon Organs

The tendon organs consist of branches of a large myelinated nerve fiber (12 to 18 micrometers in diameter [Cooper, 1960; Schoultz and Swett, 1972]) which terminate with a spray of fine endings between bundles of the collagenous fibers of tendons usually near the musculotendinous junction. To understand their function, it is essential to recognize the fact that they are arranged in series with the extrafusal muscle fibers. *Whether the muscle contracts or is stretched, the tendon organ will be stimulated*, since in both cases the tension of the tendon organ will increase (Brodal, 1981).

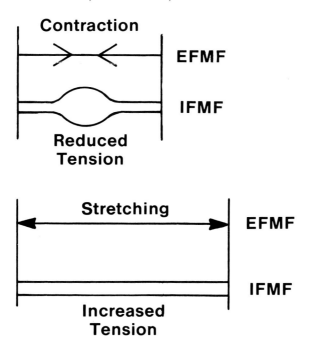

Figure XVIII-10. Schematic representation of muscle spindle function: EFMF — extrafusal muscle fibers, IFMF — intrafusal muscle fibers.

In other words, the tendon organs are tension recorders, while the muscle spindles give information about the length of the muscle (Matthews, 1933; Granit, 1955, 1975) (See Figure XVIII-9.)

For further information please refer to the chapter "The Peripheral Moto-neuron" in Neurological Anatomy in Relation to Clinical Medicine (Brodal, 1981).

c)   Alpha and Gamma Co-Activation

This is a rather complex mechanism which involves both the function of the alpha and gamma motoneurons and is of significance for manipulative medicine (Granit, 1955; 1975). Please refer to Figure XVIII-11 which is the graphic representation of the material discussed by Hassler (1981). The right side of the diagram shows the regulation of muscle length by the reflex arcs involved; the left portion of the diagram shows the regulation of muscular tension developed as a result of external force.

The myotonic reflex arc of the phasic reflex depends upon a muscle spindle with intrafusal fibers which contract due to stimulation by the gamma-1-neurons. In this fashion, the central portion of the muscle spindle (the non-contractile, central "sensory" portion) is stretched which in turn stimulates the spiral endings of the Ia-fibers which surround this central "sensory" portion. This stimulation is responsible for the elicitation of a specific automatic myotonic reflex, in which the phasic motoneurons of the alpha I fibers are stimulated via the afferent Ia-fibers along with their direct reflex collaterals thus causing contraction of the muscles involved. The gamma-1-firing then eventually causes a decrease in the length of the highly sensitive receptors in the central portion of the muscle spindle. The length of the muscle spindle and therefore the entire muscle tends to be kept constant automatically via the phasic myotonic reflex. The strength of this reflex depends on the strength of the external force as well as the firing rate of the gamma-1-fibers.

The left side of Figure XVIII-11 depicts the regulation of muscle tension. The intrafusal muscle fibers of the slender muscle spindle contract as a result of the influence of the tonic gamma-2-fibers. When the secondary sensory endings located on the intrafusal muscle fibers change their length due to external stretch these secondary endings send impulses to the ventral horn cells of type alpha-2 via afferent type II fibers and associated multisynaptic pathways. These alpha-2-motoneurons cause the slow postular musculature to contract; the length of these postural muscles is maintained as long as the spindle is kept in a certain contraction state via the gamma-2-neurons.

In addition to this tonic stretch reflex, the stretch receptors of the Golgi tendon organs take part in the regulation of muscular tension. These Golgi organs are located at the junction between muscles and tendons. Rapidly conducting I-b fibers lead from these Golgi tendon tension receptors to the spinal cord causing inhibition via several interneurons. They act on both (1) the

Normal Regulation

of Muscle Tension   of Muscle Length

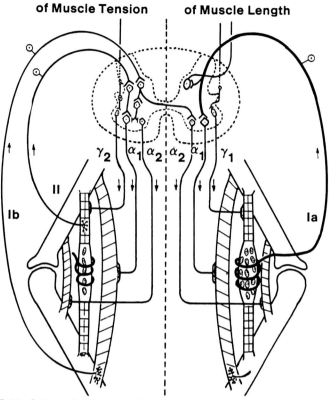

Figure XVIII-11. Schematic representation for the regulation of muscle length (right) and muscle tension (left) and the corresponding reflex arcs (from Hassler, 1981). Please see text for description.

alpha-2 neurons thereby inhibiting contraction of postural musculature which results from the tonic stretch reflex, and also (2) the motoneurons of the alpha-1 fibers and their respective fibers for the phasic extensor motions. This crossed inhibition reflex together with the extensor reflex (which originates from secondary endings) regulates the muscular tension even when it is under the influence of external stretching forces (Hassler, 1981).

In addition to impulses from the tendon organs, there is another mechanism that tends to limit the activity of the excited motoneurons, the so-called recurrent or Renshaw inhibition. When a motoneuron fires impulses, these will pass via its recurrent collaterals to Renshaw cells; these are neurons, short axons situated in the ventral horn, having an inhibitory effect on the motoneurons. The Renshaw cells, as with many other interneurons in the cord, are subjected to supraspinal control, for example from the cerebellum and the mesencephalic reticular formation (Granit, 1975).

Another experimental observation may be useful in understanding the peripheral soft tissue changes related to segmental somatic dysfunction: The muscle spindle afferents within dorsal root supplying the motoneurons mono-synaptically may spread collaterals over several segments (Rethelyi and Szentagothai, 1973). From Golgi studies of longitudinal sections of the cord Rethelyi and Szentagothai showed that these primary afferent fibers run longi-tudinally for a considerable distance near or in the dorsal columns, giving off fibers at regular intervals in a ventral direction to reach the motor nuclei. These branches are found close together in so-called micro-bundles, mainly in the transverse plane within the motor nuclei (Sterling and Kuypers, 1967). This arrangement makes it likely that afferent from one spindle may influence motoneurons in several segments of the cord.

2.2.4 Post-Contraction Sensory Discharge

Several authors have studied the phenomena of post-contraction sensory discharge experimentally (Brown et al., 1970; Eldred et al., 1976; Hnik et al., 1973) and its relation to the clinically observed phenomena of shortening of the postural muscles as well as possible explanations of several manipulative tech-nics (Buerger, 1983).

The original experiments showed by recording either from a single afferent of an individual annulospiral ending or from an entire dorsal nerve root that tetanic stimulation of gamma efferent fibers altered the frequency of firing of an afferent ending from the same muscle spindle which had been stimulated tetannically. Decreasing the length of that spindle below the length at which it had been stimulated eliminated this increase in firing. Overstretching the spin-dle abolished the effects of the tetannic stimulation. In other words, this in-creased firing after tetanic stimulation can be relieved by sudden stretching of the muscle.

The physiological cause for this post-contraction sensory discharge is not known. Eldred et al. (1976) and Granit (1976) believe the cause to be of me-chanical origin; Brown et al. (1970) hypothesize the formation of semi-permanent crossbridges between actin and myosin while Hnik (1973) feels the cause is differences in potassium concentrations.

At the present it is impossible to determine how important the experimen-tal findings discussed in sections 2.1 through 2.2.4 are in understanding the shortening of postural muscles. One may assume, however, that these phenom-ena are partially responsible for the shortening of the postural musculature as well as the transformation of fast twitch fibers to slow twitch fibers.

2.2.5 The Effect of Nociceptive Muscle Afferents on Muscle Tone

As mentioned above, the I-a fibers supply the primary muscle spindle, and I-b fibers supply Golgi-tendon organs. The II muscle afferents also innervate the muscle spindles via secondary spindle afferents. Little is known about the three-dimensional nociceptive free nerve endings and their afferents from these muscles. It can be assumed that these endings serve as receptors for noxious stimuli. Studies by Mense (1977) show that the nociceptors of these muscles do not react to one type of stimulus alone; thus they can be stimulated by mechanical or chemical means (bradykinin, potassium, serotonin). In addition, they can be activated by permanent contraction due to ischemia.

The experimental work by Schmidt et al. (1981) examines the response of alpha-motoneurons with allogenic muscles stimulation. These experiments indicate that these small nociceptive muscle afferents, which are allogenically stimulated, have a direct effect on the alpha and gamma motoneurons of the spinal cord. According to Schmidt's data this effect is rather high intensity; little myelinated muscle afferents could have significant influence on the extent and distribution of muscle tone during standing or moving.

Animal experiments demonstrate that both acute allogenic stimulation of the muscle nociceptors or the chronic stimulation of the small Type III and IV muscle afferents can lead to a permanently increased muscle tone via the gamma loop. This mechanism may be involved in the development of palpable myotendinosis in the human due to segmental dysfunction. Of interest is the work of Fassbender (1980) concerning the regressive muscle fiber damage caused by chronic myotendinosis.

Figure XVIII-12 (after Schmidt et al., 1981) schematically depicts this cycle, which can occur due to stimulation of the skeletal muscular nociceptors and activation of the gamma loop.

3. A CONCEPT OF NON-RADICULAR ARTICULAR AND MUSCULAR PAIN AND THE HISTOCHEMICAL CHANGES INVOLVED

Using the findings from the above neurophysiological studies, the author will now develop a theoretical model for the onset of pain caused by segmental dysfunction of the axial structures (Table XVIII-6).

The most important findings necessary for understanding the model are:

(1) transformation of the slow- and fast twitch fibers following different types of muscle training or conditioning (Howald, 1982; Jowett and Fidler, 1975).

(2) muscle spindles are not randomly distributed. High density in small paraspinal muscles, located closer to the slow twitch fibers (Richmond and Abrahams, 1979).

(3) post-contraction sensory discharge—increased firing Ia fibers — stimulation of alpha-motoneurons — can be relieved by sudden overstretching of the same muscle (Brown et al., 1970; Eldred et al., 1976; Buerger, 1983).

(4) palpable myotendinosis in chronic state can cause a muscle tissue damage as a result of relative hypoxemia (Fassbender, 1980).

(5) segmental dysfunction can alter the muscle tone of paraspinal and peripheral muscles (Wyke, 1975, 1979a, 1979b).

(6) allogenic irritation of the muscles results in increase of the muscle tone in the same muscle (Schmidt et al., 1981).

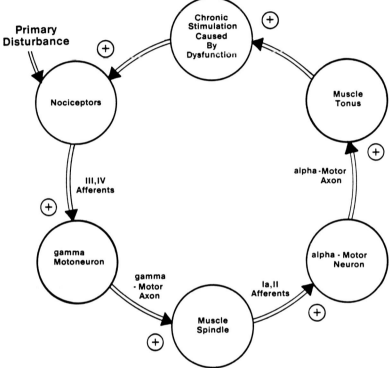

Figure XVIII-12. Increased muscle tone as a result of chronic stimulation of small size nociceptive afferents of skeletal muscle (after Schmidt, 1981).

TABLE XVIII-6
THEORETICAL MODELS FOR SEGMENTAL DYSFUNCTION

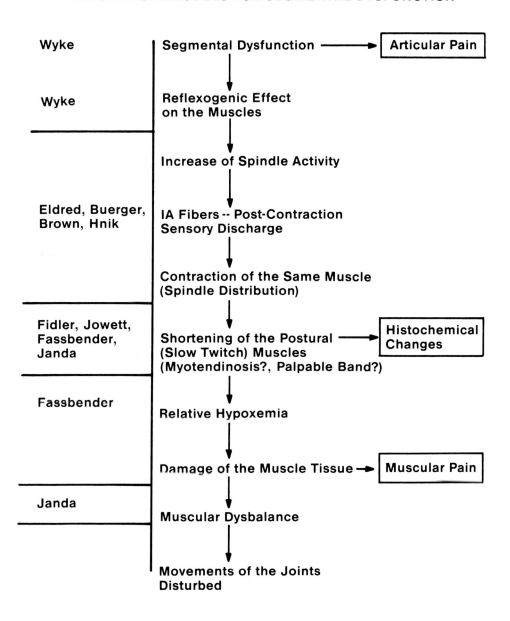

Wyke	Segmental Dysfunction ⟶ **Articular Pain**
Wyke	Reflexogenic Effect on the Muscles
	Increase of Spindle Activity
Eldred, Buerger, Brown, Hnik	IA Fibers -- Post-Contraction Sensory Discharge
	Contraction of the Same Muscle (Spindle Distribution)
Fidler, Jowett, Fassbender, Janda	Shortening of the Postural (Slow Twitch) Muscles (Myotendinosis?, Palpable Band?) ⟶ **Histochemical Changes**
Fassbender	Relative Hypoxemia
	Damage of the Muscle Tissue ⟶ **Muscular Pain**
Janda	Muscular Dysbalance
	Movements of the Joints Disturbed

REFERENCES

Billeter, R., Howald, H.: Fasertypen in der Oberschenkelmuskulatur von Schueizer Mittelstrecken- und Langstreckenlaeufern. *Jugend und Sport, 3*:89-90, 1981.

Brodal, A.: *Neurological anatomy in relation to clinical medicine.* Oxford, Oxford University Press, 3rd ed., 1981.

Brown, M.G.; Goodwin, G.M., Matthews, P.C.B.: The persistence of stable bonds between actin and myosin filaments of intrafusal muscle fibers following their activation. *Journal of Physiology, 220*:9-10, 1970.

Bruegger, A.: Pseudoradikulare Syndrome. *Documenta Geigy, Acta Rheumatologica, 19*:1-136, 1962.

Buerger, A.A.: Experimental neuromuscular models of spinal manipulative techniques. *Manual Medicine*, (in press), 1983.

Caviezel, V.H.: Beitrag zur Kenntnis des Iliosakralsyndroms. *Manuelle Medizin, 11*:102-108, 1973.

Clark, F.J.: Information signaled by sensory fibres in medial articular nerve. *Journal of Neurophysiology, 38*:1464-1472, 1975.

Clark, F.J., Burgess, P.R.: Slowly adapting receptors in cat knee joint: Can they signal joint angle? *Journal of Neurophysiology, 38*:1448-1463, 1975.

Cooper, S., Daniel, P.M.: Muscle spindles in man, their morphology in the lumbricals and the deep muscles of the neck. *Brain, 86*:563-586, 1963.

Dvorak, J., Dvorak, V.: Neurologie der Wirbelbogengelenke. *Manuelle Medizin, 20*:77-84, 1982.

Dvorak, J., Dvorak, V.: *Manuelle Medizin: Diagnostik.* Stuttgart, New York, Thieme Verlag, 1983.

Eldred, E.; Hutton, R.S., Smith, J.C.: Nature of the persisting changes in afferent discharge from muscle following its contraction. *Progress in Brain Research, 44*:157-170, 1976.

Fassbender, H.G.: Der rheumatische Schmerz. *Medizinische Welt, 31*:1263-1267, 1980.

Feinstein, B.; Langton, J.N.K., Jameson, R.M.: Experiments on pain referred from deep somatic tissues. *Journal of Bone and Joint Surgery, 36*:981-997, 1954.

Feinstein, B.: Referred pain from paravertebral structures. In: Buerger, A.A., Tobis, J.S. (eds.) *Approaches to the Validation of Manipulation Therapy.* Springfield, IL, Charles C Thomas, 1977, pp.139-174.

Freeman, M.A.R., Wyke, B.D.: The innervation of the knee joint. An anatomical and histological study in the cat. *Journal of Anatomy (London), 101*:505, 1967.

Gerstenbrand, F.; Tilscher, H., Berger, M.: Radikulare und pseudoradikulare Symptome der mittleren und unteren Halswirbelsaule. *Muenchener Medizinische Wochenschrift, 121*:1173-1176, 1979.

Glen, W.V.; Rhodes, M.L.; Altschuler, E.M.; Wiltse, L.L.; Kostanek, C., Yu, Ming Kuo: Multiplanar display computerized body tomography applications in the lumbar spine. *Spine, 4*:282-352, 1979.

Granit, R.: *Receptors and sensory perception.* New Haven, Yale Univ. Press, 1955.

Granit, R.: The functional role of the muscle spindles — facts and hypotheses. *Brain, 98*:531-556, 1975.

Grigg, P., Greenspan, B.J.: Response of primate joint afferent neurons to mechanical stimulation of knee joint. *Journal of Neurophysiology, 40*:1-8, 1977.

Gutzeit, K.: Der vertebrale Faktor im Krankheitsgeschehen. In Junghanns, H. (ed.) *Roentgenkunde und Klinik vertebragener Krankheiten.* Stuttgart, Hippokrates, 1955.

Hassler, R.: Neuronale grundlagen der spastischen tonussteigerung. In Bauer, H.J.; Koella, W.P. and Struppler, A. (ed.) *Therapie der Spastik*, Munchen, Verlag fur angewandte Wissenschaften, 1981.

Hintermann, B., Hintermann, M.: *Modifikation der Muskelfasertypen durch Ausdauer-, Interval- und Krafttraining bei eineiigen Zwillingen.* Dissertation an der Medizinischen Fakultaet der Universitaet Bern-Switzerland (in press, 1983).

Hnik, P.; Kruz, N., Vyskoci, L.: Work-induced potassium changes in muscle venous effluent blood measured by ion-specific electrodes. *Pflugers Archiv, 338*:177-181, 1973.

Howald, H.: Training induced morphological and functional changes in skeletal muscle. Int. *Journal of Sport Medicine, 3*:1-12, 1982.

Janda, V.: *Muskelfunktionsdiagnostik.* Leuven, Verlag fuer Medizin Dr. Fischer, 1979.

Jones, L.H.: *Strain and Counter Strain.* Colorado Springs, The American Academy of Osteopathy, 1981.

Jowett, R.L., Fidler, M.W.: Histochemical changes in the multifidus in mechanical derangements of the spine. *Orthopaedic Clinics of North America, 6*:145-161, 1975.

Junghans, H.: Die Bedeutung der insufficiencia intervertebralis fuer die Wirbelsaeulen forschung. *Manuelle Medizine, 12*:93-102, 1974.

Kellgren, J.H.: Observation on referred pain arising from muscle. *Clinical Science, 3*:175, 1938.

Kellgren, J.H.: The anatomical source of back pain. *Rheumatology Rehabilitation, 16*:3-12, 1977.

Korr, I.M.: Proprioceptors and somatic dysfunction. *Journal of American Osteopathic Association, 74*:638-650, 1975.

Leksell, L.: The action potential and excitatory effects of the small ventral root fibres to skeletal muscle. *Acta Physiologica Scandinavica, Supplementum 31*:1-84,1945.

Lewit, K.: *Manuelle Medizin im Rahmen der medizinischen Rehabilitation.* Muenchen, Wien, Baltimore, Urban & Schwarzenberg, 1977.

Maigne, R.: *Wirbelsaeulenbedingte Schmerzen.* Stuttgart, Hippokrates, 1970.

Mense, S.: Nervous outflow from skeletal muscle following chemical noxious stimulation. *Journal of Physiology (London), 267*:75-88, 1977.

Mitchell, F.L.; Moran, P.S., Pruzzo, M.T.: *An Evaluation and Treatment Manual of Osteopathic Muscle Energy Procedures.* Valley Park, MO, Mitchell, Moran, Pruzzo Publishers, 1979.

Mixter, W.J., Barr, J S : Rupture of intervertebral disc with involvement of spinal canal. *New England Journal of Medicine, 211*:210-215, 1934.

Polacek, P.: Receptors of the joints. Their structure, variability and classification. *Acta. Fac. Med. Univ. Brun., 23*:1-107, 1966.

Rethelyi, M., Szentagothai, J.: Distribution and connections of afferent fibers in the spinal cord. In Iggo, A. (ed.) *Handbook of Sensory Physiology.* Volume II:207-252, Berlin, Springer Verlag, 1973.

Richmond, F.J.R., Abrahams, V.C.: What are the proprioceptors of the neck? *Progress in Brain Research, 50*:245-254, 1979.

Schmidt, R.F.; Kniffki, K.D., Schomburg, E.D.: Der Einfluss kleinkalibriger Muskelafferenzen auf den Muskeltonus. In Bauer, H.J.; Koella, W.P. and Struppler A. (eds.) *Therapie der Spastik*, Munchen, Verlag fuer angewandte Wissenschaften, 1981, pp. 71-84.

Schmorl, G., Junghanns, H.: *Die gesunde und die kranke Wirbelsaule.* Stuttgart, New York, Thieme Verlag, 1968.

Schoultz, T.W., Swett, J.E.: The fine structure of the Golgi tendon organ. *Journal of Neurocytology, 1*:1-26, 1972.

Sterling,, P., Kuypers, H.G.J.M.: Anatomical organization of the brachial spinal cord of the cat: The distribution of dorsal root fibers. *Brain Research, 4*:1-15, 1967.

Simons, D.G.: Electrogenic nature of palpable bands and local twitch response associated with myofascial trigger point. *Advances in Pain Research and Therapy*. In Bonica, J.J. and Fessard, D.A. (eds.) Raven Press, 1976, pp. 913-918.

Simons, D.G.: Myofascial trigger point: A need for understanding. *Archives of Physical Medicine* and *Rehabilitation, 62*:97-99, 1981.

Sutter, M.: Versuch einer Wesensbestimmung pseudoradikularer Syndrome. *Schweiz Rundsch Med. (Praxis), 63*:842-845, 1974.

Sutter, M.: Wesen, Klinik und Bedeutung spondylogener Reflex-Syndrome. *Schweiz Rundsch Med. (Praxis), 63*:842-845, 1975.

Tilscher, H.; Steinbrueck, K.; Hicke, P. and Danielczyk, D.: Neuroorthopaedische Probleme des Ausstrahlungsschmerzes. *Orthopaedische Praxis, 7*:531-536, 1981.

Travell, J. and Rinzler, S.H.: The myofascial genesis of pain. *Postgraduate Medicine, 2*:425-434, 1952.

Travell, J.: Identificant of myofascial trigger point syndromes: A case of atypical facial neuralgia. *Archives of Physical Medicine Rehabilitation, 62*·100-106, 1981.

Walther, D.S.: *Applied kinesiology*, Pueblo, CO, SDC Publishers, (275 West Abriendo Ave., 81004), 1981.

Wyke, B.D.: Morphological and functional features of the innervation of the costovertebral joints. *Folia Morphologica (Prague), 23*:296, 1975.

Wyke, B.D.: Cervical articular contribution to posture and gait: their relation to senile disequilibrium. *Age and Aging, 8*:251-258, 1979.

Wyke, B.D.: Neurology of the cervical spinal joint. *Physiotherapy, 65*:72-76, 1979.

Zimmermann, M.: Schmerz und Schmerztherapie — neurophysiologisch betrachtet. *Schweizer Medizinische Wochenschrift, III*:1927-1936, 1981.

CHAPTER NINETEEN

A CONCEPT OF MANUAL MEDICINE

DR. HEINZ-DIETER NEUMANN, M.D.

I N manual medicine we are confronted with two facts:

1. the somatic dysfunction and,
2. its successful treatment by manual therapy.

The questions of what a somatic dysfunction actually is and how manual therapy works has been a matter of discussion since manual medicine began.

Congestion of body fluid, subluxation, pinching of a nerve, derangement of disks, sticking of the joint surfaces, asymmetric muscle spasm and nervous reflex disturbances have been among the most discussed theories.

In my opinion it is probably wrong to interpret a somatic dysfunction as being *only* of circulatory, articular muscular or nervous reflex origin.

Joint, intervertebral disk, muscles and the nervous system are parts of interrelated systems. A somatic dysfunction is most likely the dysfunction of a system which can be disturbed in *any* one of its components.

I will try to explain these thoughts with a concept in which the facet joint of the spinal column is crucial. For better understanding of the interrelation between the different functional systems, I have worked out a diagrammatic system of two interrelated circles in order to make this approach clearer (Figure XIX-1).

Each facet joint is considered part of two circuits that function together. On the one hand it is part of the Junghans (1954) mobile segment in which it has a mechanical function. On the other hand it is part of a nervous control system.

Mechanical Circuit

From the mechanical point of view, as shown in the lower circle, the facet joint is part of a spinal segment, the smallest functional unit of the spinal column. Each mobile segment has two components: the movable system (inter-

267

vertebral disk and facet joints) and the stabilizing system (ligaments and muscles). These two components are normally in equilibrium. The resistance of the disk is balanced by the elasticity of the ligaments, the tone of the muscles, and the force of gravity (Erdmann, 1967). Dysfunction of a facet joint impairs the mobility of the mobile segment and disturbs the balance of the whole spine. Somatic dysfunction, degenerative changes in disks or facet joints, ligamentous insufficiency, and muscle disturbances can be the cause or the consequence of each other. Additionally, the spine is influenced by external forces, e.g., difference in lower-limb length, asymmetry of the pelvis or vertebrae, a sacral tilt, imbalance in trunk or extremity muscles, and occupational stress.

Nervous Reflexive Circuit

In the upper circle, the figure shows the relationship of the local nervous reflexes associated with the dermatome, the myotome, the central nervous system, and the viscera. In the capsule of each joint are many receptors. We differentiate two main groups: the proprioceptors (group I, II, III) and the nociceptors (group IV). Proprioceptors are concerned with noting or feeling positions. They react to changes of tension in the joint capsule such as manipulations or traction treatments. Nociceptors are stimulated by bigger changes in the capsule such as inflammation, somatic dysfunction, etc. (Dvorak and Dvorak, 1983; Korr, 1955; Wolff, 1979; Wyke, 1967).

An irritation of the proprioceptors inhibits the nociceptors. At the *present* state of our knowledge, this mechanism is *one* of the essential concepts in manual therapy.

Proprioceptors and nociceptors are connected by the ramus dorsalis with the grey matter of the spinal cord, where afferent impulses are monitored, modulated (by inhibition or fascilitation), integrated and returned to the periphery whenever a certain threshold of sensation is exceeded. Each facet joint dysfunction has a distinct influence on the spinal muscles, the superficial trunk muscles, and the muscles of the extremities, as well as the dermatome, the vascular system and the viscera (e.g., the activity of pulmonary, cardiovascular, and gastrointestinal reflexes) (Gutzeit, 1956; Schwartz, 1974; Sutter, 1974). Stimuli exceeding the local segmental threshold are transmitted to higher centers where they are appreciated as pain.

Summation of inputs from mechanical or reflex circuits may draw attention to "silent motion restrictions" that were not causing pain. The silent motion restriction is a minor disturbance that does not cause local discomfort. It is compensated for by the body. It can often be found on an exact, systematic investigation of the locomotory system. It may be the hidden cause or consequence of functional disturbances of the viscera.

The Concept in Practice

Practice is not as easy as theory. The spinal cord is segmentally ordered by the spinal nerves, but it is not classified segmentally. Therefore the reaction of a segment on irritation may go through different pathways that are not predictable in any one case. There are several reasons for this; the joint capsule of each facet joint is innervated by the spinal nerves from different segments (cranial, caudal, or at the same level) (Wyke, 1967). There are many possibilities for inhibition or facilitation at the segmental level and on higher levels of the central nervous system. (There are nerve cells with up to 180 synapses.) In addition there are many variations in the efferent pathways of discharge through the fila radicularia and the plexus formations; that is why a confusing picture of symptoms arises; for instance the somatic dysfunction of a facet joint may lead to the fascilitation of the groups of muscles innervated by the same spinal segment, or the disturbance of the viscus may become apparent.

I have tried to describe the rather complicated pathways of the nervous reflex connections as simply and comprehensively as possible by showing the somaticovisceral or viscero-somatic reflexes in the left half of the upper circle of our scheme of the concept of manual medicine and the somaticosomatic reflexes on the right half of the upper circle in our scheme (Figure XIX-1).

Somaticosomatic Reflexes

For our diagnostic and therapeutic efforts the knowledge of the somaticosomatic reflexes is of great importance. These are the reflex connections between the facet joints, the associated muscles and the dermatome. For convenience they are divided into those mediated by the dorsal ramus of the spinal nerve and those mediated by the ventral ramus. The former innervates the erector spinae group of muscles and a hand's breadth of skin to either side of the spinous processes. Changes in tissue tension and in skin reflexes and sensation indicate this reflex route and provide a direct method of diagnosing motion restriction of the facet joint. We call this *"local segmental irritation."* It can be increased or decreased by moving the dysfunctional joint to or from the restricting barrier.

The ventral ramus of the spinal nerve supplies the ventral muscles of the trunk, the superficial muscles of the back, and the muscles of the extremities. The shift of these muscles during embryologic development in addition to the plexus formation of the ventral branch of the spinal nerves and the many possibilities of modulation of "nocireactions" in the central nervous system are the reason why peripheral segmental irritation may vary considerably and may be found far from its origin. For those untrained in manual medicine, the tracing of symptoms to the place of origin is not easy. As far as the muscles of the extremity are concerned, tracing of symptoms is facilitated by the so-called tracer muscles, which have been described by Hansen and Schliack (1962). In these muscles we find higher tension, tissue changes, and, occasionally, decreased reflexes.

We call the irritation of the superficial trunk muscles and the peripheral

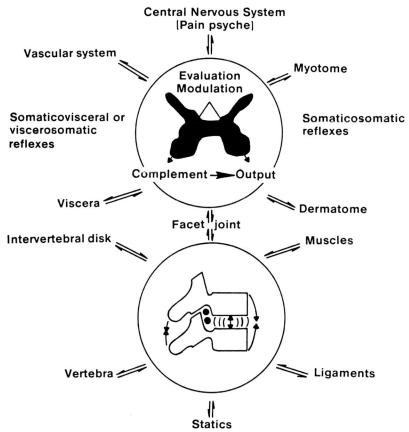

Figure XIX-1. A pictorial representation of a theory of manual medicine. Note that all arrows are double. See text for details.

muscles elicited by the ventral branch of the spinal nerve *"peripheral segmental irritation."*

It is important to emphasize that in spinal somaticosomatic reflexes, effector and affected structures are interchangeable; the reflex arc works both ways.

Clinical Signs of Somatic Dysfunction

With the help of our concept it is easy to classify the clinical signs of the dysfunction of a facet joint: motion restriction (lower circle) and local and peripheral segmental irritation (upper circle) (Figure XIX-1).

Consequently there are three possibilities for diagnosing the dysfunction of a facet joint:

1. directly, by palpating the motion restriction over the bony structure,
2. by palpating the local irritation and,
3. by palpating peripheral segmental irritation in muscles and skin.

Causes of Somatic Dysfunction

By means of our conceptional model we can also classify the causes of motion restriction in a facet joint:

1. direct cause,
2. indirect mechanical cause,
3. indirect nervous reflex cause,
4. a combination of different causes.

These can be explained as follows:

1. The motion restriction of a facet joint is occasionally caused by incorrect movement, e.g., twisting the neck when driving a car or missing a step when climbing a staircase. It may also occur when one is bending the lumbar region forward and twisting while lifting a load.
2. Frequently the motion restriction is the secondary cause of faulty posture, such as asymmetry of the vertebrae, degeneration of the vertebral disk, asymmetry of the pelvis, sacral tilt, difference in leg length, motion restriction of the lower limb joints or extremity joints, deformities of the foot, muscle disturbances, disturbance of the movement pattern, ligamentous insufficiency, or occupational strain (lower circle in Figure XIX-1).
3. Another reason for motion restriction may be the dysfunction of the nervous reflex control circuit of the spinal segment in what is called a "noci-reaction," (Wolff, 1979) e.g., a disturbance arising from a myotome, a dermatome, the psyche, the vascular system or the viscera. The motion restriction of the facet joint may be the consequence of an affliction of the somaticosomatic reflex (disturbance arising from a myotome or dermatome) or viscerosomatic affliction — e.g., musculoskeletal dysfunction at the thoracicocervical junction following a coronary (upper circle).
4. Finally a combination of the above described different causes is possible (summation of nociceptive inputs) (Korr, 1955).

The Concept in Therapy

The success of therapy depends on diagnosing the primary cause of the somatic dysfunction and the judgement of its influence in the total feature of the disease. This is what Gutmann (1957) calls the "actual pathogenic diagnosis." If the motion restriction (e.g., that caused by incorrect movement) is the primary cause of the clinical symptoms, manual treatment alone, eventually supported by a physical or medical treatment of the accompanying segmental irritation, will be successful. If the dysfunction of a facet joint is the "accompanying motion restriction" as a consequence of an affliction of mechanical (lower circle) or reflex (upper circle) disturbances of the segment, the patient will be improved after manual treatment by the taking of fascilitating inputs out of the segmental information pool. The patient may even be freed from pain, although the basic mechanical and/or reflex disturbance still exists, because the sum of fascilitating inputs to the segmental pool was reduced. Other medical or physical treatment — e.g., lift therapy, physiotherapy, heat or cold treatment, electrotreatment, infiltrations, antiphlogistics, analgesics, or tranquilizers — may be required before *lasting* relief is achieved in such a case. When psychogenic factors or occupational strain contribute to a condition, *special* attention is required.

REFERENCES

Dvorak, J. and Dvorak, V.: *Manuelle Medizin: Diagnostik*. Stuttgart, New York, Thieme, 1983.

Erdmann, H.: Grundzuege einer funktionellen Wirbelsaulenbetrachten. *Manuelle Medizin, 5*:55-63, 1967.

Gutmann, G.: Die Chiropraktik als rationelle arztliche Therapie. *Hippokrates, (Stuttgart), 28*:17, 1957.

Gutzeit, K.: Der vertebrale Faktor im Krankheitsgeschehen. *Wirbelsauele in Forschung und Praxis, Hippokrates (Stuttgart), 1*:11-21, 1956.

Hansen, K. and Schliack, H.: *Segmentle Innervation; ihre Bedeutung fuer Klinik und Praxis* (2nd ed.), Stuttgart, Thieme, 1962.

Junghanns, H.: Das Bewegungssegment der Wirbelsauele und seine praktische Bedeutung. *Arch. Orthop. Putti*, 104, 1954.

Korr, J.M. et al.: Symposium on the functional implications of segmental facilitation. *Journal of the American Osteopathic Association, 54*:265-282, 1955.

Neumann, H.-D.: *Informationskurs der Deutschen Gesellschaft fuer Manuelle Medizin*. Buhl, Kondordia, 1978.

Neumann, H.-D.: *Manuelle Medizin. Eine Einfuhrung in Theorie, Diagnose und Therapie*. Heidelberg, Berlin, New York, Tokyo, Springer-Verlag, in press.

Schwarz, E.: Manuelle Therapie und Innere Medizin. *Schweizer Rundschai fuer Medizin (Praxis), 63*:837-841, 1974.

Sutter, M.: Versuch einer Wesensbestimmung pseudoradicularer Syndrome. *Schweizer Rundschai fuer Medizin (Praxis), 63*:842-845, 1974.

Wolff, H-D.: Neurophysiologische Aspekte der Manuellen Medizin (Chirotherapie) — *(Schriftenreihe Manuelle Medizin, Volume 3)*. Heidelberg, Fischer, 1978, p. 56.

Wyke, B.: The neurology of joints. *Annals of the Royal College of Surgeons (London), 41*:25-50, 1967.

CONCLUSION

UNDER present circumstances, primarily due to historical and economic (and therefore political) reasons, it is unusual that patients with back pain receive the combined benefits of the effective treatments and the accurate diagnoses currently available. Surely they deserve a reasonable hope of effective and accurate approaches of the cause(s) of their back pain. A major objective of this volume is reducing the odds that effective treatment and accurate diagnoses could be improved by a more careful scientific examination.

The reader may have noticed that we reversed the normal order of diagnoses then treatment in the preceding paragraph. Given our present knowledge of idiopathic low back pain (which is by definition minimal), it seems worthwhile to utilize clinical trials as the primary mechanism for determining the effectiveness of treatments even if we do not fully understand the biologic reasons why these treatments appear effective. We have reached this conclusion in spite of the fact that, as explained in the section upon clinical trials, these trials are ultimately incapable of proving the effectiveness of any treatment because there is always the chance (no matter how slight) that the results occurred by chance or were due to unrecognized but related phenomena.

MANUAL MEDICINE AS AN ART

Manipulation is highly individualized both from the viewpoint of the practitioner and of the patient. It is a clinical art. To make an art a science is difficult; manipulation is still an art form. This is a major problem; any manipulative therapeutic intervention is unique to that time, that patient, that day, and hour. One can prescribe a five milligram Valium tablet and at least be sure that the range will be between 4.9 and 5.1 mg. in every sample of Valium tablets. One cannot do that with manipulation; this is one reason that it is so difficult to conduct research in manual medicine. In conclusion, until reasonable and widely accepted explanations of the predominant types of back pain and their treatments can be used to vindicate courses of treatment, the present disparity of opinion will persist.

RELIABLE AND REPRODUCIBLE MEASUREMENTS

As was mentioned earlier, one important issue which experts on the clinical aspects of back pain are only beginning to address is the development of reliable and reproducible scales for its measurement. These studies are incredibly complex. For example, it is very clear that the behavior (and therefore the attitudes) of the interviewers eliciting responses influence the responses of patients to questions, even when

(1) the interviewers are experienced clinicians, and
(2) the questionnaires are standardized (e.g., Cannel et al., 1977).

Hence, the methods of the social psychologists, as outlined, for example, in Babbie (1983), must be employed in validating any measures of back pain. One early effort is that of Hanvik (1951) and a more recent one is that of Roland and Morris (1983) but there have been several others.

In any case, the development of a sensitive index of the type defined by Babbie measuring the status of back pain patients is essential; it is probable that Roland and Morris have approximated such an index. Other measures of the ordinal type which may be usefully included in such an index are the distance a patient can walk without discomfort, and time before return to work.

SUMMARY

Those who have had extensive experience with manual medicine at the clinical level feel that manual treatments strongly correlate with improvement in symptoms. However, the major reason for this volume is presentation of the hard research data from randomized clinical trials. The people who are critics of manual medicine have strong positions because there is not sufficient data to substantiate many of the claims that have been made, except from published clinical trials.

In our view the results of the available evidence from clinical trials demonstrate the usefulness of spinal manipulation for "acute" low back pain, although we expect that the precise definition of "acute back pain" and "spinal manipulation" may require additional time for both scientific and political reasons. It seems to us that it should now be possible to design definitive clinical trials attempting to define the effects of lumbo-sacral rotational manipulation upon "acute" back pain, recognizing that the definitions of "acute low back pain", "lumbo-sacral rotational manipulation" and "definitive" are unclear. Also, other interpretations of the available data are always possible (e.g. Baker, 1983).

It is interesting that there has been a parallel interest in clinical trials by the rheumatologists, who have decided upon many of the same approaches discussed in this book. An excellent example of their concerns is *Clinical Trials in the Rheumatic Diseases* (Klippel and Decker, 1983); the first two and last chapters are of particular interest to those interested in the *design* of randomized clinical trials detailing the effects of manual medicine upon back pain. It is of particular interest that all of the problems addressed in the section of this volume on randomized clinical trials of manual medicine are also faced by those studying osteoarthritis (Altman and Hochberg, 1983).

We hope that this volume has placed in perspective the available evidence from research upon low back pain from the viewpoints of *biomechanics, epidemiology, spinal manipulation* and *clinical trials*. In persuing these objectives, the diversity of approaches to and opinions about lumbosacral pain, as well as the necessity of reliable and reproducible measures of spinal pain are formidable problems, but similar difficulties haunt any area in which clinical impressions are not yet synchronized with the basic sciences.

REFERENCES

Altman, R.D. and Hochberg, M.C.: Degenerative joint disease. In Klippel, J.H. and Decker, J.L. (ed.) Clinical trials in rheumatic diseases. *Clinics in Rheumatic Disease, 9*:681-693, 1983.

Babbie, E.R.: *The Practice of Social Research*, Belmont, CA, Wadsworth Publishing Co., 1983.

Baker, B.: Manipulation for low back pain. *Aches & Pains, 4(8)*:40-43, 1983.

Cannell, C.F., Marquis, K.H., Laurent, A.: A summary of studies of interviewing methodology. *Data Evaluation and Methods Research, 2(69)*, DHEW Publication (HRA) 77-1343, 1977, 78 pp.

Hanvik, L.J.: MMPI profiles in patients with low back pain. *Journal of Consulting Psychology, 15*:350-353, 1951.

Klippel, J.H. and Decker, J.L. (eds.) Clinical trials in the rheumatic diseases. *Clinics in Rheumatic Disease, 9*, 1983.

Roland, M., Morris, R.: A study of the natural history of back pain. Part I: Development of a reliable and sensitive measure of disability in low-back pain; Part II: Development of guidelines for trials of treatment in primary care. *Spine, 8*:141-150, 1983.

INDEX

A

Abdominal
  exercises, 150, 190
  muscles, 8-9, 19, 48, 63
  oblique, 23
  support (tube-shaped balloon), 42
  wall, 42
Accessory ligaments, 25
"Accompanying motion restriction," 271
Achilles reflex, 89, 96
Acid, uric, 101
Acromioclavicular joint, 92
Active motion tests, 109
Active range of motion, 122, 124
Activities, daily, 132
Activity levels, 132
Activity limitation, 53
"Actual pathogenic diagnosis," 271
Acupuncturists, 87
Acute back pain, 194, 207
Acute low back, xiii
Acute low back pain, 164, 177-178, 191, 237, 274
Adapting, rapidly, 249
Adnexal tissues, 107
Age, 23, 30, 32, 55, 62, 72, 135, 138, 142, 152,
  155, 160, 197, 209, 237
Aging, 31
Airplane pilots, 62
Alcohol abuse, 64
Allocation, 160
Allogenic
  irritation, 262
  stimulation, 261
Alpha and gamma co-activation, 258
Alpha-I-fibers, 258-259
Alpha-one motoneurons, 253
Alpha-motoneurons, 261
Alpha-two motoneurons, 253, 258-259
Alternative therapy, 228
Anaerobic cycle, 252
Analgesics, 229
Anesthesia, 229

Angular twist, 34
Ankle, 91
Ankyloses, 23
Ankylosing spondylitis, 185, 209
Annulospiral ending, 257, 260
Annulus, 31, 33, 36
  fibrosus, 30-31, 89
Anterior flexion tests, 206
Anterior superior iliac spine (ASIS), 96
Antropometry, 63
Aponeuroses, 48
Apophyseal
  facet, 88
  joints, 9, 244, 251
Appendicitis, 193
Arch-up, 221
Arms, 8
Arthritis, 153, 157
  inflammatory, 129
Arthrodesis, 21
Articular
  adhesion, 125
  cartilage, 22, 120
  facets, 35
  geometry, 22
  neurology, 242, 244, 252, 255
  pain, 261
  processes, 89
  rami, 244
  surfaces, 122
  tropism, 21
"Articulation," 168, 176
ASIS, 96
Assembly line industries, 61
Assessment, 155-156
  subjective, 186
Asymmetry
  spine, 268
  pelvis, 268, 271
  lower limbs, 268
ATP-ase stains, 252
Attachment, 43

Axial
  loads, 43
  traction, 121

B
Babinski test, 98
Back
  pain
    idiopathic, 107, 119
    pathophysiology, 239
    persistent, 55
    treatment, 119
Backache, 57
Back flexion, 8
Background therapy, 159
Back injuries, 73, 75, 77, 80
  payments, 80
Back muscles, 6, 8, 63
  activity, 9
Back pain, 87, 107, 193
  acute, 194
  chronic, 194, 207
  incidence, 71
  pathophysiology, 239
  payments, 71
Back school, 164, 166-167, 169-170, 175, 231
  training, 229
Back support, 55
Bending, 6, 37, 59, 61, 84, 166, 170
  lateral, 6, 61, 127
  moments, 25
  or twisting, 197, 200
  stiffness, 18
Bent-over work postures, 60
Bias, 153, 155-156
Biologic mechanism, 152
Biomechanical
  faults, 107-108
  problems, 81
Biped
  stance, 24
  standing, 25
Bipedal rats, 34
Blind, 156
  observer, 175
Blinding in clinical trials, 202
Blocked sacroiliac joint, 168
Blood pressure, 156
Body
  chart, 186
  fluid, 267
  postures, 24
Bradykinin, 261
Bragard's sign, 98
"Breaking the code," 153

Bus drivers, 62

C
Cancer, 129
Capsular barrier of resistance, 124
Capsule, subsynovial, 251
Carrying, 61
Cartilaginous endplates, 30
Cases, dismissed, denied, or withdrawn, 72
Cauda equina involvement, 188
Causal associations, 170
Causes, low back pain, 119
Cavitation, 122
Central spinal stenosis, 133
  syndrome (C.S.S.S.), 129, 134, 138
Cervical
  collar, 183
  dysfunction, 111
  muscle, 109
  pain, 183
  region, 109
  sidebending, 109, 116
  spine, 110
Changes, degenerative, 142
Chemical irritation, 251
Chiropractic, 182
  clinicians, 55
Chiropractors, 87, 241
Chondroitin sulfate, 32
Chronicity, 160
Cineradiographs, 183
Clinical art, 271
Clinical trials, 150, 152, 228, 239, 271, 274-275
  controlled, 228
  cross-over, 228
  design, 106, 228
  double blind, 228
  exclusions of patients, 209
  of manipulation, 183
    design, 179
  parallel group, 228
  patient selection, 209
  prospective, 228
  single blind, 228
Co-activation, 258
Coaptation, 121
Codeine, 159
Collagen, 30-31, 37, 43, 46
Collaterals, recurrent, 259
Compensatory changes, 183
Complaint of pain, 117
  subjective, 107
Compression, 6, 18, 37
Compressive load, 6, 25, 34
Computer model, 47

Confidentiality, 153
"Confounding factors," 154
Conservative therapies, 150
Conservative treatment, 130
Construction, 76
"Contracted postural muscles," 168
Contractions, lateral, 46
Control group, 176
Corpuscles
  fusiform, 250
  vater-Pacinian, 246, 254
Corsets, 208, 210, 229
Cost of low back pain, 179
Counter-rotation, 124
Crack, 122
"Cracking," 123
Cracking noise, 121
Crafts, 77
Creep, 36
  properties, 31
Criteria, 120
  for manipulation, 179
  objective, 205
  subjective, 120, 205
Crossed inhibition reflex, 259
Cross-over, 229
  design, 157, 159, 162
Cross-sectional
  design, 55
  surveys, 55
C.S.S.S., 134
CT-scan, 20-21, 103, 133, 138, 140, 241
Cultures, two, 71
Cyclic loading, 21, 36

D

Deformity, 31
Demographic
  factors, 152
  features, 162
Demyelinating disease, 129
Dermal scar tissue, 47
Dermatomal distribution of pain, 137
Dermatome, 268-269
Designs, paired, 157
Deyo, 150
Diabetic, 101
Diagnostic
  level, 111
  signs, 107
Diathermy, 150
  detuned short wave, 178, 229
Diminished sensation, 137
Disability, 55
  low back rating scale, 130

Disease
  malignant, 209
  Paget, 185
Disc (also spelled "Disk") 6, 8, 267
  bending, 35
  degeneration, 31, 64-65
  expansion, 5
  herniation, 30, 55, 60-61
  intervertebral, 18, 30, 88, 89, 229, 234, 241, 251
    center, 20
    degenerative, 30
    properties, 20
    "sequestrated", 89
  pressure, 8
    measurement, 5
  prolapse, 56, 60
  protrusion, 21, 237
  self-healing, 34
  thoracic, 31
  vertebral, 271
Discectomy, 34
Discogenic radiculopathy, 90
Discograms, 31
Discography, 102-103
Divorces, 64
Doran and Newell, 150
Double-blind, 153, 156, 228
  clinical trials (*see also* Blinding), 202
  controlled trial, 186
Dressing, 198
Drug abuse, 64
Dura mater, 88
Dynamic strength tests, 212
Dysfunctional
  levels, 134
  segments, 144

E

Edema, 18
Education level, 64
Educational Council of Osteopathic Principles (ECOP), xiv
Elasticity, 25
Electromyography (EMG), 5, 9, 33, 47, 101, 110, 133, 138, 166
  activity, 8
  asymmetry, 116
  frequency of discharge, 116
  studies, 47
  symmetry, 116
Employees
  female, 77
  male, 77
"Employer's Basic Report of Injury" (Form 100),

71-72
Employment, 57
Encoding systems, 77
End-plate fracture, 34
Energy demand, 60
Epidemiology, 156
  of low back pain, 53
  studies, 166
Epidural venography, 102
Epidurography, 102
Equivocal outcome, 158
Erector spinae group, 269
Erector spinae, lateral, 23
Ergonomics, 82
  analysis, 170
  counseling, 167
  instruction, 150
  principles, 175
Erythrocyte sedimentation rate (ESR), 101
Ethics, 153
Etiology, 170
Examination
  physical, 91
  subjective, 187
Exercises, 33, 208, 210
  flexor, 210
  extensor, 210
  lateral flexor, 210
  rotator, 210
Extension, 6, 9, 20, 127-128
  longitudinal, 46
  lumbar spine, 46
    from flexed position, 9
Extensor
  hallucis longus, 90
  moment, 7, 43
  reflex, 259
External force, 258
Extrafusal muscle fibers, 256-257
"Extruded" intervertebral disk, 89
Eye, 249, 251
  muscles, 249

F

Fabere test, 96
Facet
  failure, 35
  interaction, 37
  joints, 19, 88-89, 126, 267, 269, 271
Farrell and Tohmey, 150
Fatigue, 253
Femoral stretch, 89
Fetus, 22
Fibers
  fast twitch, 252-254, 256, 261

fusimotor, 257
  gamma, 257-258
  efferent, 260
  I-a, 260-261
  I-b, 260
  intrafusal, 256, 258
  slow twitch, 252-256
Fibrotic nucleus, 34
Fibrous
  adhesion, 125
  joint capsule, 247-249
Finance, insurance and real estate, 76
Firefighters, 63
Flexion, 6, 9, 122, 128
  extension, 35
  forward, 7, 9
    trunk, 24
  hip, 213
  lateral, 35, 123
  moment, 7, 25, 31
  of back, 8
  relaxation, 9
Fluid content, 108
  pressure, 30
Foot, 91
  eversion, 206
Foramen
  intervertebral, 88
Foraminal-anterior-posterior distance, 214
  narrowing, 65
Forceful, 59
  movements, 61, 166
Forces, oncotic, 32
Forward bending, 46
Fractures, 90
Functional muscular balance, 254

G

"Gapping," 168
Gas bubble, 122
Gastrocnemius, 91
Generalizability, 152
General practitioner, 175, 185, 233
Getting up, from chair, 198, 201
Glover, 149
Glucose, 252
Gluteal region, 165
Gluteus
  major, 23
  maximus, 9
  muscle, 26
Glycogen, 252
Glycosamine, 32
Glycosaminoglycan, 32
Golgi

corpuscles, 250
 organs, 251, 254, 257-258, 260
Goniometer, 213
Gutmann, 271
Gynecological disorders, 209

H

Hamstring test, passive, 155
Handling tasks, manual, 61
Harrington hook, 21
"Hartspann," 244
Health insurance data, 54
Heel-walk, 91
Herniation, 35
Heterogeneity, 160
High velocity, 124
Hip joint, 9, 25
 rotation, 213
History, 90
Heat treatment, 168
Hospitalization, xiii
Hospital patients, 155, 185
Human leukocyte antigen test, 101
Hyaluronic acid, 32
Hydrostatic
 pressure, 33
 properties, 6
Hydroxylysine, 32
Hypermobility, 100, 127, 134, 168
Hypomobility, 100, 134, 168, 254
Hypotheses, 162
 diagnostic, 107
Hysteresis, 31, 36

I

"Ileitis," 193
Ilia, 26
Iliac
 cartilage, 23
 spine, 92
Incidence, 56
Industrial
 classification, 72
 groups, 75
 surveys, 57
Inflammation, 18
Informed consent, 153
Inhibition, 259
 of nociceptive afferent receptors, 249
 of motoneurons, 250
 recurrent, 259
Injuries, male, 78
Irritation, local, 270
 zone of, 243
Instruction

ergonomic principles, 175
Interaction, 43
Interarticular distance, 214
Inter-examiner reliability, 106, 108, 110, 116
International Federation of Manual Medicine
 (FIMM), xiv
Interneurons, 258-259
Interpedicular distance, 214
Intervertebral insufficiency, 252
Ischemia, 261
Ischial tuberosities, 99
Isometric tension, 6

J

Jaw, 249, 251
Joint
 blockage, xv
 capsule, 122, 249-251, 268
 disease, degenerative, 125
 dysfunction, 125-126, 128, 145
 fixation, 124
 lumbosacral, 101
 manipulation, 120, 122
 metacarpophalangeal, 120
 paravertebral, 243
 sacroiliac, 101
 zygoapophseal, 19
Junction, 43

K

Kinematic findings
 findings, 116
 studies, 24
Knee, 91
Kyphosis, 63

L

Laborers, 77
Lactic acid production, 252
Lasegue's sign, 98
Lateral tilt fixation, 127
Leg length, 271
 discrepancy, 63
Leg pain, 137, 146
 distal, 146
Length, lower limb, 268
Length, pedicular, 215
Lesion, manipulable, xv, 120, 125
Lever, arm, 42, 47
Life-time
 incidence, 56
 prevalence, 56
Lifting, 59, 61, 83-84, 166
 advice, 190
 heavy manual, 61

movement, 170
techniques, 167
Ligament
 dorsal, 26
 interosseous, 22
 interspinous, 19, 44, 46
 intertransverse, 19, 46
 longitudinal, 89
 stiffness, 27
Ligamentous sheet, 45
Ligamentum, flavum, 21, 88
 lateral, 21
Ligamentum posterior longum, 22
Limb, 249, 251
Lind, 151
Load, 6
 on disc, 33
 on lumbar spine, 5
 separation curve, 121
 sharing, 20
Lordoses, 63, 127
Low back
 pain, 30
  acute, 237, 274
  chronic, 274
  disease versus symptoms, 180
  duration, 168, 219
  mechanical factors, 164
  natural history, 160
  onset, 188
  prognosis, 177
  psychological factors, 164
  relapses, 168
  remission, 160
  sick leave, 168
  social factors, 164
  symptoms versus disease, 180
  three digit rubrics, 162
 scale, 197
 school, 131, 149
Lumbago, 60
Lumbar
 apophyseal joints, 9
 artery, 19
 disc, 6
 injections, 131
 instability, 134
 intervertebral disc, 36
 lateral mobility, 125, 213
 manipulation, 123, 179, 228
 operation, 136
 posterior joints, 119
 radiographs, 133
 sagittal mobility, 213
 spine, 9, 33, 124, 127

 flattening, 8
 support, 8, 131
 surgery, 130, 142
 traction, 131, 208-209
 vertebra, 88
Lumbosacral
 pain, 91
 spine, 175
Lymphatic fluids, 34

M
Maitland techniques, 189
Malignancy, 188
Manipulable patients, selection of, 179
Manipulation, 112, 119, 121-122, 143, 174, 208-
 209, 271
 clinical trials, 194, 228
 criteria, 116, 120, 129, 194, 205
 diagnoses of manipulable patients, 237
 definition of, 120
 duration of effect, 236
 duration of treatment, 195
 early effects, 236
 non-specific, 144
 number of treatments, 195
 responsive diagnoses, 237
 techniques, 143
 treatment, 132
 types
  direct thrust, 182
  long lever, 182
  oscillatory, 182
  vertebral, 182
Marathon runner, 254
Marital status, 152
Matching, 155, 160
 randomized clinical trial, 196
Mathematical structural models, 27
Manufacturing, 73, 76
Measurements
 objective, 186
 quantifiable, 149
 reproducibility, 215
Mechanical circuit, 267
 fault, 88
 stress, 88
Mechanism, pathophysiological, 161
Mechanoreceptors, 248-249, 252, 255
Medial malleoli, 96
Medications, 131
Medicine, manipulative, 258
Menstrual period, 209
Metastases, 209
Metrizamide, 103
Micro-bundles, 260

Microstructure, 43
Microwave, minimal, 190
Midsagittal diameter, 214
Mini-mult, 197
Mining, 76
Minnesota Multiphasic Personality Inventory (MMPI), 103
Mobile unit, 107, 114
Mobility, 107-109, 221
  spine, 177
  tests, 212
Mobilization, 121-122, 143, 150, 168, 185, 191, 229, 231, 233
Models, 36, 47
Moment
  loads, 18, 23
  stiffness, 26
  tests, 19
Monotonic or linear, 6
Monotony, 59
  at work, 62
Motion
  assessment, 133, 145
  asymmetry, 112
  function, 108
  limitation, 107
  restriction, 270-271, 268
  segment, 6, 34-35, 124
  test, 109-111
Motion restrictions, silent, 268
Motoneurons, 253, 258, 260
Motor nuclei, 260
Motor units, 116
Movements, 59, 115, 255
Muscle
  contractions, 25
  fiber types, 252
  hamstring, 9, 90
    tightness test, 206
  iliopsoas, 8
  intertransverse, 255
  latissimus dorsi, 47
  multifidous, 254
  oblique, 8
  pain, 261
  phasic, 252, 256
  postdural, 252, 256, 258, 260
  Quadricepts, 100
  spasm, 125, 267
  spindles, 251, 253-256, 258, 260-261
  strength, 63
  suboccipital, 255
  tension, 107-108, 258-259
    regulation, 258
  tone, 244, 262

tracer, 269
training, 261
transverse, 8
wasting, 185
weakness, 137
Musculature, postural, 259
Musculature, voluntary, 255
Musculo-fascial tissue, 243
Musculoskeletal dysfunction, 107
  problem, 111
  system, 87, 167
Myelogram, 237
Myelographic studies, 30
Myelography, 102-103, 133, 140, 229, 241
Myoelectric
  activity, 7, 9, 109
  findings, 116
Myotendinosis, 243-244, 252, 261-262
Myotome, 268
Myotonic reflex, 258

N

Neck, 249, 251
  sidebending, 109
  sprain, 109
Nerve
  compression, 134, 137, 141, 144, 146, 254
  endings, 26, 254
  pinching, 267
  root entrapment, 119, 133
    syndrome (N.R.E.S.), 129, 134, 137
  vascular supply, 138
Nervous misinformation 244
Neurological
  deficits, 129, 134, 136-137, 139
  examination, 175
  signs, 176
  status, 132
Neurologists, 87
Neurosurgeons, 55, 87
Nociceptors, 88, 251-252, 254, 261, 268
  muscle afferents, 260
Nocireactions, 269
North American Academy of Manipulative Medicine (NAAMM), xiv
N.R.E.S., 134
Nuclear extrusion, 34
Nucleus pulposus, 30-31, 33, 89, 119, 129
Numbness, 90
Nutrition, 32

O

Obesity, 64
Occiput, 111
Occupation, 27, 72, 152

back injuries, 71
factors, 170
groups, 77
hazards, 72
injuries, 73, 80
medicine, 71
safety, 72
strain, 271
Onset, of attack, 188
Operatives, 77
Orthopaedic
clinics, 185
surgeons, 55, 87, 165
Orthotropic nature, 36
Osteoarthritis, 23, 64-65, 209
Osteopathic
lesion, xv
management, 112
physicians, 55, 241
Osteopathy, 182
Osteoporosis, 65
Osteitis condensans, ilii, 209
Osteophyte, 137
formation, 23
Out-patients, 209
Oxygen consumption, 252

P

Pain, 55, 87, 89-91, 101, 104, 107-108, 111, 117,
129, 132, 134-136, 139, 146, 152, 165, 193,
220
buttock, 136
chronic, 107
dermatomal distribution, 137
drawing, 104
duration, 135, 138
free direction, 176
multi-dermatomal, 139
non-dermatomal, 134
non-radicular, 242, 261
proximal, 146
pseudo radicular syndrome, 241
"quasi-objective," 206
scale, 212
scores, 160, 232
stiffness, 125
subjective, 125
Palpation, 106, 115, 189, 193, 243-244, 252, 261-
262, 270
Palpatory
cues, 116
findings, 114, 120, 126
signs, 108-109
tests, 106-107, 111
Pantopaque, 103
Parallel group, 229

Paraphysiological
space, 123
zone, 121
Paraspinal musculature, 255
Paravertebral
muscle, 116
region, 165
spasm, 125
structures, 242
Pars interarticularis, 21
Parturition, 27
Patellar reflex, 96
Patient
assessment, 155
examination, 167
experience, 87
grading of, 132
population, 174
primary care, 155
recruitment, 153
Patrick or Fabere Test, 96
Pedicles, 19, 101
Pelvis, 8-9, 91, 268
girdle motion, 25
Periosteum, 255
Peripheral segmental irritation, 270
Physical fitness, 63
Physical therapy, 231
Physiotherapeutic management of sciatic symp-
toms, 208
Physiotherapist, 175
Physiotherapy, 164, 167, 169-170, 188, 229
Piriformis, 23
syndrome, 99
P.J.S., 134
Placebo, 168
Plexiform nerve endings, 251
Point prevalence, 56
Popliteal nerves, 138
"Popping," 123
Position, flexed, 9
Post-contraction sensory discharge, 260-261
Posterior elements, 18, 21, 35, 124
Posterior facet, 119, 134, 138
Posterior facetectomy, 35
Posterior joints, 119, 133
Posterior joint syndrome (P.J.S.), 129, 133-134,
146
Posterior ligamentous system, 48
Posterior longitudinal ligament, 88
Posterior spinous processes, 46
Posterior superior iliac spines, 92, 95, 99
Posterior thoracolumbar fascia, 43
Posture, 33, 63, 92
correction, 190
Predictive value of tests, 156, 162

Pregnancy, 27, 185, 209
Present attack, 188
Pressure, 8, 251
  abdominal, 7, 33
  gastric, 7
  intestinal, 7
  intra-abdominal, 7, 33, 42
    measurements, 5
  intra-discal, 6, 33
    measurements, 33, 166
  measurement needle, 6
  oscillatory, 189
  peak, 20
  peritoneal, 7
  sensitive
    film, 20
    radio pill, 7
  thoracic, 7
  trunk, 7
Prevalence, 53, 58, 60, 65
  back pain, 57
  rate, 55
  studies, 53
Problems, family, 64
  psychiatric, 64
Process, degenerative, 35
Prognosis, 177
Prolapse, 32, 35
  intervertebral disc, 89, 234
Proprioceptors, 268
Proteoglycans, 32
PSIS, 96
PSOAS muscle, 8, 23, 33
Psychogenic factors, 271
Psychological
  disturbances, 185
  examination, 132
  factors, 59, 64
  profile, 129
Psychologists, 87
Public administration, 75-76
Pubic bone, 26
Pubic tubercles, 96
Public service, 71
Public utilities, 75
Pulling, 61, 84
Pushing, 61
Push and draw 176

Q
Quadratus lumborum, 23

R
Radiation
  below the knee, 164
  lowest level microwave, 229

Radicular
  failure, 241
  pain syndrome, 241-242
Radiography, 23, 31, 55, 64, 103, 120, 122, 126,
    132, 134, 142, 175, 182-183, 241
  anteroposterior, 127
  CT scan, 20
  lateral views, 128
  stereo-photometric techniques, 20
Radiographic changes, 62
Radiographic measurements, 212-213
Radiology, 88
Radiolucent articular cartilages, 120
Radiolucent cavity, 122
Radiopaque markers, 31
Rami, dorsal, 244
Ramus, dorsal, ventral, 268-269
Randomization, 154, 162
Randomized clinical trial, 174, 193, 239, 274
Randomized controlled trial, 151
Random sample, 72
Range of motion, passive, 122, 124
Reaching, 197
Receptor
  slowly adapting, 249
  Type I, II, III, IV, 248-251
Reclining, 8
Recumbent positioning, 25
Rectus abdominis muscle, 8
Rectus femoris muscle, 255
Referred pain syndrome, 133-134, 141, 144, 146
Reflex
  inhibition, 9
  loss, 137
  nervous, 267
  phasic effect, 249
  tonic stretch, 249, 258
Reflexogenic pathway, 244
Regions
  Abdominal, 8
  cervical, 8, 87
  lumbar, 8, 87, 90
  sacroiliac, 90
  thoracic, 8
Reliable, 274
Relapses, 168
Renshaw cells, 259
Renshaw inhibition, 259
Repetitive work, 59, 61
Reproducibility, 106, 162, 274
  subjective measures, 149
  tests, 156
Results
  best, 87
  non-significant, 158
Retail trade, 73

Reticular formation, 259
Retrospective studies, 168
Return of function, 149
Rheumatic diseade, 3 digit rubric, 163
Rheumatism, 242
Rheumatoid arthritis, chronic, 153
Rheumatological department, 175
Rheumatologists, 87, 275
Rheumatology clinics, 185
Risk factors, 55
R.O.M., 124
Root compression, 176
Rotation, 122-123, 127
Rotational
  articulation, 176
  fixation, 127
Rotational manipulation, 23, 176, 193, 229
  lumbosacral spine, 194
  Rasmussen, 176
Ruffinian corpuscles, 246

S

Sacral
  cartilage, 23
  nerve roots, 89
  pain, 136
  promontory, 25
  tilt, 268
Sacroiliac, 133
  capsule, 27
  disease, 209
  joint, 18, 22-24, 88, 119, 126, 136-137
    accessory ligaments, 22
    articular geometry, 22
    innervation, 22
    shear stiffness, 26
  ligaments, 22
  loading, 26
  syndrome (S.-I.S.), 129, 134, 136
Sacrilization, 65
Sacrospinous, 26
  ligament, 22, 26
Sacrotuberous, 26
  ligament, 22, 99
Sacrum, 26, 99
Sample size, 156, 161
Sampling, 162
  procedure, 72
Scales
  for low back disability, 130
  reliable, 274
  reproducible, 274
Scar tissue, 47
Scheuermann's disease, 65
Schmarl's nodes, 34

Schober's Test, 149, 175, 177
Sciatic
  distribution, 209
  nerve, 137
  notch, 137
  pain, 229
  radiation of pain, 132, 141
  symptoms, 208
Sciatica, 21, 55, 60, 63, 142, 220
  distal, 141
  proximal, 142
Scoliosis, 63, 65, 254
  idiopathic, 254
Scurvy, 151
Secondary sensory ending (flower-spray), 257-258
Segmental
  dysfunction, xv, 116, 242-244, 261-262
  findings, 111
  instability, 128
  irritation, 270
Segments
  fixed, 134
  spinal, 145
  unstable, 134
Self-sealing effect, 35
Segmental motion tests, 115
Segmental threshold, 268
Sensitive index, 274
Sensitivity, 162
Sequential
  cross-over, 162
  design, 157
  trials, 157, 162
Serotonin, 261
Service workers, 77
Severity of low back pain, 55
Sex, 62, 72, 77-78, 152, 155, 160
Sham manipulation, 228, 231
Shear, 6, 20
  forces, 18
  loads, 22-23, 26, 35
  strength, 26
  tests, 19
Shearing, deep pressure, 111
Short amplitude thrust, 124
Short-wave, 231
  apparatus, 168
  diathermy, 174, 210
  therapy, 164
  treatment, 169-170, 177
Sick leave, 168
  listing, 55
Sickness-absence
  episodes, 54

rate, 61
Sidebending, 92, 109
Side-flexion, 176
Side-lying, 176
"Single blind," 156, 228
Sino-vertebral nerve, 89
S.-I.S., 134
Sitting, 7, 8, 60
Sitting down, 198, 201
Sitting up from lying position, 198
Sit-up test, 221
"Six film study," 101
Skeletal defects, 65
Skin, 47
  hyperesthesia, 155
Small amplitude high velocity thrust, 189
Social problems, 64
Social psychologists, 274
Social security payments, 179
Social workers, 87
Socioeconomic
  class, 162
  status, 152
Soft tissue, 121, 242
  changes, 242, 260
  contracture, 125
  massage, 194, 196, 228-229
  technique, 176
  treatment, 175-176
Somatic
  dysfunction, xv, 106-110, 116, 260, 267, 269-271
  pain, 106, 108
  system examination, 107
  system function, 106
Somaticosomatic reflexes, 269-271
Specificity, 162
Spina bifida occulta, 65
Spinal
  extension, 233
  flexion, 233
  joint dysfunction, 144
  ligaments, 25
  manipulation, 119, 122-123, 128, 274
  mobility, 64, 122
  motion, 42, 124
  segment, 144, 267
  stenosis, 65, 119
  surgery, previous, 185
Spine, manual treatment, 241
Spinous processs, 19, 44, 127, 175
Spirit goniometer, 213
Spondylogenic reflex syndromes, 241-242, 244-245
Spondylolisthesis, 65, 209

Spondylolysis, 21, 133, 88
Spontaneous
  recovery, 229
  remission, 157, 160
  resolution, 191
Sports, 63
Sprains, 73
Stabilization exercises, 168
Stabilizing system, 268
Stance
  biped, uniped, 24
Standing, 7-8, 25
Static work postures, 59-60
Statistician, 157
Statistics
  insurance, 53
  labor, 73
  national, 53
Stiffness, 20, 31
Stimulation, tetanic, 260
Straight leg raising, 89, 134, 136, 206, 213, 233-234
  tests, 96, 98, 149
Strains, 31, 73
Stratification, 154-155
Stress, 88
  failure, 25
  fiber, 31
Stretching exercises, 167-168
Stride, 91
Subluxation, xv, 267
Superior articular process, 137
Supraspinous ligament, 19, 44, 46
  direction of fibers, 19
Surgery, 107
Surgical intervention, xiii
Swiss School for Manipulative Medicine, 242
Sympathetic nerve fibers, 251
Symphysis pubis, 234, 27
Symptoms, duration of, 132, 142
Synovial
  capsule receptors, 255
  fluid, 122
  joint, 136
  membrane, 22
System function, 106
Systematic myotendinoses, 244, 252

T
Tallness, 63
Taxes, lost, 179
Team approach, 87
Telemetry, 7
Tenderness, deep, 55
Tendinoses, 244

Tensile forces, 33
  stiffness, 36
Tension, 6
Terminology, xiv
Tibialis anterior, 91
Tests
  axial rotation, 109
  failure, 26
  head side bending, 109
  medial shear, 27
  neck sidebending, 109
  sagittal flexion, 109
  tissue, 111
  validation, 155
Therapy
  manual, 167, 267
  manipulative, 131
  pharmaceutical, 241
Thermal properties, 108
Thoracic
  spinal region, 111
  spinal segment, 116
  support, 33
Thoracolumbar fascia, 9, 19, 42-43
  attachment, 43
  circumferential force, 45
  microstructure, 43
  interaction, 43
  junction, 43
  ligamentous deformable sheath, 45
  middle layer, 43
  posterior layer, 43
Tingling, 90
Toe-walk, 91
Torsion, 6, 20, 31, 37
  strength, 35
Traction, 120, 122, 175, 209
Techniques, 176, 191
Tractor drivers, 62
Transportation, 75
Transverse processes, 45-46
Treatment, low voltage short wave, 164
Trials, fixed size, 156
"Triple blind," 156
Trochanters, 92
Truck drivers, 62
Trunk
  flexion, 24
  load, 8
  moment, 9
  muscle activity, 25

Tuberculosis, 151
Tumor surgery, 26
Twisting, 59, 61, 84, 166, 170
Two cultures, 71

U
Uniped stance, 24

V
Vertebral
  body, 138
  bony position, 114
  collapse, 185, 209
  end-plate, 32
  force, 33
  fracture, 251
  ligaments, 43, 46-47
  motion, 88
  segments, 244
  unit, 243
    inner function, 242
Vibration, 36, 59-60, 62
Viscera, 269

W
Walking, 92, 197
Wasting, 137
Weakness, 90
With force, 6
Work
  absence, 60
  accidents, cost, 78
  condition, 167
  days lost, 81
  dissatisfaction, 59, 62
  heavy, 59, 60, 64
  injuries, 79
  physical, 59
  posture, 60
  psychological, 62
  situation, 63
  site visits, 167
  transfer, 167
Workplace, 7
  environment, 72
  factors, 59
  modification, 149

X
X-rays, 183